Anti-Mycotoxin Strategies for Food and Feed

Anti-Mycotoxin Strategies for Food and Feed

Edited by

Deepa Nagaraju
Molecular Mycotoxicology Laboratory, Department of Studies in Microbiology, University of Mysore, Mysuru, Karnataka, India.

Sreenivasa Marikunte Yanjarappa
Molecular Mycotoxicology Laboratory, Department of Studies in Microbiology, University of Mysore, Mysuru, Karnataka, India.

Premila N. Achar
Department of Molecular and Cellular Biology, Kennesaw State University, Kennesaw, GA, USA.

and

Angel Medina Vaya
Director of Environment and Agrifood, Cranfield University, Cranfield, Bedford, U.K.

WILEY

Registered Offices
John Wiley & Sons, Inc., 111 River Street, Hoboken, NJ 07030, USA
John Wiley & Sons Ltd, The Atrium, Southern Gate, Chichester, West Sussex, PO19 8SQ, UK

For details of our global editorial offices, customer services, and more information about Wiley products visit us at www.wiley.com.

Wiley also publishes its books in a variety of electronic formats and by print-on-demand. Some content that appears in standard print versions of this book may not be available in other formats.

Library of Congress Cataloging-in-Publication Data
Names: Nagaraju, Deepa, editor. | Sreenivasa, M. Yanjarappa (Marikunte Yanjarappa), editor. | Achar, Premila N., editor. | Medina Vaya, Angel, editor.
Title: Anti-mycotoxin strategies for food and feed / edited by Deepa Nagaraju, Sreenivasa M. Yanjarappa, Premila N. Achar and Angel Medina Vaya.
Description: Hoboken, NJ : Wiley, [2024] | Includes bibliographical references and index.
Identifiers: LCCN 2023039034 (print) | LCCN 2023039035 (ebook) | ISBN 9781394160792 (hardback) | ISBN 9781394160808 (adobe pdf) | ISBN 9781394160822 (epub)
Subjects: MESH: Mycotoxins–adverse effects | Fungi–pathogenicity | Food Contamination–prevention & control | Animal Feed–microbiology
Classification: LCC RA1242.M94 (print) | LCC RA1242.M94 (ebook) | NLM QW 630.5.M9 | DDC 615.9/5295–dc23/eng/20231106
LC record available at https://lccn.loc.gov/2023039034
LC ebook record available at https://lccn.loc.gov/2023039035

Cover Design: Wiley
Cover Image: © Kateryna Kon/Shutterstock, Evgeniy Kazantsev/Shutterstock, Nopparat/Adobe Stock Photos

Set in 9.5/12.5pt STIXTwoText by Straive, Pondicherry, India

Contents

List of Contributors

Premila N. Achar
Department of Molecular and Cellular Biology
Kennesaw State University
Kennesaw, GA, USA

G. Adithi
Applied Mycology Laboratory
Department of Studies in Microbiology
University of Mysore
Mysuru, India

Dominic Agyei
Department of Food Science
Division of Sciences
University of Otago
Dunedin, New Zealand

Kadaiah Ajithkumar
Main Agricultural Research Station
University of Agricultural Sciences
Raichur, Karnataka, India

Azam Ali
Center for Bioengineering and Nanomedicine, Division of Health Sciences
University of Otago
Dunedin, New Zealand

Ali Atoui
Laboratory of Microbiology
Department of Life and Earth Sciences
Faculty of Sciences, Hadath Campus
Lebanese University
Beirut, Lebanon

Thippeswamy Basaiah
Department of Post-Graduate Studies and Research in Microbiology
Jnanasahyadri
Kuvempu University
Shivamogga, Karnataka, India

Priyanthi Chandravarnan
Department of Food Science
Division of Sciences
University of Otago
Dunedin, New Zealand

Center for Bioengineering and Nanomedicine
Division of Health Sciences
University of Otago
Dunedin, New Zealand

Department of Biosystems Technology
University of Jaffna
Jaffna, Sri Lanka

Rouaa Daou
Centre d'Analyses et de Recherche (CAR)
Unité de Recherche Technologies et
Valorisation Agro-Alimentaire (UR-TVA)
Faculty of Sciences
Saint-Joseph University of Beirut
Campus of Sciences and Technologies
Mar Roukos, Lebanon

Regina S. Dass
Fungal Genetics and Mycotoxicology
Laboratory, Department of Microbiology
School of Life Sciences
Pondicherry University
Pondicherry, India

N. Deepa
Molecular Mycotoxicology Laboratory
Department of Studies in Microbiology
University of Mysore
Mysuru, Karnataka, India

S. Divyashree
Applied Mycology Laboratory
Department of Studies in Microbiology
University of Mysore
Mysuru, India

Andre El Khoury
Centre d'Analyses et de Recherche (CAR)
Unité de Recherche Technologies et
Valorisation agro-Alimentaire (UR-TVA)
Faculty of Sciences
Saint-Joseph University of Beirut
Campus of Sciences and Technologies
Mar Roukos, Lebanon

Quenton Kritzinger
Department of Plant and Soil Sciences
University of Pretoria
Hatfield, South Africa

Theresa S.R. Mahadevarao
Postgraduate Department of Microbiology
Maharani's Science College for Women
(Autonomous)
JLB Road, Mysuru
Karnataka, India

Pavagada K. Maheshwar
Department of Microbiology
Yuvaraja's College, University of Mysore
Mysore, Karnataka, India

Manjunath K. Naik
Department of Plant Pathology
College of Agriculture
University of Agricultural Sciences
Raichur, Karnataka, India

Ankita B. Nayak
Department of Post-Graduate Studies and
Research in Microbiology Jnanasahyadri
Kuvempu University
Shivamogga, Karnataka, India

Monica C. Paul
Fungal Genetics and Mycotoxicology
Laboratory, Department of Microbiology
School of Life Sciences
Pondicherry University
Pondicherry, India

Raghavendra M. Puttaswamy
Postgraduate Department of
Microbiology
Maharani's Science College for Women
(Autonomous)
JLB Road, Mysuru
Karnataka, India

Matapati Renuka
Main Agricultural Research Station
University of Agricultural Sciences
Raichur, Karnataka, India

Santosh Sharma
The Biotechnology Research
Ghaziabad, Delhi, India

Attihalli S. Savitha
Department of Plant Pathology
College of Agriculture
University of Agricultural Sciences
Raichur, Karnataka, India

B. Shruthi
Applied Mycology Laboratory
Department of Studies in Microbiology
University of Mysore
Mysuru, India

Agriopoulou Sofia
Department of Food Science and Technology
University of the Peloponnese
Kalamata, Greece

M.Y. Sreenivasa
Molecular Mycotoxicology Laboratory
Department of Studies in Microbiology
University of Mysore
Mysuru, Karnataka, India

Prakash Sumalatha
Department of Microbiology
Yuvaraja's College, University of Mysore
Mysore, Karnataka, India

Angel M. Vaya
Director of Environment and Agrifood
Cranfield University
Cranfield, Bedford, UK

Sowmya H. Veeranna
Department of Post-Graduate Studies and Research in Microbiology Jnanasahyadri
Kuvempu University, Shivamogga
Karnataka, India

Preface

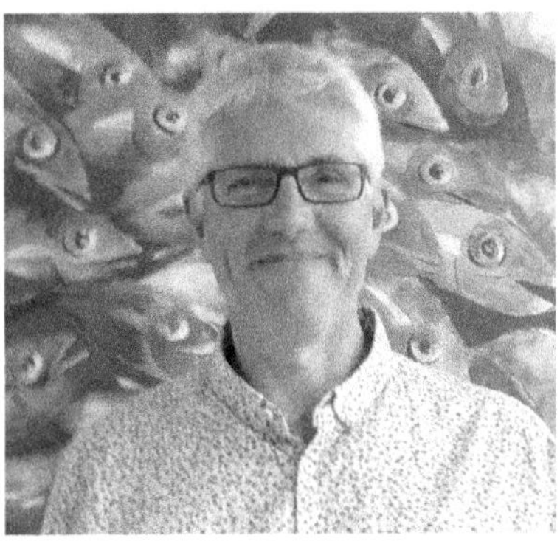

Prof. Dr. Laurent Dufossé
Université de La Réunion, France
Laboratoire CHEMBIOPRO (Chimie et Biotechnologie des Produits Naturels),
ESIROI agro-alimentaire,
île de la Réunion,
France

Mycotoxins are toxic compounds produced by toxigenic fungi that accumulate in food and feed on possessing health hazards to humans and animals. We need to accept that the use of current traditional methods to control fungi and mycotoxins production is not effective, hence mycotoxins still enter our food chain. Several research groups across the globe have developed novel strategies to keep control on mycotoxigenic fungi and their negative impact on food and feed products. This book highlights several advanced and promising approaches to curb economically important mycotoxins and covers the information regarding the recent methods used against mycotoxins. Authors have discussed strategies to control health risk mycotoxins associated with foods and feeds. Each individual chapter is carefully designed and offered a breath of information elucidating various anti-mycotoxin strategies that include physical, chemical, and biological methods. Special attention has been paid to diseases caused by mycotoxigenic fungi and their destructive effect during preharvest, post-harvest, or storage. Moreso, of global concerns, the mycotoxins pose a long term health risk to humans and animals, if the contaminated food or feed enters our food chain. Current information on mycotoxin management strategies is presented and discussed at length in different chapters.

The book *Anti-Mycotoxin Strategies for Food and Feed* forms to be a combined approach of advanced novel techniques used against mycotoxigenic species and mycotoxins that will be helpful to study the strategies for different mycotoxins. The chapters are arranged by considering all the most important mycotoxins reported worldwide that needs major attention to control. Each chapter describes a recent strategy used for controlling/detoxification/degradation/binding methods and biosynthesis with graphical representations of protocols and figures used for each mycotoxin and also future perspectives. Authors have provided information on recent developments to control important mycotoxigenic fungi and their dangerous toxins. Overall, the book presents advanced methods and strategies used to control the economically important mycotoxigenic fungi persisting in agriculture and food chain.

Introduction

Fungi are a diverse group of eukaryotic organisms ranging from unicellular to more complex multicellular forms. They consist of mass of branching intertwined filaments called hyphae and mass of such hyphae is known as mycelium. The hyphal growth allows the fungus to colonize a food and feed source as well as to grow from one food source to another (Sietsma et al. 1995). As a consequence of growth and colonization, fungi cause decay and spoilage of food and feed grains.

Fungi commonly associated with cereal food grains are broadly separated into field fungi and storage fungi (Table 1) (Deepa and Sreenivasa 2019). Of the fungi involved, the most important field fungi are *Fusarium*, *Alternaria*, *Curvularia*, and *Cladosporium*, while *Penicillium* and *Aspergillus* are important storage fungi (Christensen and Kaufmann 1969; Lacey and Magan 1991; Frisvad 1994; Samson et al. 1996; Pitt and Hocking 1997; Deepa and Sreenivasa 2019). These fungi, when grown on stored grains, can reduce the germination along with loss of carbohydrate, protein, and oil content; increase the moisture content and the quantity of free fatty acid; and also bring about several other biochemical changes (Wilson et al. 1995; Deepa and Sreenivasa 2017). The fungal growth also causes discoloration of grain, dry matter loss, mustiness, heating, and several secondary metabolite productions such as mycotoxins. Mycotoxins on consumption are potentially hazardous to humans and animals (Christensen and Kaufmann 1969; Bhattacharya and Raha 2002; Deepa et al. 2021a,b).

These fungal species in cereals, cereals-based food and feed matrix, fruits, and vegetables include many species that are pathogenic to crops and responsible for range of diseases, and among them some are mycotoxigenic and some cause opportunistic contagions in humans and farm animals (Munkvold and Desjardins 1997; Rebell 1981; Nelson et al. 1981; Marasas et al. 1984; Burgess 1985; Joffe 1987; Marasas and Nelson 1987; Deepa and Sreenivasa 2022). Mycotoxigenic fungal species cause destructive diseases in some of the world's most agriculturally important food crops such as maize, wheat, potato, cassava, palm, banana, pine, and numerous vegetables and fruits (Sreenivasa et al. 2011; Leslie et al. 1990; Summerell et al. 2003). Mycotoxigenic fungi are associated with food and feed in moderate and semi-tropical areas, as well as all European crop-growing areas. They cause root, stem, and ear rot diseases (Table 2), with severe reductions in crop yield, often

Anti-Mycotoxin Strategies for Food and Feed, First Edition. Edited by Deepa Nagaraju, Sreenivasa Marikunte Yanjarappa, Premila N. Achar, and Angel Medina Vaya.

Table 1 Fungi and the commodities they affect.

Commodity	Field fungi	Storage fungi	Mycotoxigenic fungi
Maize	*Nigrospora; Cuvularia; Lasiodiplodia; Bipolaris; Arthrinium; Rhizopus; Phoma; Rhizoctonia*	*Aspergillus; Chaetomium; Penicillium citrinum; P. funiculosum; A. wentii*	*Aspergillus flavus; Fusarium moniliforme* (=*F. verticillioides*); *F. semitectum*
Peanuts	*Cladosporium cladosporioides; Lasiodiplodia theobromae; Pestalotiopsis guepinii*	*Aspergillus niger; Penicillium pinophilum; Chaetomium* species	*Aspergillus flavus*
Rice	*Bipolaris maydis; Fusarium semitectum; Cladosporium cladosporioides; Nigrospora oryzae; Curvularia lunata; C. genticulatus; C. oryzae; C. eragrostidis; C. pallescens; Phoma* species; *Colletotrichum* species	*Aspergillus* species; *Penicillium* species; *Alternaria* species	*Altenaria padwickii; A. alternata; A. longissima; Fusarium* species
Sorghum	*Bipolaris maydis; Fusarium semitectum; Cladosporium cladosporioides; Nigrospora oryzae; Curvularia lunata; C. pallescens; Phoma* species; *Setosphaeria rostrata*	*Aspergillus niger; Eurotium chevalieri; E. rubrum; Chaetomium* species	*Aspergillus flavus; Fusarium moniliforme; Penicillium citrinum; Alternaria longissima; A. alternata*
Soybean	*Arthrinium phaeospermum; Lasiodiplodia theobromae; Fusarium semitectum; Cladosporium cladosporioides; Nigrospora oryzae; Curvularia lunata; C. pallescens; Phoma* species; *Epicoccum nigrum; Pestalotiopsis guepinii*	*Aspergillus niger; A. wentii; A. restrictus; A. penicillioides; Eurotium rubrum; Eupen cinnamopurpureum; Chaetomium* species	*Aspergillus flavus; Fusarium moniliforme; Penicillium citrinum; Alternaria alternata*
Fruits and vegetables	*Paecilomyces; Xylaria; Bysochlamys; Peacylomyces; Eupenicillium* species	*Penicillium species, Aspergillus species*	*Penicillium expansum Aspergillus species*

Source: Adapted from Champ et al. (1991)

appraised at between 10% and 30%. Consumption of such contaminated food and feed affects humans and animals among which some mycotoxins are considered to be carcinogenic and life-threatening (Deepa and Sreenivasa 2017; Logrieco et al. 2002).

Mycotoxins are secondary metabolites produced by several species of fungi. It has been estimated that up to 50% of the world's food crops are affected by mycotoxins (Charmley et al. 1995; Bullermann 1996; Eriksen and Alexander 1998; Fandohan et al. 2003; Sreenivasa et al. 2012). Mycotoxins establish a varied range of compounds molded from different forerunners and pathways that are gathered together based on their harmfulness to higher animals and humans. Some mycotoxins are produced by only a few fungal species, while others are produced by a large number of species from several genera (Smith et al. 1984).

Table 2 Common diseases caused by mycotoxigenic fungi species in cereals, humans, and animals.

Commodities	Diseases
Cereal crops (Wheat, Paddy, Maize, Sorghum, Barley, Feed-matrix)	Crown rot (=foot rot), Root rot, Ear rot, Seed-rot, Seedling blight, Dryland root rot, Pink snow mold, Scab (=head blight), Pecky rice (kernel spotting), Kernel rot, Gibberella ear rot, Stalk rot, Damping-off, Pokkah Boeng (twisted top), Rusts (Scab)
Fruits and vegetables	Anthracnose, Botrytis rot, Downy mildew, Powdery mildew, Rust, Rhizoctonia rot, Sclerotia rot, Fusarium rot, Oak root, Sappy bark, Phytophthora root, Crown rot
Animals and birds (Horse, Swine, Rats, Rabbit, Chicken, primates)	Equine leukoencephalomalacia, Porcelain pulmonary edema, Hepatotoxicosis, Lesions in liver and lungs, Targets to pancreas, Heart, Oesophagus, Kidney, Hepatic nodules, Adenofibrosis, Hepatocellular carcinoma, Cholangiocarcinoma, Hepatotoxins, Anorectic, lethargic, Erythrocyte formation, Lymphocyte cytotoxic effects, Weight reduction, Biliary hyperplasia, Thymic cortical atrophy, Oesophageal cancer, Reduction in WBC and RBC
Humans	Esophageal cancer, Skin lesions, Wounds, Keratitis

Source: Adapted from The American Phytopathological Society, http://www.apsnet.org/online/common/toc.asp

They are chemically diverse and occur in a wide diversity of substrates. They cause illness/death of humans and animals. If food or feed containing them is consumed, it may also cause economic losses in livestock through disease and reduced efficiency of production (Deepa and Sreenivasa 2017). Many of the fungi that produce the toxins are also frequent contaminants of food and feed-based products (Table 3). These comprise members of the genera *Fusarium*, *Aspergillus*, *Penicillium*, and *Alternaria* producing mycotoxins such as aflatoxins, fumonisins, citrinin, patulin, trichothecenes, deoxynivalenol, T-2 toxin, HT-2 toxins, nivalenol, ochratoxin, and zearalenone.

In current days, molecular-based techniques have been used as advanced technologies for the accurate detection of mycotoxins since identification and detection of mycotoxigenic fungi by conventional methods are labor- and time-consuming tasks that require expertise in fungal taxonomy and chemical analysis. Nowadays variations among PCR techniques, immunological and serological methods, nanotechnology base methods, and aptamers have become faster alternatives as the early identification method even though DNA from fungus present in the food and feed samples are extracted prior to its incubation period. Killed fungi can also be detected which might be an additional advantage (Deepa et al. 2021a,b, 2022).

The eradication of the growth of mycotoxigenic fungi and associated mycotoxins in food and feed is of supreme importance because of consumption of significant quantities of these cereals by humans. Managemental strategies are required and need to be practiced by detecting at an early stage for the improvement of crop yield, food safety, and economic development. Most of the traditional methods from drying, sorting, and heating involving physical methods like separation, washing, adsorption, and irradiation play a role in the management of mycotoxins. Certain chemical methods such as ozone treatment, alkaline treatment, and many biological methods involving microorganisms, essential oils, plant products, genetic engineering, resistant varieties, and commercial products are in recent days practice as strategies for mycotoxin control (Shruthi et al. 2022). Advanced methods

Table 3 Mycotoxins most commonly found in food and feed.

S. No.	Toxin	Fungus	Food commonly affected
1	Aflatoxin	*Aspergillus flavus, A. parasiticus.*	Maize, groundnuts, cottonseeds, feeds
2	Fumonisins	*F. moniliforme, F. proliferatum, F. nygamai*	Maize, sorghum, feed matrix
3	Ochratoxin	*Aspergillus ochraceus, Penicillium viridicatum*	Maize, wheat, barley, oats, poultry feed matrix
4	Patulin	*Bysochlamys, Eupenicillium, Penicillium, Aspergillus* and *Peacylomyces*	Apples, apricots, kiwis, plums, peaches, cereal-based food
5	Trichothecenes/T-2/HT-2/Nivalenol	*F. graminearum, F. asiaticum, F. culmorum, F. cerealis, F. pseudograminearum, F. sporotrichioides, F. sibiricum F. langsethiae, F. acuinatum* and *F. poae*	Wheat, barley, maize
6	Citrinin	*Penicillium, Aspergillus* and *Monascus*	Food grains, beans, fruits, vegetables, black olive, roasted nuts, sunflower seeds, spices, herbs and spoils dairy products
7	Zearalenone	*F. graminearum*	Wheat, maize, barley, sorghum
8	Deoxynivalenol	*Fusarium graminearum*	Wheat, barley, oats, maize, rye, feeds
9	Ergot alkaloids	*Claviceps purpurea, C. Africana, A. fumigatus, Pencillium sp.*	Rye, triticale, wheat, barley, millet, oats

Source: Adapted from www.mycotoxin.org

like cold plasma, nanoparticles, pulsed electric fields, and molecular strategies are in practice against mycotoxins associated with foods and feeds. These methods are applicable with their respective advantages and disadvantages in managing mycotoxins. Presently, degradation and detoxification strategies as adsorbents of the mycotoxins are in much practice.

Our edited book "Anti-Mycotoxin Strategies in Food and Feed" consists of eleven chapters discussing various strategies for degradation and decontamination of mycotoxins in food and feed. We have hereby covered all the major mycotoxins such as Aflatoxins, Fumonisins, Ochratoxin, Patulin, Citrinin, Trichothecenes, Zearalenone, Deoxynivalenol, Nivalenol, T-2/HT-2, and Ergot alkaloids. Our contributors have discussed each mycotoxin, its occurrence and distribution, and effects of particular mycotoxin during both pre- and post-harvest stages including effects on humans and animals on consumption of such mycotoxin-associated foods and feed. The authors have majorly discussed all the recent advanced strategies involved such as physical, chemical, and biological methods and have mainly concentrated on detoxification, degradation, and other binding methods against respective mycotoxins. Further aspects of reading and study questions pertaining to each mycotoxin have been discussed in each of the chapters.

References

Bhattacharya, K. and Raha, S. (2002). Deteriorative changes of maize, groundnut and soybean seeds by fungi in storage. *Mycopathologia* 155: 135–141.

Bullermann, L.B. (1996). Occurrence of *Fusarium* and fumonisins on food grains and in foods. In: *Fumonisins in Food* (ed. L.S. Jackson, J.V. De Vries, and L.B. Bullerman), 27–38. New York: Plenum Press.

Burgess, L.W. (1985). Mycotoxigenic species of *Fusarium* associated with grain diseases in Eastern Australia. In: *Trichothecenes and Other Mycotoxins* (ed. J. Lacey). New York: John Wiley and Sons Ltd.

Champ, B.R., Highley, E., Hocking, A.D., and Pitt, J.I. (1991). *Fungi and Mycotoxins in Stored Products: Proceedings of an International Conference*. ACIAR Proceedings No. 36. Bangkok, Thailand. Australian Centre for International Research.

Charmley, L.L., Trenholm, H.L., Prelusky, D.A., and Rosenberg, A. (1995). Economic losses and decontamination. *Nat. Toxins* 3: 199–203.

Christensen, C.M. and Kaufmann, H.H. (1969). *Grain Storage: The Role of Fungi in Quality Loss*. Minneapolis, USA: University of Minnesota Press.

Deepa, N. and Sreenivasa, M.Y. (2017). Fumonisins: a review on its global occurrence, epidemiology, toxicity and detection. *J. Vet. Med. Res.* 4 (6): 1093.

Deepa, N. and Sreenivasa, M.Y. (2019). Chapter 13: "Biocontrol strategies for effective management of phytopathogenic fungi associated with cereals". In: *New and Future Developments in Microbial Biotechnology and Bioengineering-Microbial Biotechnology in Agro-Environmental Sustainability*, 177–189. Elsevier.

Deepa, N. and Sreenivasa, M.Y. (2022). Molecular approaches for the early detection of mycotoxigenic fungi in feeds and feed matrix. Mycotoxinsite.com.

Deepa, N., Achar, P., and Sreenivasa, M.Y. (2021a). Current perspectives of biocontrol agents for management of *Fusarium verticillioides* and its fumonisin in cereals – a review. *J. Fungi* 7: 776.

Deepa, N., Adkar-Purushothama, C.R., and Sreenivasa, M.Y. (2021b). Chapter 6: "Molecular technologies for the early detection of fungal phytopathogens associated with cereal crops". In: *Microbial Genomic Technologies to Combat the Problems of Farming Lands. Microbes in Land Use Change Management*, 137–154. Elsevier.

Deepa, N., Chennappa, G., Deepthi, B.V. et al. (2022). Antifungal potential of *Azotobacter* species and its metabolites against *Fusarium verticillioides* and biodegradation of fumonisin. *J. Appl. Microbiol.* 133 (4): 2430–2444.

Eriksen, G.S. and Alexander, J. (1998). *Fusarium* toxins in cereals – a risk assessment. 146 pp. TemaNord 1998:502. Nordic Council of Ministers. Ekspressen Tryk and Kopicenter, Copenaghen, Denmark.

Fandohan, P., Hell, K., Marasas, W.F.O., and Wingfield, M.J. (2003). Infection of maize by *Fusarium* species and contamination with fumonisin in Africa. *Afri. J. Biotechnol.* 2: 570–579.

Frisvad, J.C. (1994). Mycotoxins and mycotoxinogenic fungi in storage. In: *Stored Grain Ecosystems* (ed. D.S. Jayas, N.D.G. White, and W.E. Muir), 251–288. New York, USA.

Joffe, A.Z. (1987). *Fusarium poae* and *F. sporotrichioides* as principal causal agents of alimentary toxic aleukia. In: *Mycotoxic Fungi, Mycotoxins, Mycotoxicoses: An Encyclopaedic Handbook*, 3e (ed. T.D. Wyllie and L.G. Morehouse), 21–86. New York, USA.

Lacey, J. and Magan, N. (1991). Fungi in cereal grains: their occurrence and water and temperature relationships. In: *Cereal Grain Mycotoxins, Fungi and Quality in Drying and Storage*, 77–118. Amsterdam: Elsevier Science.

Leslie, J.F., Pearson, C.A.S., Nelson, P.E., and Toussoun, T.A. (1990). *Fusarium* spp. from corn, sorghum, and soybean fields in the Central and Eastern United States. *Phytopathology* 80: 343–350.

Logrieco, A., Mule, G., Moretti, A., and Bottalico, A. (2002). Toxigenic *Fusarium* species and mycotoxins associated with maize ear rot in Europe. *Eur. J. Plant Pathol.* 108: 597–609.

Marasas, W.F.O. and Nelson, P.E. (1987). *Mycotoxicology*. Pennsylvania: Pennsylvania State University Press, University Park, USA.

Marasas, W.F.O., Kriek, N.P.J., Fincham, J.E., and Van Rensburg, S.J. (1984). Primary liver cancer and oesophageal basal cell hyperplasia in rats caused by *Fusarium moniliforme*. *Int. J. Cancer* 34: 383–387.

Munkvold, G.P. and Desjardins, A.E. (1997). Fumonisins in maize: can we reduce their occurrence? *Plant Dis.* 81: 556–565.

Nelson, P.E., Toussoun, T.A., and Cook, R.J. (1981). *Fusarium Diseases, Biology and Taxonomy*. University Park, USA: Pennsylvania State University Press.

Pitt, J.I. and Hocking, A.D. (1997). *Fungi and Food Spoilage*, 2e. London, UK: Chapman and Hall.

Rebell, G. (1981). *Fusarium* infections in human and veterinary medicine. In: *Fusarium: Diseases, Biology, and Taxonomy* (ed. P.E. Nelson, T.A. Toussoun, and R.J. Cook). University Park, USA: Pennsylvania State University Press.

Samson, R., Hoekstra, E., Frisvad, J., and Filtenborg, O. (1996). *Introduction to Food-borne Fungi*, 5e. Netherlands: Centraal bureau voor Schimmel cultures. Baarn.

Shruthi, B., Deepa, N., Rakesh, S. et al. (2022). Exploring biotechnological and functional characteristics of probiotic yeasts: a review. *Biotechnol. Rep.* 34: e00716.

Sietsma, J.H., Wosten, H.A.B., and Wessels, J.G.H. (1995). Cell wall growth and protein secretion in fungi. *Can. J. Bot.* 73: 388–395.

Smith, J.E., Lewis, C.W., Anderson, J.G., and Solomons, G.L. (1984). Mycotoxins in human nutrition and health. In: *EUR 16048 EN. European Commission*. Agro-Industrial Research Division.

Sreenivasa, M.Y., Dass, R.S., Raj, A.-P.C. et al. (2011). Assessment of the growth inhibiting effect of some plant essential oils on different *Fusarium* species isolated from sorghum and maize grains. *J. Plant Dis. Prot.* 118 (6): 208–213.

Sreenivasa, M.Y., Raj, A.-P.C., Dass, R.S., and Janardhana, G.R. (2012). Diversity of *Fusarium* species associated with Maize and Sorghum grains grown in Karnataka, India. *Fungal Sci.* 26 (2): 111–123.

Summerell, B.A., Salleh, B., and Leslie, J.F. (2003). A utilitarian approach to *Fusarium* identification. *Plant Dis.* 87: 117–128.

Wilson, J.P., Cooper, H.H., and Wilson, D.M. (1995). Effect of delayed harvest on contamination of pearl millet grain with mycotoxin producing fungi and mycotoxins. *Mycopathologia* 132: 27–30.

1

Strategies for the Control of Aflatoxigenic *Aspergillus* Species in Contaminated Food and Feed

Premila N. Achar[1], Quenton Kritzinger[2], and Santosh Sharma[3]

[1] Department of Molecular and Cellular Biology, Kennesaw State University, Kennesaw, GA, USA
[2] Department of Plant and Soil Sciences, University of Pretoria, Hatfield, Pretoria, South Africa
[3] The Biotechnology Research, Ghaziabad, India

CONTENTS

Abstract

Aspergillus flavus and *Aspergillus parasiticus* are pathogenic to a variety of crops, including maize, groundnuts, and sorghum. Contamination occurs during pre- and post-harvest and storage. Current strategies against *Aspergillus* spp. in grains include physical and chemical methods. Extensive use of chemicals may produce side effects, such as carcinogenicity, teratogenicity, and toxicity to consumers due to toxic residues in food products. Due to an increased global

Anti-Mycotoxin Strategies for Food and Feed, First Edition. Edited by Deepa Nagaraju, Sreenivasa Marikunte Yanjarappa, Premila N. Achar, and Angel Medina Vaya.

awareness of the use of chemicals, there is an increased interest in sourcing alternate natural products against pathogenic fungi. It is proven that natural products are less toxic, environmentally safer, and most importantly, biodegradable as opposed to synthetic fungicides. In this chapter, we highlight the anti-aflatoxigenic strategies of plant extracts and essential oils against *Aspergillus* spp. to reduce or prevent aflatoxin contamination in food and feed. Emphasis will be placed on the feasibility of plant biologicals as alternative control methods, highlighting the research gaps.

Keywords *Aspergillus spp., aflatoxin, food and feed, plant extracts, essential oils and control strategies*

Graphical Representation

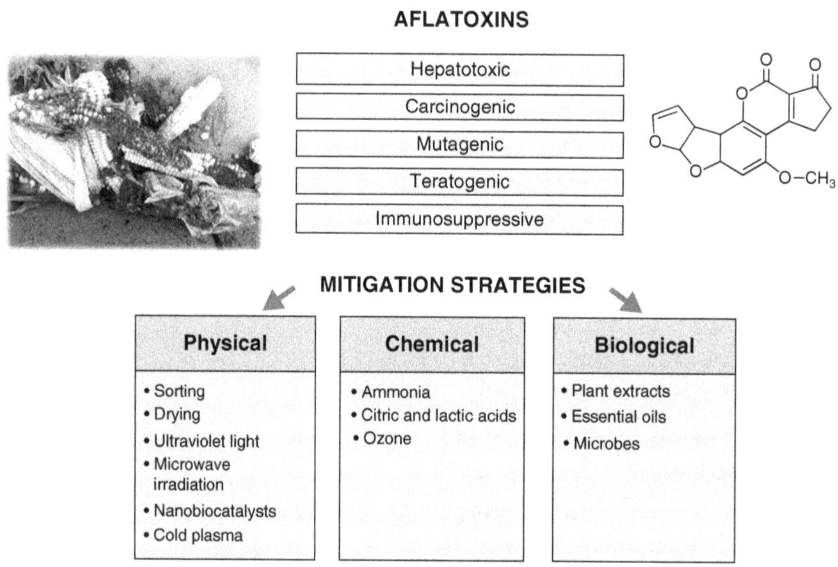

1.1 Introduction

Mycotoxins are secondary metabolites produced by fungi, detected in our food and feed that ultimately lands in our food chain. These toxic chemical compounds are produced by certain fungi and are associated with diseased or moldy crops. According to the Food and Agriculture Organization (FAO) of the United Nations, one-fourth of the world's crops are affected by mycotoxins (Deepa et al. 2016a, b; Eskola et al. 2020; Nazhand et al. 2020). However, the mycotoxins of importance and of greatest significance in human foods and animal feeds are aflatoxins produced by *Aspergillus* species.

1.2 *Aspergillus* Species and Aflatoxin Types in Food and Feed

Aspergillus species have been reported as one of the serious contaminants of plants, plant products, food, and feed (Kumar et al. 2022a) and in various agricultural crops before harvesting or during storage (Saini and Kaur 2012). Aflatoxins are produced by many fungal species though mainly by various species of *Aspergillus* section Flavi. These include *Aspergillus flavus*, *Aspergillus parasiticus*, *Aspergillus nomius*, *Aspergillus pseudotamarii*, *Aspergillus parvisclerotegenus*, and *Aspergillus minisclerotigenes* (Ahmad et al. 2014; Pleadin et al. 2014; Olana 2022). Of all the *Aspergillus* species, *A. flavus* and *A. parasiticus* (Figure 1.1) are known as the most toxigenic strains (Ajmal et al. 2022; Shabeer et al. 2022). Recent reports indicate at least 28 species of the genus *Aspergillus* have been identified to produce aflatoxins (Frisvad et al. 2019; Ajmal et al. 2022). The type of aflatoxins detected in various food sources around the world between 2010 and 2022 and the method of detection using various techniques are documented at length (Kumar et al. 2022b). The most common and important ones are aflatoxin-B1 (AFB1), aflatoxin-B2 (AFB2), aflatoxin-G1 (AFG1), aflatoxin-G2 (AFG2) (Benkerroum 2020), aflatoxin-M1 (AFM1), and aflatoxin-M2 (AFM2) (MdQuadri et al. 2012). While B1, B2, G1, and G2 are found in food crops or their products, M1 (metabolite of B1) and M2 (metabolite of B2) are found in the animals' by-products such as dairy products (Serraino et al. 2019; Shabeer et al. 2022). In addition, aflatoxins have been found in animal urine (Lalah et al. 2020). Aflatoxin B1 has been classified as a class I human carcinogen by the International Agency for Research on Cancer (IARC) and is reportedly the most toxic (World Health Organization and International Agency for Research on Cancer 1993; IARC 2012; Deepa and Sreenivasa 2017; Deepa et al. 2021).

1.3 Distribution of Aflatoxin Contamination Across the Globe

Aflatoxigenic fungi are worldwide in distribution, and due to their ubiquitous nature, about 4.5 billion of the world's population is subjected to aflatoxin contamination (Sreenivasa et al. 2008, 2011a; Tola and Kebede 2016; Shabeer et al. 2022). According to the latter author, aflatoxin contamination is most prevalent in Asia and Africa, where climatic conditions favor the development of aflatoxigenic strains in both field and storage conditions. Due to global climate change, aflatoxin is an emerging threat in regions that were previously free from this menace, though there have been a few reports of aflatoxin in different regions of Europe (Nagaraja et al. 2016; Jallow et al. 2021; Ajmal et al. 2022). Moreover, aflatoxin contamination of food and feed is still of global significance and remains a food safety issue since it poses significant health risks to humans and animals. Increased mortality in farm animals and the marketability of food products are adversely affected by aflatoxin contamination (Reiter et al. 2009; Sreenivasa et al. 2011b; Rajarajan et al. 2013; Ajmal et al. 2022). Even with the best prevention strategies, according to researchers (Peles et al. 2021), aflatoxins can end up in the food chain given that they are universal worldwide and that ever-changing environmental conditions prevent strict elimination. Singh et al. (2021) reported challenges in the supply chain and socio-economic hardships caused by the ongoing COVID-19 pandemic. In addition, the numbers of those affected may rise with increased consumption of aflatoxin-contaminated foods and due to political instability (World Bank 2022).

1.4 Aflatoxin Limits in Food and Feed

International agencies have enacted regulations to minimize the levels of aflatoxins in food and feed. The FAO has provided regulations on mycotoxin concentration in both food and feeds, and the Food and Drug Administration (FDA) has assigned specific limits

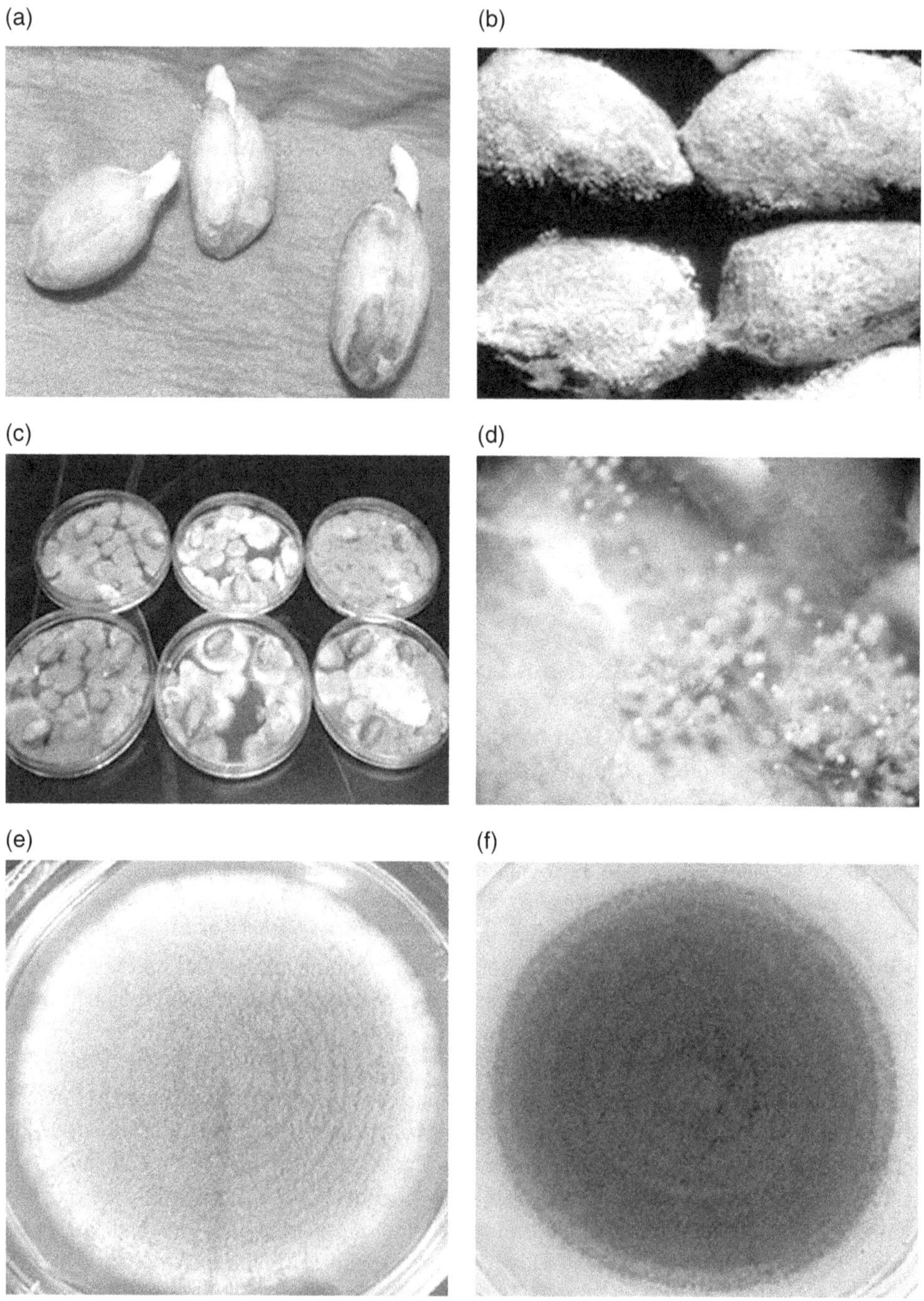

Figure 1.1 (a) Healthy peanuts; (b) *Aspergillus flavus* on infected peanuts; (c) *A. flavus*-contaminated peanuts on Potato Dextrose Agar (PDA) after seven days of incubation; (d) seed coat cracked by sporulating *A. flavus*; (e) *A. parasiticus* and (f) *A. flavus* culture on PDA.

for aflatoxin consumption. For humans' and animals' consumption, the maximum limit for aflatoxins in food and feed has been set to 20 ppb by the European Commission (FDA 2019; Commission Directive 2003), a limit to 4 ppb by the European Union, and 0.5 ppb in food and dairy products, respectively (Kodape et al. 2022). According to the Rapid Alert System for Food and Feed (RASFF 2022) database, most of the aflatoxin contamination was reported in nuts such as peanuts, pistachios, hazelnuts, and almonds; spices; and dried figs with up to 1000 µg/kg. Pickova et al. (2021) suggested that this high concentration of aflatoxins was mainly due to poor food management practices of the COVID-19 pandemic. Hence, an increase in health concerns related to it could also be expected.

1.5 Aflatoxin Biosynthesis

Aflatoxins are furanocoumarin derivatives produced by a polyketide pathway by many strains of *A. flavus* and *A. parasiticus*; in particular, *A. flavus* is a common contaminant in agriculture (Bennett and Klich 2003). A detailed review of biosynthesis and regulation of aflatoxins, for reducing human exposure to aflatoxins as well as how aflatoxin impacts human health, was reported (Roze and Linz 2013). The biosynthesis of aflatoxins involves an elaborate series of at least 15 post-polyketide synthase steps, yielding a series of increasingly toxigenic metabolites (Figure 1.2) (Nazhand et al. 2020).

1.6 Aflatoxin Mitigation

Due to the harmful effect of aflatoxins on the health of humans and animals worldwide, the control of aflatoxins is essential (Shabeer et al. 2022). It is imperative that researchers understand the role of various abiotic and biotic factors that predispose the infection of the host with aflatoxigenic fungi and the conditions that encourage their formation in order to minimize or prevent aflatoxin contamination in crops (Paterson and Lima 2010; Udomkun et al. 2017). To minimize aflatoxin contamination in plants, several strategies have been developed, including traditional and innovative techniques to control *Aspergillus* spp. in food and feed.

Innovative control technologies can enhance sustainable agricultural productivity (Filazi and Sireli 2013; Prietto et al. 2015). However, the first step is to understand pre- and post-harvest management techniques (Olana 2022). Conventional approaches for mycotoxin reduction include both prevention and decontamination strategies. These strategies can be grouped into physical, chemical, and biological processes (Table 1.1). In addition, the development and future perspective of nanoenzymes in aflatoxin degradation (Figure 1.3) have been reported (Deepa and Sreenivasa 2019a, b; Guo et al. 2021).

Each group represents its own advantages and limitations regarding implementation and overall efficacy. In the following sections, each process is briefly discussed, providing an overview of current and novel technologies and methods with regard to aflatoxin decontamination of grain, food, and feed.

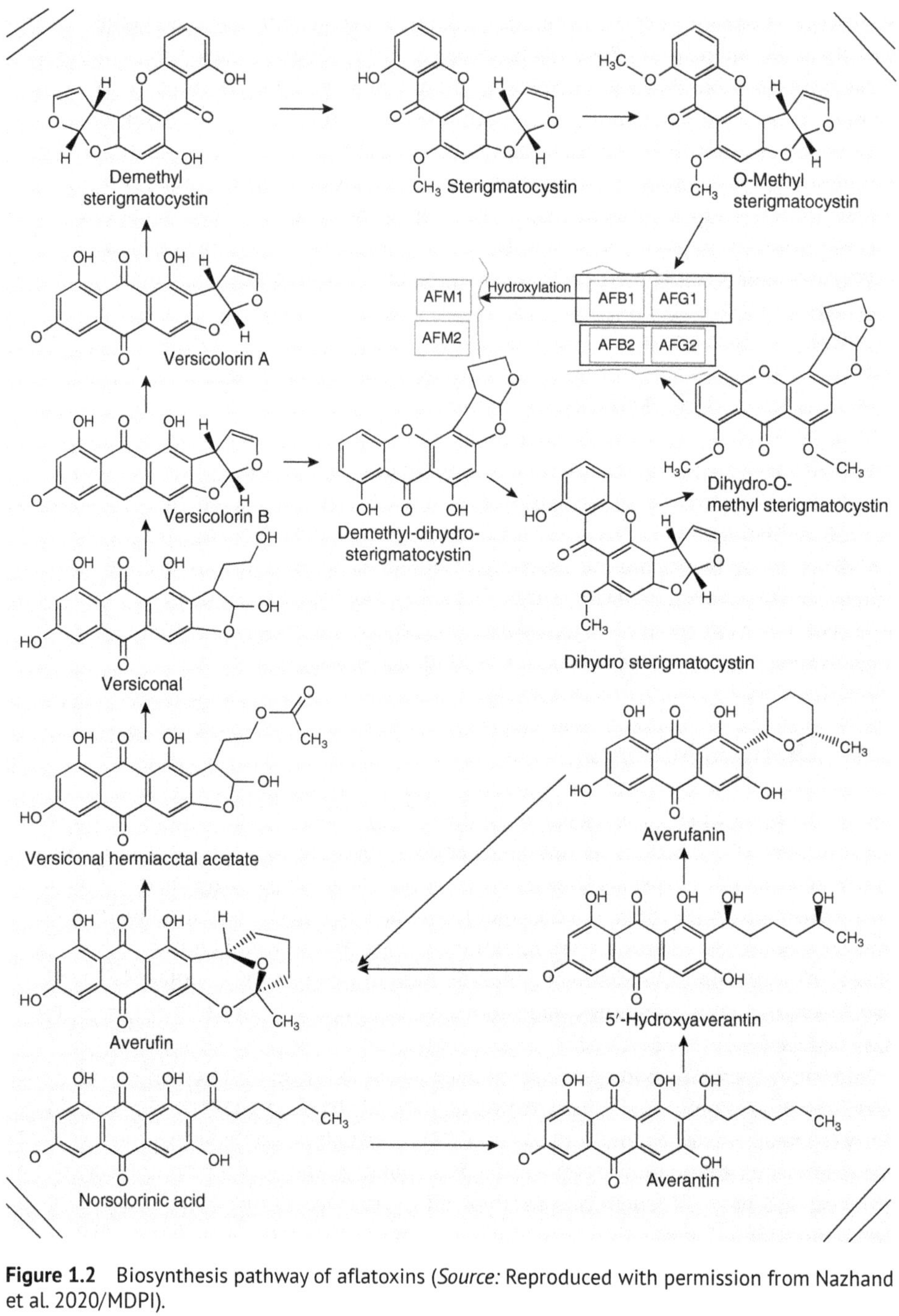

Figure 1.2 Biosynthesis pathway of aflatoxins (*Source:* Reproduced with permission from Nazhand et al. 2020/MDPI).

Table 1.1 Physical, chemical, and biological strategies for the reduction of aflatoxins.

S. No.	Aflatoxin reduction strategy		Methodology	Percentage reduction	References
1.	Physical	Sorting	Bright greenish yellow fluorescence (BGYF) test	AFB 85–90%	Marshall et al. (2020)
		High-temperature treatments	Heating in an oven	AFB1 50% and 90% at 150 and 200 °C, respectively	Hussain et al. (2011)
2.	Chemical	Citric acid	Combination of citric acid and pulsed light treatments	AFB 98.2% AFB1 98.9%	Abuagela et al. (2019)
		Lactic acid	Lactic acid in combination with heating for 120 minutes	AFB1 85%	Aiko et al. (2016)
		Ozone	Ozonated-roasted	AFB1 100%	Kaur et al. (2022)
			Ozonated only	AFB1 80.95%	
			Roasted only	AFB1 57.14%	
			40 minutes treatment with 90 mg/L ozone	AFB1's decrease from 77.6 to 21.42 mug/kg	Luo et al. (2015)
			2.8 and 5.3 mg/L of ozone stream at room temperature for up to 240 minutes in poultry feed samples	AFB1 74.3–86.4%	Torlak et al. (2016)
			2.8 and 5.3 mg/L of ozone stream at room temperature for up to 120 minutes in poultry feed samples	AFB1 53.3–70.2%	
3.	Biological	Plant extracts	Oil extract from *Cymbopogon citratus*	AFB1 100% at 0.1 mg/mL	Paranagama et al. (2003)
			Punica granatum	AFB1 100% at 5 mg/mL	Mostafa et al. (2011)
			Zingiber officinalis and *Olea europaea*	AFB1 100% at 15 mg/mL	
			Prosopis rusciflolia (methanol extract of aerial parts)	AFB1 100% at 47 μg/mL	Gomez et al. (2020)
			Turmeric (25% ethanolic extract)	AFB1 90.78%	Behiry et al. (2022)

(*Continued*)

Table 1.1 (Continued)

S. No.	Aflatoxin reduction strategy	Methodology	Percentage reduction	References
		Peel wastes:		Ismail et al. (2021)
		Eggplant (50% diethyl ether extract)	AFB1 96.11%	
		Sugar apple (75% ethanol extract)	AFB1 94.85%	
		Pomegranate (25% diethyl ether extract)	AFB1 78.83%	
	Essential oils	Various concentrations of different EOs (antifungal activities of EOs – disc diffusion, poisoned food technique, MIC)	Up to 100%	Thanaboripat et al. (2016) Kahkha et al. (2014) Gemeda et al. (2014) Gupta et al. (2011) Yooussef et al. (2016)
			Over 90%	Achar et al. (2020)
			67.53–72.7%	Abd El-Aziz et al. (2015) Xiang et al. (2020)
			Potent antifungal	Hyldgaard et al. (2012) Alizadeh et al. (2010) Sulieman et al. (2016) Wang et al. (2018)
	Microbes	Binding ability to cell wall of *Saccharomyces cerevisiae*	AFB1 3.96 ppb reduction when viable yeast cells used	Sahebghalam et al. (2013)
		Lactobacillus spp.	AFB1 (29.9–44.5%)	Oluwafemi et al. (2010)
		Atoxigenic *A. flavus* strains	AFB1 90%	Xu et al. (2021)

1.7 Physical Strategies to Control *Aspergillus* Species and Aflatoxins

Hand sorting is the most common physical decontamination process that can be labor-intensive and time-consuming. Grain that looks moldy, discolored, deformed, wrinkled, or unhealthy should be removed and discarded. Marshall et al. (2020) remarked that the combination of fluorescence-based sorting to remove highly contaminated produce paired with a secondary decontamination process is believed to offer great potential in reducing

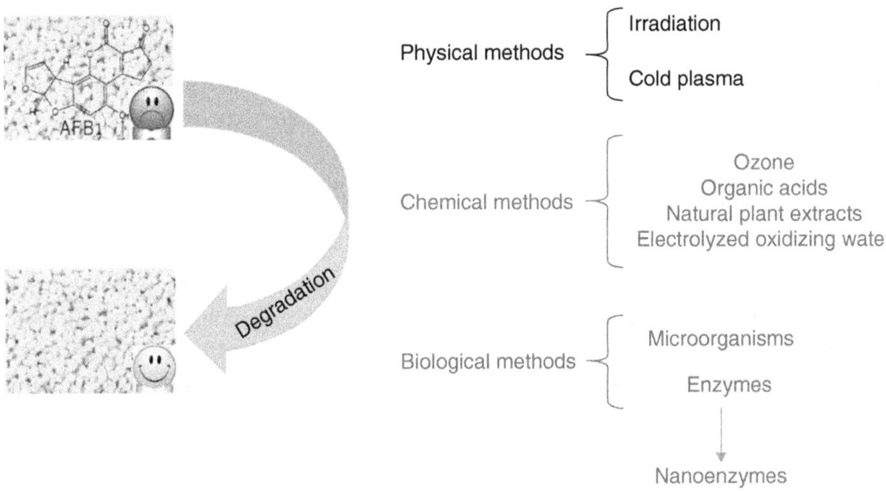

Figure 1.3 Novel strategies for degradation of aflatoxins in food and feed (*Source:* Reproduced with permission from Guo et al. (2021)/Elsevier).

aflatoxin contamination in grain but also not negatively affecting the sensorial and nutritional profile. The bright greenish yellow fluorescence (BGYF) test is based on the fluorescent properties of kojic acid (formed by *A. flavus* or *A. parasiticus*) or the mycotoxin itself and peroxidase enzyme present in the plant tissues. A camera using hyperspectral fluorescence data with an LED-based UV lighting system can detect and sort contaminated grain at a remarkable speed (Marshall et al. 2020).

An effective strategy to prevent aflatoxin contamination of food crops and foodstuff is the ability to manipulate the storage environment to prevent fungal growth. Drying is the basic but fundamental process of moisture removal from grain. More conventional types of drying include mechanical driers and solar drying. Sun-drying, where grain is heated by solar radiation, is regarded as the cheapest process. On sunny days, the drying process can normally take two to three days depending upon the spreading density and the climatic conditions. It is important that all processes after drying (e.g. packaging, transport, storage) be followed with care to ensure that the grain remains dry.

Naturally, the storage container and conditions are of utmost importance. Clean and dry storage containers, for example, drums, metallic silos, or polyethylene bags, are essential. To prevent mycotoxin contamination, grain should be stored under anaerobic conditions since most fungal species are obligate aerobes. Airtight containers or hermetically sealed bags, for example, Purdue Improved Crop Storage (PICS), can be used to decrease moisture and oxygen levels (Walker et al. 2018).

Various field management practices may also prevent aflatoxin contamination in crops. These include the use of resistant varieties, correct planting time, fertilizer application, weed control, insect control, and avoiding stress (e.g. water or mineral stress) (Hell and Mutegi 2011). Basically, good management practices can lead to reduction of aflatoxin contamination in the field.

It is well known that aflatoxins are highly thermostable and therefore do not decompose during cooking or processing. However, high-temperature treatments of 100 and 150 °C did reduce AFB1 levels significantly in soybean (*Glycine max*) milk (Su 2019). Furthermore, it is reported that high-pressure cooking is more effective than conventional cooking to remove AFB1.

There are numerous reviews that focus on the control and decontamination of aflatoxins in food and feed using physical methods (Peng et al. 2018; Marshall et al. 2020; Guo et al. 2021; Kutasi et al. 2021; Sipos et al. 2021; Abou Dib et al. 2022). Recently, Hamad et al. (2023) published a comprehensive review of innovative strategies for controlling mycotoxins in foods, highlighting cold plasma (CAP), magnetic materials, and nanoparticles as part of the physical methods. CAP is a novel non-thermal technology used to inactivate fungal pathogens and mycotoxins, which is regarded as being eco-friendly, highly efficient, and low cost (Guo et al. 2021; Sipos et al. 2021; Wu et al. 2021). According to Misra et al. (2019), CAP is a result of atmospheric dielectric discharge, causing the ionized gas to contain metastable atoms and molecules with a nearly zero net electrical charge. The mycotoxin degradation is attributed to the free radicals of O and OH.

Other physical approaches that have been reviewed include ultraviolet (UV) light (Sipos et al. 2021), gamma rays (Tahir et al. 2018; Sipos et al. 2021), and microwave irradiation. Awan et al. (2022) found that AFB_1 concentration in pine nuts was reduced through UV-based detoxification. Microwave irradiation resulted in a 3-log reduction in aflatoxin producing *A. parasiticus* contamination of hazelnuts (*Corylus avellana*) after 120 seconds of treatment, without any noticeable change in nutritional and sensorial properties of the nuts (Basaran and Akhan 2010). The authors also proposed a hybrid process where UV-C surface treatment and vacuum-assisted microwaves can be combined with air drying to increase the shelf life and quality of the nuts. On the other hand, Hussain et al. (2011) found that AFB1 reduction was directly proportional to washing time in contaminated wheat (*Triticum aestivum*) varieties. However, the concentration of AFB1 was reduced more by heating than washing; AFB1 levels decreased by 50% and 90% by heating in an oven at 150 and 200 °C, respectively. Kutasi et al. (2021) reported that processes including freezing, cooking, and pressurizing have little effect on aflatoxins. Furthermore, they commented that methods such as irradiation with UV photons, pulses of extensive white radiation, and gaseous plasma are propitious but further studies are needed to understand the exact mechanisms of how these techniques degrade aflatoxins.

New advances include the use of novel combined proteinous nanobiocatalysts. Lyagin et al. (2022) developed enzymatic nanobiocatalysts that can destroy mycotoxins, including AFB1. The treatment of contaminated feed with these enzymes (belonging to hydrolases, oxidoreductases, and lyases) stabilized within polyelectrolyte complexes with poly(glutamic acid) significantly decreased the negative effects of mycotoxin mixtures on blood biochemical parameters, which were indicative of severe damage to liver and kidneys of Sprague-Dawley rats (Lyagin et al. 2022).

In addition to the reviews mentioned earlier, Pankaj et al. (2018) discussed the advantages and limitations of decontamination technologies including microwave heating, gamma and electron beam irradiation, UV and pulsed light, and electrolyzed water and CAP. For instance, pulsed light, electrolyzed water, and CAP have shown complete degradation of aflatoxin on various substrates. However, the application of food products needs further research due to their interaction with food components and the toxicology of the degradant.

1.8 Chemical Strategies to Control *Aspergillus* Species and Aflatoxins

Chemical treatment has been used as one of the most effective means for the removal of mycotoxins from contaminated commodities. Ammonia, as an anhydrous vapor and aqueous solution, has attracted the widest interest and has been exploited commercially by the feed industry for the destruction of aflatoxin (Peng et al. 2018). On-farm procedures involve spraying with aqueous ammonia followed by storage at ambient temperature for approximately two weeks in large silage bags (Coker 1994).

However, chemicals used as grain protectants or to protect stored produce have become expensive and are also perceived as being harmful to the environment and human health. Furthermore, the contamination of grain and foodstuff by chemicals can cause diseases or death in animals or humans. Chemical exposure does not only apply to people eating contaminated grains but it also applies to people working in the agricultural sector such as sprayers and farm workers. The use of chemicals has been reported to have adverse effects on the environment by causing toxic build-up, infertility, and groundwater contamination (Schoumans et al. 2014). Moreover, chemical pesticides tend to affect non-target organisms and increase the likelihood of resistance to pathogens (Zaker 2016; Walia et al. 2017). Azole fungicides such as prochloraz and tebuconazole are commonly used on important grains like maize against multiple *Aspergillus* spp. These fungicides inhibit the biosynthesis of ergosterol in fungi and yeast (Zarn et al. 2003). Ergosterol is important in the regulation of the fluidity and permeability of membranes (Jordà and Tuig 2020). However, the inhibition of fungi by azole fungicides has led to several teratogenic effects noted in humans (Chambers et al. 2014; Chennappa et al. 2014, 2016).

Abuagela et al. (2019) studied the effect of citric acid and pulsed light treatments (physical and chemical treatments) combined to degrade AFBs in groundnuts. Aflatoxins reduced by 98.2% with the combined treatment when compared to untreated groundnuts. Of significance, AFB1 was reduced by up to 98.9%. However, there were changes in color parameters in the groundnuts and further investigations are required to deliver a commercially preferred product. Another study has shown lactic acid to be the most efficient in degrading AFB1 when compared to acetic and citric acids (Aiko et al. 2016). Approximately, 85% degradation of AFB1 was achieved in combination with heating for 120 minutes. Although two degradation products were formed, namely AFB(2) and AFB(2a), AFB(2a) showed much reduced cytotoxicity on HeLa cells when compared to AFB1.

Ozone (O_3) treatment has been identified as a process that contributes to improved quality and safety of food (Mohamed et al. 2022). Studies using ozone as an aflatoxin detoxification treatment on food and feed have shown varying results. Mohamed et al. (2022) reported that ozone treatments eliminated or significantly reduced aflatoxins in raw and ready-to-eat meat products with minor changes in physicochemical properties. Kaur et al. (2022) found that groundnut kernels that underwent ozonation and roasting had a

100% reduction in AFB1 when compared to kernels that just received ozonation or roasting. In addition, these authors found that the combined ozonation-roasting treatment had enhanced the functional compounds, structure, and texture of the kernels. Luo et al. (2015) found that AFB1 contents in maize with a moisture content of 20.37% decreased from 77.6 to 21.42 mug/kg after 40 minutes of treatment with 90 mg/L ozone. The degradation rate was found to be 72.4% (Luo et al. 2015). Contrary to these reports, Baazeem et al. (2022) found that AFB1 production in raw pistachio nuts was stimulated in *A. flavus* colonies after ozone treatment and storage for a period of 10 days and in nuts inoculated with conidia prior to ozone exposure.

Ozone proved to be an efficient chemical control method in poultry feed with a high AFB1 elimination percentage of up to 86.4% and did not affect the quality of the grain (Torlak et al. 2016). It is important that the application of ozone follows proper ozonation parameters to prevent ozone from decomposing into hydroxyl, hydroperoxyl, and superoxide radicals (Torlak et al. 2016), which can have negative effects on the grain. It is not known to be highly toxic to humans when used at concentrations effective as a fungicide (Sciorsci et al. 2020). However, the use of ozone by smallholder farmers may be limited due to costs or ease of access. A basic Google search on industrial ozone generators showed an average cost of between $400 and $900 per unit, which may be a high price to pay for small, already financially struggling farmers. In addition, a lack of knowledge on the usage of ozone by smallholder farmers may prove to be a major setback (El-Desouky et al. 2012).

1.9 Biologicals as a Control Strategy Against *Aspergillus* spp. and Aflatoxins

In this section, biological approaches include plant extracts, essential oils (EOs), and the use of microorganisms as biodegradation agents to control aflatoxin production in food and feed.

1.9.1 Plant Extracts

Plant extracts were introduced when chemical methods for controlling fungi were criticized for their pathogen resistance or toxicity to the environment and physical methods were criticized for their efficiency. Plant extracts as botanical fungicides could offer a unique alternative and opportunity to combat issues faced in agriculture and animal and human health due to aflatoxin contamination. Bearing this in mind, for successful implementation of such a strategy, both positive and negative aspects need to be considered. Plant extracts are considered environmentally friendly, safe, and more efficient in controlling fungi infection and mycotoxin production (Copping and Menn 2000; Peng et al. 2018). Moreover, plant extracts are advantageous over chemical fungicides as they have a narrow target range with a more specific mode of action. So, they are less likely to have harmful effects on non-target organisms in the environment and humans (Zaker 2016). Other advantages include being biodegradable, easy to prepare, and reduced costs in storage and disposal (Onaebi et al. 2019).

There are several examples where plant extracts are reported to control fungal infection and aflatoxin contamination. For example, leaf powder of *Withania somnifera* and peel powder of *Citrus sinensis* were proven to be efficient in controlling the production of AFB1 in soybean seeds infected with *A. flavus* (Krishnamurthy and Shashikala 2006). The oil extract of lemongrass (*Cymbopogon citratus*) was also proven to be efficient in inhibiting the growth, sporulation, and mycotoxin production of *A. flavus* in rice (*Oryza sativa*) at a specific concentration (Paranagama et al. 2003). *Punica granatum* methanolic extract inhibited AFB1 production at a concentration of 5 mg/mL, while it totally inhibited the growth of *A. flavus* at 10 mg/mL (Mostafa et al. 2011). Gomez et al. (2020) reported that methanolic extracts of the native northwest Argentinian plant *Prosopis ruscifolia* and indolizidine alkaloids showed strong antifungal activity against *A. flavus* and *A. parasiticus*. Moreover, they completely suppressed the synthesis of aflatoxins. Other extracts from ginger, *Olea europaea*, *Bidens pilosa*, pomegranate, sugar apple, eggplant peel, and turmeric have been reported to control or inhibit *A. flavus* growth and have aflatoxin detoxification potential (Saraswathy et al. 2020; Ismail et al. 2021; Behiry et al. 2022). However, many smallholder farmers are discouraged from using plant extracts because of the level of acceptance in the market. This is because the shelf-life and durability of plant extracts in the environment are limited, and they perform differently in different storage systems or areas (Copping and Menn 2000). However, other farmers use them quite frequently because of their belief in organic farming or producing organic food.

The use of plant extracts as an alternative is not flawless. To date, a major setback has been the lack of research on application of plant extracts in field trials. In addition, levels of cytotoxicity of potential natural fungicides developed from plant extracts in the laboratory and used in field trials need to be determined to ensure they are safe for human or animal ingestion. Plant extracts have a generally beneficial effect if consumed, but this is largely dependent on the dose. An incorrect dose can be toxic. Other elements for consideration include shelf-life, limited persistence in the environment, and variable field performance. However, with extensive research and development, plant extracts as botanical fungicides can become a leading alternative, especially for farmers in developing countries (Zaker 2016).

1.9.2 Essential Oils

Natural products could potentially serve as effective alternatives to synthetic chemicals for the control of food contamination by *Aspergillus* spp. (Hyldgaard et al. 2012). Among these, EOs from various aromatic plants are gaining interest as food additives and are widely accepted by consumers because of their relatively low toxicity, high volatility, transient nature, and biodegradability (Gupta et al. 2011). In this section, we have summarized the biological control of *Aspergillus* spp. and aflatoxins with potent antifungal EOs in foods and feeds (Yooussef et al. 2016; Achar et al. 2020). Abd El-Aziz et al. (2015) identified cinnamon and thyme EOs as having stronger antimicrobial potential in cashew seeds than garlic, mint, and rosemary. In addition, they found that 11 EOs, including cinnamon, oregano, lemongrass, clove, citronella, basil, thyme, *Litsea cubeba*, peppermint, mugwort, and rosemary, were anti-aflatoxigenic in maize. Xiang et al. (2020) reported cinnamon, oregano, and lemongrass EOs, in vapor state, with optimal antifungal effects. Essential oil from *Carum copticum* (Ajwain) was also reported as a potential candidate for the protection of foodstuff and feeds from toxigenic fungal growth and aflatoxin contamination (Kahkha et al. 2014). Thanaboripat et al. (2016) established that anise star EO had an inhibitory effect on both *A. flavus* and *A. parasiticus* with significant differences followed by cinnamon, cajuput, and ginger. Alizadeh et al. (2010) also reported that *Zateria multiflora*, *Carum capticum*, *Satureja hortensis*, and *Thymus migricus* EOs showed emerging effects against aflatoxin-producing species including *A. flavus*, *A. parasiticus*, *Aspergillus niger*, *Aspergillus ochraceus*, and *Aspergillus terreus*, whereas *Foeniculum vulgare EO* was not effective against any of these strains.

Gemeda et al. (2014) observed that *Cymbopogon martinii*, *F. vulgare*, and *Trachyspermum ammi* EOs showed antifungal properties such as inhibiting spore germination, growth, and mycotoxin production of *A. niger* and *A. flavus*, respectively. Of all EOs tested, *T. ammi* showed maximum antifungal effect and significant anti-aflatoxigenic potency by totally inhibiting aflatoxin production. In addition, *C. martinii*, *F. vulgare*, and *T. ammi* oils were found to be superior to synthetic preservatives. On the other hand, Sulieman et al. (2016) observed clove EO with optimum antifungal properties than six other EOs tested against mycelial growth of *A. flavus* and aflatoxin production. Similarly, Achar et al. (2020) demonstrated that clove EO could be a promising natural fungicide for an effective bio-controlled, non-toxic, bio-preservative, and an eco-friendly alternative to synthetic additives against *A. flavus* in peanuts. Since *Cinnamomum cassia*, *L. cubeba*, *C. martini*, and *Thymus mongolicus* showed stronger inhibitory effects and lower minimal inhibitory concentrations against *A. flavus*, *Penicillium viridicatum*, and *Aspergillus carbonarius*, Wang et al. (2018) suggested that these four EOs showed potential as novel natural antifungal alternatives for preventing fungal contamination.

1.9.3 Microbes

Certain microbes are exploited as biological treatments for the detoxification of aflatoxins. Oluwafemi et al. (2010) investigated the use of *Lactobacillus* spp. (lactic acid-producing species) for the detoxification of AFB_1 in maize grains. Five different lactic acid bacteria showed significant reductions in AFB1 on artificially inoculated maize grains, with *Lactobacillus plantarum* being most efficient (Rao et al. 2017). The authors stated that lactic acid bacteria should be considered bio-detoxification agents since they are already classified as Generally Regarded As Safe (GRAS) (www.fda.gov). Hell and Mutegi (2011) further commented that lactic acid and probiotics can be incorporated into the diet of consumers to reduce AFB1 toxic effects related to AFB1 ingestion. In another study, contaminated feed was inoculated with *Saccharomyces cerevisiae* cell cultures as three treatments: heat treated, acid treated, and no treatment (Sahebghalam et al. 2013). Average reduction of AFB_1 for different treatments showed viable yeast cells resulting in highest reduction, followed by heat-treated cells and then acid-treated cells. Furthermore, most reduction of toxin was observed within the first four hours of incubation, which indicates that aflatoxin binding reaches saturation rather quickly. Their results indicated that yeast cells, whether viable or non-viable, are suitable for detoxification of contaminated animal

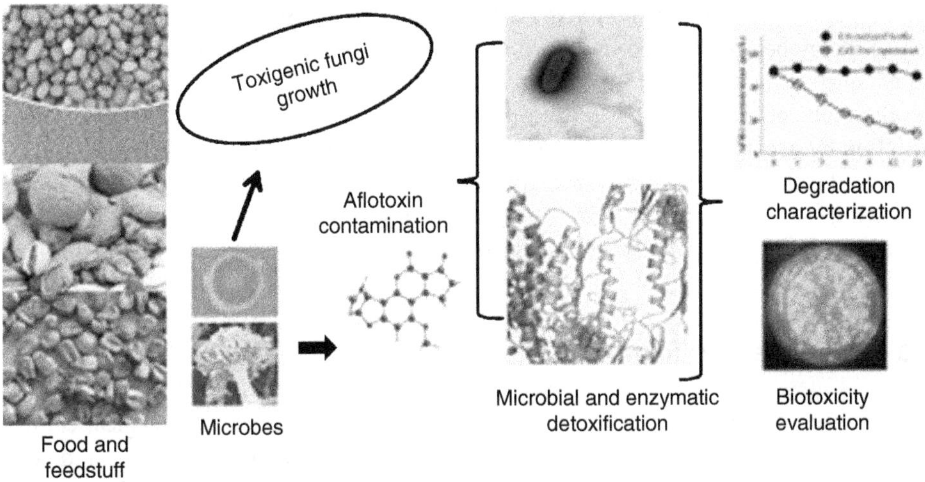

Figure 1.4 Detoxification of aflatoxin B1 by *Stenotrophomonas* sp. CW117 and characterization of the thermophilic degradation process (*Source:* Reproduced from Cai et al. 2020/with permission of Elsevier).

feeds. Cai et al. (2020) indicated that *Stenotrophomonas* sp. CW117 degraded AFB1 via a combination of enzymes and micro-molecule oxides, suggesting its potential significance to detoxification development on food and feedstuff (Figure 1.4). Although there are commercial products based on living microbes for the detoxification of trichothecenes and ochratoxin A, there are thus far no commercially microbe-based products to detoxify aflatoxins (Loi et al. 2023).

The use of atoxigenic fungi to competitively displace toxigenic fungi is well known (Xu et al. 2021). These strains are believed to act by "competitive exclusion" of the native strains, reducing the amount of aflatoxin in the harvested crop (King et al. 2011). Several atoxigenic strains have been registered in the United States to reduce aflatoxins in maize and groundnuts. Afla-Guard®, containing the non-aflatoxigenic *A. flavus* strain NRRL 21882, was the first product to be commercialized in groundnuts and maize, respectively. Xu et al. (2021) isolated and characterized two atoxigenic strains (L morphotype) from groundnuts and both were able to reduce AFB_1 levels, in both culture media and groundnut kernels, by up to 90%.

1.10 Summary

We have presented several methods such as traditional, physical, chemical, and biological to mitigate aflatoxins in food and feed. Combinations of these methods have proven efficient in reducing both pre- and post-harvest aflatoxin contamination. Different management strategies such as good agricultural manufacturing and storage practices have also been used to control aflatoxin contamination in food and feed across the globe. In addition, newer processing technologies in combination with data generated by genetic engineering, combined with disease development, and climatic change, have the potential to control *Aspergillus* infection and the contamination of carcinogenic aflatoxins in food and feed, which land in the food chain. Researchers across the globe are engaged in developing aflatoxin-resistant varieties, however, with no conclusive data to control *Aspergillus* spp. and free our crops from infection. The development of aflatoxin-resistant crops is perhaps the preferred solution to prevent infection by *Aspergillus* spp. However, this route of mitigation may not be cost-effective in underdeveloped countries where grains form part of their staple diet. These novel technologies should also not compromise the nutrient value of our food and feed products while keeping consumers safe worldwide.

1.11 Future Implications

Further studies should generate conclusive data on a combination of biological control methods and genetic engineering to develop disease-resistant crops against pre- and post-infection by *Aspergillus* spp. and prevent aflatoxin contamination in our food chain.

1.12 Study Questions

1) Health risks of aflatoxins in food and feed.
2) Biosynthesis of aflatoxins.
3) How to integrate cost-effective biological control methods in large crop fields?
4) Novel techniques for detoxification of aflatoxins across the globe.

Author Contributions

Conceptualization, coordinating, writing, and editing, P.N.A.; supervision, writing, and editing, Q.K. and S.S.

Acknowledgments

We would like to thank the Department of Molecular and Cellular Biology, Kennesaw State University (KSU), United States, and the Department of Plant and Soil Sciences, University of Pretoria, South Africa, for partial funding of the research on *Aspergillus* spp. We thank our research students Mullis, E. and Boyo, M. (KSU) for providing *Aspergillus* pictures, and Roberson, K., graduate writing coach, Writing Center (KSU) for professional editing of the manuscript.

Conflict of Interest

The authors confirm that they have no conflicts of interest.

References

Abd El-Aziz, A.R.M., Mahmoud, M.A., Al-Othman, M.R., and Al-Gahtani, M.F. (2015). Use of selected essential oils to control aflatoxin contaminated stored cashew and detection of aflatoxin biosynthesis gene. *Sci. World J.* 2015: 958192.

Abou Dib, A., Assaf, J.C., El Khoury, A. et al. (2022). Single, subsequent, or simultaneous treatments to mitigate mycotoxins in solid foods and feeds: a critical review. *Foods* 11 (20): 3304. https://doi.org/10.3390/foods11203304.

Abuagela, M.O., Iqdiam, B.M., Mostafa, H. et al. (2019). Combined effects of citric acid and pulsed light treatments to degrade B-aflatoxins in peanut. *Food Bioprod. Process.* 117: 396–403. https://doi.org/10.1016/j.fbp.2019.08.011.

Achar, P.N., Quyen, P., Adukwu, E.C. et al. (2020). Investigation of the antifungal and anti-aflatoxigenic potential of plant-based essential oils against *Aspergillus flavus* in peanuts. *J. Fungi* 6 (4): 383.

Ahmad, M., Ali, A., Hamid, R. et al. (2014). Detection *of Aspergillus flavus* and *Aspergillus parasiticus* from aflatoxin-contaminated peanuts and their differentiation using PCR-RFLP. *Ann. Microbiol.* 64: 1597–1605.

Aiko, V., Edamana, P., and Mehta, A. (2016). Decomposition and detoxification of aflatoxin B-1 by lactic acid. *J. Sci. Food Agric.* 96 (6): 1959–1966. https://doi.org/10.1002/jsfa.7304.

Ajmal, M., Bedale, W., Akram, A., and Yu, J.-H. (2022). Comprehensive review of aflatoxin contamination, impact on health and food security, and management strategies in Pakistan. *Toxins* 14 (12): 845. https://doi.org/10.3390/toxins14120845.

Alizadeh, A., Zamani, E., Sharaifi, R. et al. (2010). Antifungal activity of some essential oils against toxigenic *Aspergillus* species. *Commun. Agric. Appl. Biol. Sci.* 75 (4): 61–767.

Awan, H.S., Ahmad, K.S., Iram, S. et al. (2022). Analysis and quantification of naturally occurring aflatoxin B_1 in dry fruits with subsequent physical and biological detoxification. *Nat. Prod. Res.* 36 (12): 3100–3104.

Baazeem, A., Medina, A., and Magan, N. (2022). Impacts of gaseous ozone (O_3) on germination, mycelial growth, and aflatoxin B_1 production *in vitro* and *in situ* contamination of stored pistachio nuts. *Toxins* 14 (6): 416. https://doi.org/10.3390/toxins14060416.

Basaran, P. and Akhan, U. (2010). Microwave irradiation of hazelnuts for the control of aflatoxin producing *Aspergillus parasiticus. Innov. Food Sci. Emerg. Technol.* 11 (1): 113–117. https://doi.org/10.1016/j.ifset.2009.08.010.

Behiry, S.I., Hamad, N.A., Alotibi, F.O. et al. (2022). Antifungal and antiaflatoxigenic activities of different plant extracts against *Aspergillus flavus. Sustainability* 14 (19): 12908.

Benkerroum, N. (2020). Aflatoxins: producing-molds, structure, health issues and incidence in Southeast Asian and Sub-Saharan African countries. *Int. J. Environ. Res. Public Health* 17 (4): 1215.

Bennett, J.W. and Klich, M. (2003). Mycotoxins. *Clin. Microbiol. Rev.* 16 (3): https://doi.org/10.1128/CMR.16.3.497-516.

Cai, M., Qian, Y., Chen, N. et al. (2020). Detoxification of aflatoxin B1 by *Stenotrophomonas* sp. CW117 and characterization the thermophilic degradation process. *Environ. Pollut.* 261: 114178.

Chambers, J.E., Greim, H., Kendall, R.J. et al. (2014). Human and ecological risk assessment of a crop protection chemical: a case study with the azole fungicide epoxiconazole. *Crit. Rev. Toxicol.* 44 (20): 176–210.

Chennappa, G., Adkar-Purushothama, C.R., Umdale, S. et al. (2014). Impact of pesticides on PGPR activity of *Azotobacter* sp. isolated from pesticide flooded paddy soils. *Greener J. Agric. Sci.* 4 (4): 117–129.

Chennappa, G., Naik, M.K., Adkar-Purushothama, C.R. et al. (2016). PGP, abiotic stress tolerant and antifungal activity of *Azotobacter* sp. isolated from paddy soils. *Indian J. Exp. Biol.* 54 (5): 322–331.

Coker, N.R.I. (1994). Biodeterioration of grain and the risk of mycotoxins. In: *Grain Storage Techniques: Evolution and Trends in Developing Countries*, FAO Agricultural Services Bulletin, vol. 109 (ed. D.L. Proctor), 27–38.

Commission Directive (2003). 2003/100/EC of 31 October 2003 amending annex I to directive 2002/32/EC of the European Parliament and of the council on undesirable substances in animal feed. *OJEU* 285: 33–37.

Copping, L.G. and Menn, J.J. (2000). Biopesticides: a review of their action, applications and efficacy. *Pest Manag. Sci.* 56: 651–676.

Deepa, N. and Sreenivasa, M.Y. (2017). Fumonisins: a review on its global occurrence, epidemiology, toxicity and detection. *J. Vet. Med. Res.* 4 (6): 1093.

Deepa, N. and Sreenivasa, M.Y. (2019a). Biocontrol strategies for effective management of phytopathogenic fungi associated with cereals. In: *New and Future Developments in Microbial Biotechnology and Bioengineering* (ed. J.S. Singh and D.P. Singh), 177–189. Elsevier. ISBN: 9780444641915. 10.1016/B978-0-444-64191-5.00013-4.

Deepa, N. and Sreenivasa, M.Y. (2019b). Molecular methods and key genes targeted for the detection of fumonisin producing *Fusarium verticillioides* - an updated review. *Food Biosci.* 32: 100473. https://doi.org/10.1016/j.fbio.2019.100473.

Deepa, N., Nagaraja, H., and Sreenivasa, M.Y. (2016a). Prevalence of fumonisin producing *Fusarium verticillioides* associated with cereals grown in Karnataka (India). *Food Sci. Human Well.* 5: 156–162. https://doi.org/10.1016/j.fshw.2016.07.001.

Deepa, N., Charith Raj, A.P., and Sreenivasa, M.Y. (2016b). Multiplex PCR method for the early detection of fumonisin producing *Fusarium verticillioides*. *Food Biosci.* 13: 84–88.

Deepa, N., Achar, P.N., and Sreenivasa, M.Y. (2021). Current perspectives of biocontrol agents for management of *Fusarium verticillioides* and its Fumonisin in cereals—a review. *J. Fungi* 7: 776. https://doi.org/10.3390/jof7090776.

El-Desouky, T.A., Sharoba, A., El-Desouky, A.I. et al. (2012). Effect of ozone gas on degradation of aflatoxin B1 and *Aspergillus flavus* fungal. *J. Environ. Anal. Toxicol.* 2 (2): 1000128.

Eskola, M., Kos, G., Elliott, C.T. et al. (2020). Worldwide contamination of food-crops with mycotoxins: validity of the widely cited 'FAO estimate' of 25%. *Crit. Rev. Food Sci. Nutr.* 60: 2773–2789.

Filazi, A. and Sireli, U.T. (2013). Occurrence of aflatoxins in food. In: *Aflatoxins-Recent Advances and Future Prospects* (ed. R.M. Abyanehin), 408. London: IntechOpen Book Series https://doi.org/10.5772/51031.

Food & Drug Administration (FDA). (2019). CPG Sec. 683.100 Action levels for aflatoxins in animal feeds. https://www.fda.gov/regulatory-information/search-fda-guidance-documents/cpg-sec-683100-action-levels-aflatoxinsanimal-feeds (accessed 17 February 2023).

Frisvad, J.C., Hubka, V., Ezekiel, C. et al. (2019). Taxonomy of *Aspergillus* section *Flavi* and their production of aflatoxins, ochratoxins and other mycotoxins. *Stud. Mycol.* 93: 1–63.

Gemeda, N., Woldeamanuel, Y., Asrat, D., and Debella, A. (2014). Effect of essential oils on *Aspergillus* spore germination, growth, and mycotoxin production: a potential source of botanical food preservative. *Asian Pac. J. Trop. Biomed.* 4 (Suppl 1): S373–S381.

Gomez, A.A., Baptista, Z.P.T., Mandova, T. et al. (2020). Antifungal and antimycotoxigenic metabolites from native plants of Northwest Argentina: isolation, identification and potential for control of *Aspergillus* species. *Nat. Prod. Res.* 34 (22): 3299–3302.

Guo, Y., Zhao, L., Ma, Q., and Ji, C. (2021). Novel strategies for degradation of aflatoxins in food and feed: a review. *Food Res. Int.* 140: 109878. https://doi.org/10.1016/j.foodres.2020.109878.

Gupta, A., Sharma, S., and Naik, S.N. (2011). Biopesticidal value of selected essential oils against pathogenic fungus, termites, and nematodes. *Int. Biodeterior. Biodegrad.* 65: 703–707.

Hamad, G.M., Mehany, T., Simal-Gandara, J. et al. (2023). A review of recent innovative strategies for controlling mycotoxins in foods. *Food Control* 144: 109350. https://doi.org/10.1016/j.foodcont.2022.109350.

Hell, K. and Mutegi, C. (2011). Aflatoxin control and prevention strategies in key crops of Sub-Saharan Africa. *Afr. J. Microbiol. Res.* 5 (5): 459–466.

Rapid Alert System for Food and Feed (RASFF). (2022). RASFF-window. https://webgate.ec.europa.eu/rasff-window/screen/search (accessed 9 February 2022).

Hussain, A., Lutfulla, G., and Khan, S. (2011). Reduction of aflatoxin B-1 contamination in Pakistani wheat varieties by physical methods. *Pak. J. Sci. Ind. Res. B Biol. Sci.* 54 (1): 23–28.

Hyldgaard, M.T., Mygind, T., and Meyer, R.L. (2012). Essential oils in food preservation: mode of action, synergies, and interactions with food matrix components. *Front. Microbiol.* 3: 12.

International Agency for Research on Cancer (IARC) (2012). *Review of Human Carcinogens: Chemical Agents and Related Occupations.* Geneva: World Health Organization.

Ismail, I.A., Qari, S.H., Shawer, R. et al. (2021). The application of pomegranate, sugar apple, and eggplant peel extracts suppresses *Aspergillus flavus* growth and aflatoxin B1 biosynthesis pathway. *Horticulturae* 7 (12): 558.

Jallow, A., Xie, H., Tang, X. et al. (2021). Worldwide aflatoxin contamination of agricultural products and foods: from occurrence to control. *Compr. Rev. Food Sci. Food Saf.* 20: 2332–2381.

Jordà, T. and Tuig, S. (2020). Regulation of ergosterol biosynthesis in *Saccharomyces cerevisiae*. *Genes* 11 (7): 795.

Kahkha, M.M.R., Amanloo, S., and Kaykhaii, M. (2014). Antiaflatoxigenic activity of *Carum copticum* essential oil. *Environ. Chem. Lett.* 12 (1): 231–234.

Kaur, G., Sidhu, G.K., Kaur, P., and Kaur, A. (2022). Influence of ozonation and roasting on functional, microstructural, textural characteristics, and aflatoxin content of groundnut kernels. *J. Texture Stud.* 53 (6): 908–922. https://doi.org/10.1111/jtxs.12713.

King, E.D., Bassi, A.B. Jr., Ross, D.C., and Druebbisch, B. (2011). An industry perspective on the use of "atoxigenic" strains of *Aspergillus flavus* as biological control agents and the significance of cyclopiazonic acid. *Toxin Rev.* 30 (2–3): 33–41. https://doi.org/10.3109/15569543.2011.588818.

Kodape, A.R., Raveendran, A., Shivegowda, C., and Babu, V. (2022). Aflatoxins: a postharvest associated challenge and mitigation opportunities. In: *Aflatoxins - Occurrence, Detection and*

Novel Detoxification Strategies (ed. J.C. Assaf), 188. London: IntechOpen Book Series https://doi.org/10.5772/intechopen.106333.

Krishnamurthy, Y.L. and Shashikala, J. (2006). Inhibition of aflatoxin B1 production of *Aspergillus flavus*, isolated from soybean seeds by certain natural plant products. *Lett. Appl. Microbiol.* 43 (5): 469–474.

Kumar, A., Pathak, H., Bhadauria, S., and Sudan, J. (2022a). Aflatoxin contamination in food crops: causes, detection, and management: a review. *Food Prod. Process. Nutr.* 3 (17): 1–9.

Kumar, P., Gupta, G., Mahato, D.K. et al. (2022b). Aflatoxins in cereals and cereal-based products: occurrence, toxicity, impact on human health, and their detoxification and management strategies. *Toxins* 14: 687. https://doi.org/10.3390/toxins14100687.

Kutasi, K., Recek, N., Zaplotnik, R. et al. (2021). Approaches to inactivating aflatoxins-a review and challenges. *Int. J. Mol. Sci.* 22 (24): https://doi.org/10.3390/ijms222413322.

Lalah, J.O., Omwoma, S., and Orony, D.A.O. (2020). Aflatoxin B1: chemistry, environmental and diet sources and potential exposure in humans in Kenya. In: *Aflatoxin B1 Occurrence, Detection and Toxicological Effects* (ed. X.D. Long), 220. London: IntechOpen Book Series.

Loi, M., Logrieco, A.F., Pusztahelyi, T. et al. (2023). Advanced mycotoxin control and decontamination techniques in view of an increased aflatoxin risk in Europe due to climate change. *Front. Microbiol.* 13: 1085891.

Luo, X., Wang, R., Wang, L. et al. (2015). Efficiency and kinetics of ozone degradation of aflatoxin B1 in corn. *Food Sci.* 36 (15): 45–49. https://doi.org/10.7506/spkx1002-6630-201515010.

Lyagin, I., Maslova, O., Stepanov, N., and Efremenko, E. (2022). Degradation of mycotoxins in mixtures by combined proteinousnanobiocatalysts: *in silico*, *in vitro* and *in vivo*. *Int. J. Biol. Macromol.* 218: 866–877. https://doi.org/10.1016/j.ijbiomac.2022.07.179.

Marshall, H., Meneely, J.P., Quinn, B. et al. (2020). Novel decontamination approaches and their potential application for post-harvest aflatoxin control. *Trends Food Sci. Technol.* 106: 489–496. https://doi.org/10.1016/j.tifs.2020.11.001.

MdQuadri, S.H., Niranjan, M., Chaluvaraju, K. et al. (2012). An overview of chemistry, toxicity, analysis, and control of aflatoxins. *Int. J. Chem. Life Sci.* 2: 1071–1078.

Misra, N.N., Yadav, B., Roopesh, M.S., and Jo, C. (2019). Cold plasma for effective fungal and mycotoxin control in foods: mechanisms, inactivation effects, and applications. *Compr. Rev. Food Sci. Food Saf.* 18: 106–120.

Mohamed, M.H., Ammar, M.A.M., Zaki, Z.M., and Youssef, A.E.K. (2022). Ozone as a solution for eliminating the risk of aflatoxins detected in some meat products. *Curr. Res. Nutr. Food Sci.* 10 (1): 334–348.

Mostafa, A.A., Al-Rahmah, A.N., and Abdel-Megeed, A. (2011). Evaluation of some plant extracts for their antifungal and antiaflatoxigenic activities. *J. Med. Plant Res.* 5 (17): 4231–4238.

Nagaraja, H., Chennappa, G., Rao, P.C.R.K. et al. (2016). Diversity of toxic and phytopathogenic fusarium species occurring on cereals grown in Karnataka state, India. *3 Biotech* 6: 57.

Nazhand, A., Durazzo, A., Lucarini, M. et al. (2020). Characteristics, occurrence, detection and detoxification of aflatoxins in foods and feeds. *Foods* 9: 644.

Olana, A. (2022). Aflatoxin producing fungi and its management: a review. *J. Plant Pathol. Microbiol.* 13: 641.

Oluwafemi, F., Kumar, M., Bandyopadhyay, R. et al. (2010). Bio-detoxification of aflatoxin B_1 in artificially contaminated maize grains using lactic acid bacteria. *Toxin Rev.* 29 (3–4): 115–122. https://doi.org/10.3109/15569543.2010.512556.

Onaebi, C., Onyeke, C., Osibe, D. et al. (2019). Antimicrobial activity of *Ocimumgratissimum* L. and *Carica papaya* L. against postharvest pathogens of avocado pear (*Persea americana* Mill.). *J. Plant Pathol.* 102: 319–325.

Pankaj, S.K., Shi, H., and Keener, K.M. (2018). A review of novel physical and chemical decontamination technologies for aflatoxin in food. *Trends Food Sci. Technol.* 71: 73–83. https://doi.org/10.1016/j.tifs.2017.11.007.

Paranagama, P.A., Abeysekera, K.H.T., Abeywickrama, K., and Nugaliyadde, L. (2003). Fungicidal and anti-aflatoxigenic effects of the essential oil of *Cymbopogon citratus*(DC.) Stapf. (lemongrass) against *Aspergillus flavus* Link. isolated from stored rice. *Lett. Appl. Microbiol.* 37: 86–90.

Paterson, R.R. and Lima, N. (2010). How will climate change affect mycotoxins in food? *Food Res. Int.* 43 (7): 1902–1914.

Peles, F., Sipos, P., Kovács, S. et al. (2021). Biological control and mitigation of aflatoxin contamination in commodities. *Toxins* 13: 104.

Peng, Z., Chen, L., Zhu, Y. et al. (2018). Current major degradation methods for aflatoxins: a review. *Trends Food Sci. Technol.* 80: 155–166. https://doi.org/10.1016/j.tifs.2018.08.009.

Pickova, D., Ostry, V., Toman, J., and Malir, F. (2021). Aflatoxins: history, significant milestones, recent data on their toxicity and ways to mitigation. *Toxins* 13: 399.

Pleadin, J., Vulić, A., Perši, N. et al. (2014). Aflatoxin B1 occurrence in maize sampled from Croatian farms and feed factories during 2013. *Food Control* 40: 286–291.

Prietto, L., Moraes, P.S., Kraus, R.B. et al. (2015). Post-harvest operations and aflatoxin levels in rice (*Oryza sativa*). *Crop Protect.* 78: 172–177. https://doi.org/10.1016/j.cropro.2015.09.011.

Rajarajan, P.N., Rajasekaran, K.M., and Asha Devi, K. (2013). Aflatoxin contamination in agricultural commodities. *Indian J. Pharm. Biol. Res.* 1 (4): 148–151.

Rao, P.K., Deepthi, B.V., Rakesh, S. et al. (2017). Anti-aflatoxigenic potential of cell free supernatant from *Lactobacillus plantarum* MYS44 against *Aspergillus parasiticus*. *Probio Antimicroprot.* 11 (1): 55–64.

Reiter, E., Zentek, J., and Razzazi, E. (2009). Review on sample preparation strategies and methods used for the analysis of aflatoxins in food and feed. *Mol. Nutr. Food Res.* 53: 508–524. https://doi.org/10.1002/mnfr.200800145.

Roze, L.V., Hong, S.-Y., and Linz, J.E. (2013). Aflatoxin biosynthesis: current frontiers. *Annu. Rev. Food Sci. Technol.* 4: 293–311. https://doi.org/10.1146/annurevfood-083012-123702.

Sahebghalam, H., Sani, A.M., and Mehraban, M. (2013). Bio-detoxification of AFB_1 in animal feeds using *Saccharomyces cerevisiae*. *J. Innov. Food Sci. Technol.* 5 (3): Pe99–Pe104.

Saini, S.S. and Kaur, A. (2012). Aflatoxin B1: toxicity, characteristics and analysis. *Glob. Adv. Res. J. Chem. Mater. Sci.* 1: 63–70.

Saraswathy, S.D., Mershiba, S., and Sahayamary, S. (2020). Exploring the antimycotoxigenic potential of *Acalypha indica* and *Bidens pilosa*. *Int. J. Life Sci. Pharma Res.* 10: 13–18.

Schoumans, O., Chardon, W., Bechmann, M. et al. (2014). Mitigation options to reduce phosphorus losses from the agricultural sector and improve surface water quality: a review. *Sci. Total Environ.* 468: 1255–1266.

Sciorsci, R.L., Lillo, E., Occhiogrosso, L., and Rizzo, A. (2020). Ozone therapy in veterinary medicine: a review. *Res. Vet. Sci.* 130: 240–246.

Serraino, A., Bonilauri, P., Kerekes, K. et al. (2019). Occurrence of aflatoxin M1 in raw milk marketed in Italy: exposure assessment and risk characterization. *Front. Microbiol.* 10: 2516.

Shabeer, S., Asad, S., Jamal, A., and Ali, A. (2022). Aflatoxin contamination, its impact and management strategies: an updated review. *Toxins* 14: 307. https://doi.org/10.3390/toxins14050307.

Singh, U., Gupta, S., and Gupta, M.A. (2021). A review study on biological ill effects and health hazards of aflatoxins. *Asian J. Adv. Med.* 3 (1): 1–8.

Sipos, P., Peles, F., Brasso, D.L. et al. (2021). Physical and chemical methods for reduction in aflatoxin content of feed and food. *Toxins* 13 (3): https://doi.org/10.3390/toxins13030204.

Sreenivasa, M.Y., Dass, R.S., Charith Raj, A.P., and Janardhana, G.R. (2008). PCR-based detection of genus *Fusarium* and Fumonisin-producing isolates from freshly harvested Sorghum grains grown in Karnataka, India. *J. Food Saf.* 28: 236–237.

Sreenivasa, M.Y., Dass, R.S., Charith Raj, A.P., and Janardhana, G.R. (2011a). Mycological evaluation of maize grains produced in Karnataka (India) for the post harvest fungal contamination. *World Appl. Sci. J.* 13 (4): 688–692.

Sreenivasa, M.Y., Dass, R.S., Adkar-Purushothama, C.R. et al. (2011b). Assessment of the growth inhibiting effect of some plant essential oils on different *Fusarium* species isolated from sorghum and maize grains. *J. Plant Dis. Protect.* 118 (6): 208–213.

Su, Q.-Y. (2019). The toxification and detoxification mechanisms of aflatoxin B1: an update. In: *Aflatoxin B1 Occurrence, Detection and Toxicological Effects* (ed. X.D. Long), 195. London: IntechOpen Book Series, IntechOpen Ltd https://doi.org/10.5772/intechopen.

Sulieman, A.M.E., Abdel-Rahim, A.M., and Mohammed, H.A. (2016). Impact of some essential oils on inhibition of aflatoxin production by *Aspergillus flavus*. *J. Food Process. Technol.* 7 (9 (Suppl)): 48.

Tahir, N.I., Hussain, S., Javed, M. et al. (2018). Nature of aflatoxins: their extraction, analysis, and control. *J. Food Saf.* 38 (6): https://doi.org/10.1111/jfs.12561.

Thanaboripat, D., Sarutipaisan, C., Puangtong, C. et al. (2016). Effects of four essential oils on the growth of aflatoxin producing fungi. *KMITL Sci. Tech. J.* 16 (2): 64–71.

Tola, M. and Kebede, B. (2016). Occurrence, importance and control of mycotoxins: a review. *Food Sci. Technol.* 2: 1191103. https://doi.org/10.1080/23311932.2016.1191103.

Torlak, E., Akata, I., Erci, F., and Uncu, A.T. (2016). Use of gaseous ozone to reduce aflatoxin B1 and microorganisms in poultry feed. *J. Stored Prod. Res.* 68: 44–49.

Udomkun, P., Wiredu, A.N., Nagle, M. et al. (2017). Innovative technologies to manage aflatoxins in foods and feeds and the profitability of application: a review. *Food Control* 76: 127–138.

Walia, S., Saha, S., Tripathi, V., and Sharma, K.K. (2017). Phytochemical biopesticides: some recent developments. *Phytochem. Rev.* 16: 989–1007.

Walker, S., Jaime, R., Kagot, V., and Probst, C. (2018). Comparative effects of hermetic and traditional storage devices on maize grain: mycotoxin development, insect infestation and grain quality. *J. Stored Prod. Res.* 77: 34–44.

Wang, H., Yang, Z., Ying, G. et al. (2018). Antifungal evaluation of plant essential oils and their major components against toxigenic fungi. *Ind. Crops Prod.* 120: 180–186.

World Bank. (2022). Food security update/World Bank response to rising food insecurity (accessed 27 March 2023).

World Health Organization and International Agency for Research on Cancer (1993). Some naturally occurring substances: Food items and constituents, heterocyclic aromatic amines and mycotoxins. In: *IARC Monographs on the Evaluation of the Carcinogenic Risk of Chemicals to Humans*, vol. 56. Geneva: World Health Organization.

Wu, Y., Cheng, J.H., and Sun, D.W. (2021). Blocking and degradation of aflatoxins by cold plasma treatments: applications and mechanisms. *Trends Food Sci. Technol.* 109: 647–661. https://doi.org/10.1016/j.tifs.2021.01.053.

Xiang, F., Zhao, Q., Zhao, K. et al. (2020). The efficacy of composite essential oils against aflatoxigenic fungus *Aspergillus flavus* in maize. *Toxins* 12 (9): 562.

Xu, J., Wang, P., Zhou, Z. et al. (2021). Selection of atoxigenic *Aspergillus flavus* for potential use in aflatoxin prevention in Shandong Province, China. *J. Fungi* 7: 773. https://doi.org/10.3390/jof7090773.

Yooussef, M.M., Quyen, P., Achar, P.N., and Sreenivasa, M.Y. (2016). Antifungal activity of essential oils on *Aspergillus parasiticus* isolated from peanuts. *J. Plant Protect. Res.* 56 (2): 139–142.

Zaker, M. (2016). Natural plant products as eco-friendly fungicides for plant diseases control - a review. *Agriculturists* 14 (1): 134–141.

Zarn, J.A., Brüschweiler, B.J., and Schlatter, J.R. (2003). Azole fungicides affect mammalian steroidogenesis by inhibiting sterol 14α-demethylase and aromatase. *Environ. Health Perspect.* 111: 255–261.

Further Reading

World Bank. (2023). Sharp, long-lasting slowdown to hit developing countries hard.

Beltran, A.O. and Bandyopadhyay, R. (2023). Aflatoxin biocontrol in practice requires a multidisciplinary, long-term approach. *Front. Sustain. Food Syst.* 7: 2023.

2

Advanced Anti-Fumonisin Strategies in Food and Feed

N. Deepa[1], Angel M. Vaya[2], and M.Y. Sreenivasa[1]

[1] *Molecular Mycotoxicology Laboratory, Department of Studies in Microbiology, University of Mysore, Mysuru, Karnataka, India*
[2] *Director of Environment and Agrifood, Cranfield University, Cranfield, Bedford, UK*

CONTENTS

Abstract

Fumonisins are toxic secondary metabolites produced by *Fusarium* species which is commonly found in food and feed. Species of *Fusarium* grow on a variety of different food crops and feedstuffs including cereals and cereal-based products like feeds, nuts, spices, dried fruits, apples, and coffee beans. Fumonisin-contaminated food and feed are known to produce adverse health effects leading to grave risk to humans, animal health, and livestock inducing acute and long-term chronic toxic effects being carcinogenic, mutagenic, cytotoxic, neurotoxic, teratogenic, nephrotoxic, immunosuppressant, and estrogenic. Fumonisins may be carried over into meat and eggs when poultry are fed with contaminated feed. Currently, the idea of monitoring

Anti-Mycotoxin Strategies for Food and Feed, First Edition. Edited by Deepa Nagaraju, Sreenivasa Marikunte Yanjarappa, Premila N. Achar, and Angel Medina Vaya.

fumonisin-producing *Fusarium* species is being challenged using recent biological control methods which play an important role in sustainable agriculture on food and feed. Recent innovative strategies like cold plasma, enzymes, nutrients, nanoparticles, ozone treatment, microbial antagonists techniques may be applied alone or integrated. As said, the strategies may be applied in the integrated form with endophytes, plant products, Plant Growth Promoting Rhizobacteria (PGPR), polyphenols, probiotics, and with several atoxigenic strains of organisms. These techniques are applied in recent days as anti-fumonisin strategies in food and feed which emerged as a promising approach on managing fumonisin contamination.

Keywords *Carcinogen, fumonisin, strategy, contamination, detoxification, degradation*

Graphical Representation

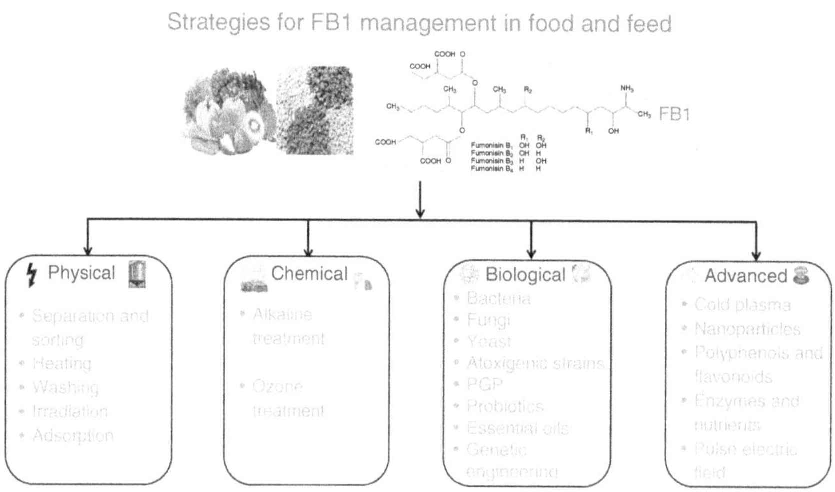

2.1 Introduction

Fumonisins referred to as *Fusarium* toxins were first discovered in 1988 at the Programme on Mycotoxins and Experimental Carcinogenesis (PROMEC) of the Medical Research Council (MRC) in Tygerberg, South Africa (Deepa and Sreenivasa 2017a, b). Fumonisins are toxic secondary metabolites produced in food and feed commodities by *Fusarium* species namely *Fusarium verticillioides* and *Fusarium proliferatum* (Rheeder et al. 2002). Fumonisins are mainly associated with corn and corn-based products, rice, wheat, rye, barley, millet, oat, tortillas, corn flakes, and feeds (Cendoya et al. 2018). In addition, *Aspergillus niger* also produces fumonisins in raisins, grapes, maize, sorghum, coffee, beer, wine, and peanut samples (Scott 2012; Kumar et al. 2017). Nearly, more than 28 fumonisin homologues are characterized, namely fumonisin A, fumonisin B, fumonisin C, P, and Py (Rheeder et al. 2002). Fumonisin B analogues include FB1, FB2, FB3, and FB4, whereas FB1 is reported to be the most toxic form as it is found with highest concentrations when compared to other forms (Alberts et al. 2016; Deepa and Sreeniasa 2017b; Braun and Wink 2018; Damiani et al. 2019). Chemical structure of fumonisins was first explicated by

Bezuidenhout et al. (1988) in a collaborative effort between PROMEC and Council for Scientific and Industrial Research (CSIR) in Pretoria (Deepa and Sreenivasa 2017b).

2.2 Occurrence and Distribution

Fumonisins are universal in nature and distribution. They are frequently associated in fields with freshly harvested, stored agricultural commodities, foods, feeds, and coffee from several parts of the world (Alberts et al. 2016). FB1 comprises 70% and is the most prominent fumonisin toxin when compared to the other forms FB2, FB3, and FB4 with 30% (Wang et al. 2008). FB1 contamination in maize-based products such as cereals, cornmeal, and corn flakes is being increasing in day-to-day life (Sreenivasa et al. 2011a, b; Alberts et al. 2016), popcorn (Bullerman and Tsai 1994), tortillas, and tortilla chips in Italy (Doko and Visconti 1994), sweet corn in Italy (Trucksess et al. 1995) but are also found to be allied in rice, sorghum, pearl millet, beans, wheat noodles, curry, chili pickle, cowpea, triticale, asparagus (Corpas-Hervias et al. 2006), soya beans in Japan (Aoyama et al. 2010), red wine in Italy (Logrieco et al. 2009, 2010), beer (Shephard et al. 2005), Cameroon in China (Njobeh et al. 2010), onion (Boonzaaijer et al. 2008), black tea (Omurtag and Yazicioglu 2004), cassava products in Tanzania (Manjula et al. 2009), garlic (Seefelder et al. 2002; Boonzaaijer et al. 2008), black radish (Di Mavungu et al. 2009), sugarcane (Mohammadi et al. 2012), figs in Turkey (Senyuva and Gilbert 2008; Karbancioglu-Guler and Heperkan 2009), peanuts in Ivoire, cow's milk in Italy (Gazzotti et al. 2009), meat (Prelusky et al. 1996), eggs (Vudathala et al. 1994), dietary and therapeutic plants in South Africa, flowers of linden and chamomile in Portugal, orange leaves (Martins et al. 2001), mint, sage leaves, stinging nettle in Turkey (Munkvold and Desjardins 1997), valerian root in Spain (Santos et al. 2009), banana (Anthony et al. 2004), corn-based brewing adjuncts (Desjardins et al. 2000), wheat (Desjardins et al. 2007), and sorghum (Tesso et al. 2004).

Maize grain samples were screened in Brazil and documented nearly 96% frequency of *F. verticillioides* (Rocha et al. 2011). In India, certain intelligence predicted contamination of fumonisins among poultry feeds, maize, and other cereal samples with *F. verticillioides* (Jindal et al. 1999). A study from Karnataka reported 59.20% of relative density with association of *F. verticillioides* from cereal samples collected in which 29 maize samples were infected with the *F. verticillioides* out of 61 maize samples (Deepa et al. 2016a, b). Nearly, 80 poultry feed mixtures and 114 animal feeds made of constituent maize pellets and wheat bran were analyzed for fumonisin contamination which reported uppermost prevalence of *F. verticillioides* (Dass et al. 2009). Cereal samples such as maize were infected with 103 fum-producing *Fusarium* species whereas sorghum cereal samples were associated with 64 fumonisin producers (Sreenivasa et al. 2007, 2008a, b). *F. proliferatum* is the second most *Fusarium* species reported with 108 feed sample contamination reporting 45.37% of feed assortments in fumonisin production (Deepthi et al. 2017).

2.3 Toxicity and Its Effects

Fumonisins resemble sphingosine structurally due to its polyhydric alcohol moiety. The mechanism of fumonisin involves a key enzyme ceramide synthase inhibition which disrupts the entire sphingolipid metabolism in tissues, cells, renal cells, neurons, and hepatocytes by

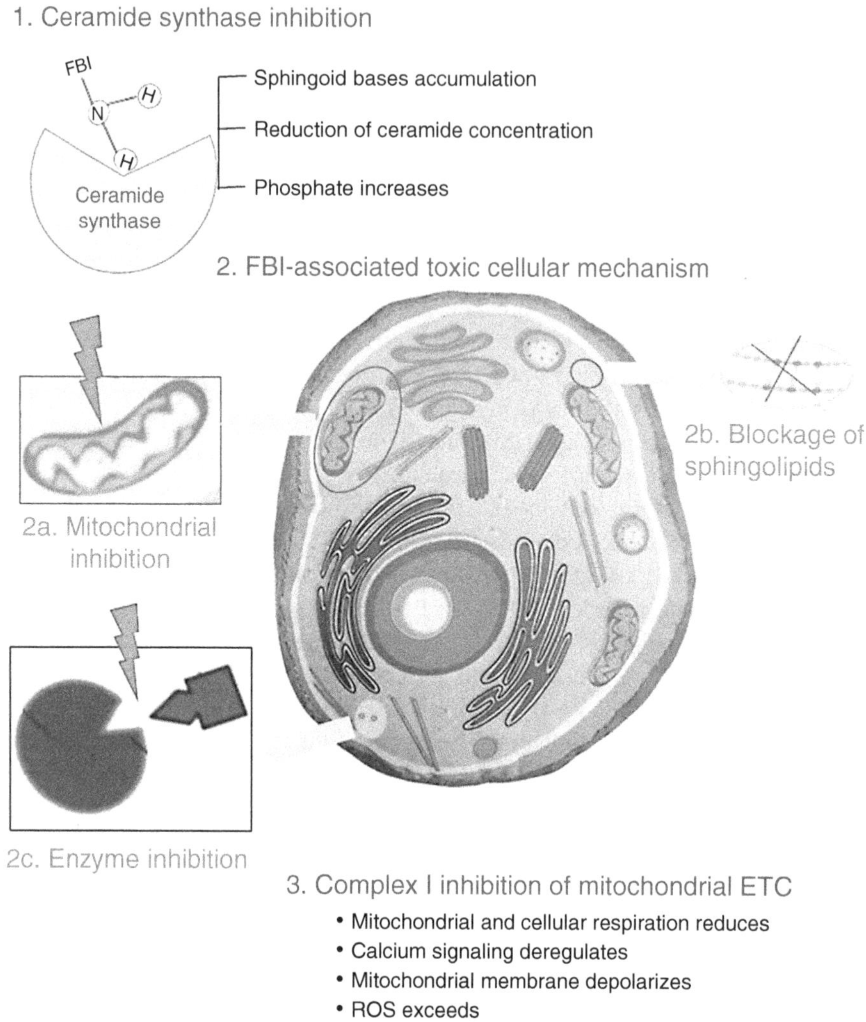

Figure 2.1 Representation of inhibition of ceramide synthase by Fumonisin B1.

Smith and Merrill (1995). FUM gene is the collection of fumonisin biosynthetic gene that is responsible for exploring the fum biosynthesis in *Aspergillus* and *Fusarium* (Alexander et al. 2009). This gene synthesis causes certain toxicological effects among humans, animals, and poultry. Accumulation of free sphinganine in liver, kidney, and lungs leads to cytotoxicity affecting the protein kinase activity causing apoptosis, cell growth, and cell differentiation subjecting to carcinogenesis with DNA damage (Domijan et al. 2007) (Figure 2.1).

Fumonisin B1 consumption mainly targets the kidney, liver, and lungs among animals and humans with wounds, oncotic necrosis, skin lesions, increased apoptotic, and hyperplasia in liver (Deepa and Sreenivasa 2017a; Sreenivasa et al. 2012). Hydrolyzed FB1 (HFB1) hinders sphingolipid metabolism without reporting any neural defects but blood-brain barrier was infused in young carp and mouse models (Kovacic et al. 2009). Studies

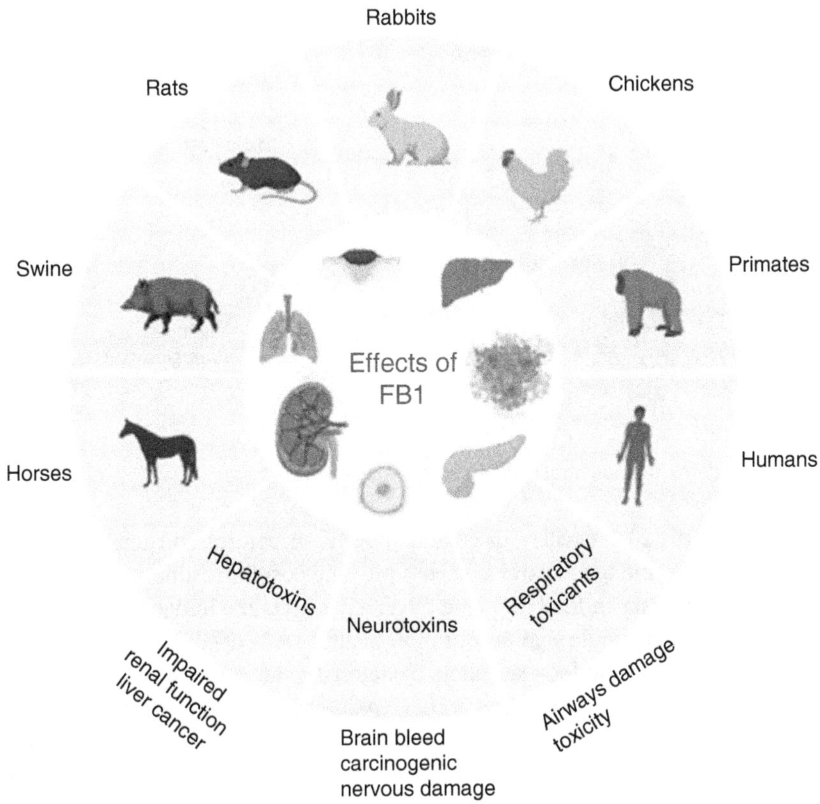

Figure 2.2 Post-effects of fumonisins on humans and animals.

reported the pigs and horses fed with fumonisin-contaminated corn and corn-based foods and feeds were subjected to Pulmonary Edema Syndrome (PES) and leukoencephalomalacia (LEM), respectively (Voss et al. 2009). Among humans, enormous reports of esophageal cancer were reported in Linxhian, China, Northern Italy (Fransceschi et al. 1990), South Africa, Transkei (Thiel et al. 1992), Golestan, South-eastern United States, and Iran (Alizadeh 2012) (Figure 2.2).

FB1 is associated with different health issues among humans and animals throughout the world, in Asia (85%), and in Europe (51%) (Correa et al. 2018) with suppression and stimulation of the immune system, hepatocarcinoma, flaws in neural-tube, and other ailments as explained. The International Agency for Research on Cancer (IARC) categorized FB1 as group 2B carcinogen in humans and animals like mice, rats, horses, and rabbits (IARC and the World Health Organization (WHO) 2002). Further, the WHO and the Joint Food and Agriculture Organization (FAO) set a bearable daily consumption for fumonisins to 2 μg/kg bw/day with a lack of any opposing things in nephrotoxicity among male rats (Joint FAO and WHO Expert Committee on Food Additives 2019).

The control of fumonisin contamination can be practiced either by its detoxification or its prevention of production (Ben Taheur et al. 2019). Generally, for elimination, fumonisin from feed and food follows many chemical, physical, and biological methods (Kumar et al. 2017;

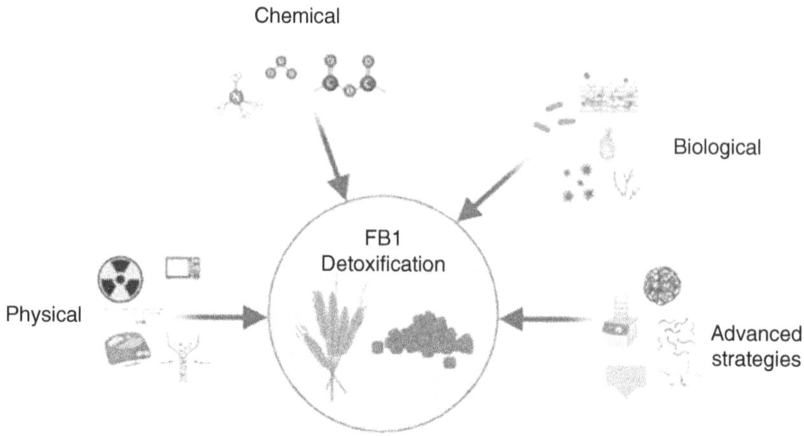

Figure 2.3 Fumonisin detoxification strategies in food and feed.

Deepa and Sreenivasa 2019a, b). We will be discussing prevention, control, and detoxification/decontamination strategies among food and feed both pre- and post-harvesting.

Contamination of fumonisin in food and feed adversely affects the budget and international craft along with effects on animal and human health. Developed countries uphold the high standards of retailers and food suppliers by deterring the regulatory controls that involve Hazard Analysis and Critical Control Point (HACCP) production, best agricultural managing practices, and storage management, together with physical, chemical and biologically based treatments which could reduce fumonisin degradation effectively in local marketing of fumonisin contaminated cereals and cereal-based food and feed-based products. Whereas developing countries' regulatory trials are poorly imposed by simple, practical, farming communities involving certain culturally acceptable hand-sorting methods due to food insecurity which proved to be effective as a former mark of defense for reducing fumonisin exposure resulting in increased mycotoxin exposure (Pitt et al. 2012; Alberts et al. 2016; Deepa et al. 2021). Management of fumonisin includes prevention, regulation, monitoring, avoidance, decontamination, detoxification, and animal treatments. Many studies have looked at both pre- and post-harvest control and prevention strategies for preventing development and secondary metabolite toxin production among *Fusarium* species when crops are still in the field condition by applying physical, chemical, biological, and other advanced methods like breeding resistant crop varieties, application of plant extracts, introduction of biocontrol microorganisms, expressing fumonisin-degrading enzymes, and many recent innovation strategies like cold plasma and many more (Nagaraja et al. 2022; Deepa et al. 2021) (Figure 2.3).

2.4 Physical Detoxification Strategies Against Fumonisin

Decontamination or degradation by physical techniques includes sorting, separation, heating, adsorption, washing, solvent extraction, and irradiation (Shapira and Paster 2004; Matumba et al. 2015).

2.4.1 Sorting and Separation

Fumonisins are not regularly spread among food and feed; they mainly appear in discolored broken parts (Mutungi et al. 2019). One of the safest and preliminary methods against mold growth by drying grains which are the major ingredient in food and feed is by freshening of grains on lowering the moisture content which can be further stored safely for longer duration (Bankole and Adebanjo 2003). Usually, the specific gravity of the fumonisin-contaminated cereal grains used for food and feed will be relatively lower than the normal ones. Based on this, aspiration, sieving, gravity separation, image processing, and photoelectric separation methods are used to separate the physically damaged and infected foods and feed matrix from healthy ones which serve as feasible and efficient techniques for reducing fumonisin contamination (Reddy et al. 2008). Matumba et al. (2015) reported dehulling, hand sorting, and flotation remove nearly 93% of fumonisins from shelled white maize and stated 98% of fumonisin can be removed on a combination of all these methods. Optical visual sorting strategies can be used to detect wheat kernels and moldy maize with more than 92% accuracy in minimizing the detoxification of fumonisin (Karlovsky et al. 2016; Shi et al. 2018; Hu and Wu 2019; Liu et al. 2020). The separation and segregation techniques are suitable only for small-scale applications and seem to be costly (Table 2.1).

2.4.2 Heating

This is the main physical factor carried out during food processing to withstand the temperature >150 °C which degrades the fumonisin stability and hence is considered to be used as leaching on removal of fumonisin (Jackson Di et al. 1996). Heating is being in practice as a thermal treatment for decontamination of fumonisin among food and feed. The method mainly concentrates on the chemical structure and concentration of fumonisin, moisture content, duration, temperature, ionic concentration, and pH during the thermal treatment (Kabak et al. 2006). Fumonisin B1 is a heat-stable compound with 150 °C decomposition temperature which appears difficult to eliminate by heating. Drying rice from 150 to 200 °C for 40 minutes, frying chips at 190 °C for 15 minutes, and cooking rice at 100 °C for 10 minutes reduced FB1 by 67%, 70%, and 80%, respectively (Becker-Algeri et sal. 2013). Due to its use of excessive amount of energy and high temperature, it reduces the feed ingredients' nutritional value and acts as limitation factor to claim the method on lessening the fumonisin among food and feed industry (Pankaj et al. 2018) (Table 2.1).

2.4.3 Washing

Fumonisin can be decontaminated by washing with water based on its water-soluble or fat-soluble property. 73–74% of FB1 is removed by floating and washing with water from the food and feed commodities (Matumba et al. 2015). Karlovsky et al. (2016) reported corn and wheat on washing with water solution consisting of 10–30% NaCl, 1 mol/L sodium carbonate, and 30% sucrose and its floating property increases the fumonisin removal rate. Hand sorting and washing techniques in combination reduce nearly 84% of fumonisin (Westhuizen et al. 2011). The strategy is expensive due to drying and outcomes such as loss of nutrients by limiting their large-scale application (Table 2.1).

Table 2.1 Strategies on detoxification of fumonisin B1.

S. No.	Anti-fumonisin strategy		Methodology	Percent of reduction (%)	References
1.	Physical	Sorting and separation	Sieving, aspiration, photoelectric separation, gravity separation, image processing	93	Liu et al. (2020), Matumba et al. (2015), and Shapira and Paster (2004)
		Heating	High temperature, high voltage	80	Pankaj et al. (2018)
		Washing	Solvent extraction (methanol, ethanol, acetone, isopropanol, acetonitrile)	73–74	Karlovsky et al. (2016) and Westhuizen et al. (2011)
		Irradiation	X-rays, γ-rays, electron beams, UV rays, infrared, and microwave	63–100	Pleadin et al. (2019) and Deepthi et al. (2017)
		Adsorption	Hydrated sodium, calcium, aluminosilicate	84–92	Vila-Donat et al. (2020), Adamovic et al. (2011), and Adunphatcharaphon et al. (2020)
			Lactobacillus plantarum B7, *L. pentosus*	52–58	
			X8	99	
			Chitosan polymer		
2.	Chemical	Ozone treatment	Ammonium hydroxide	89	Jalili and Son 2011
		Alkaline treatment	Calcium hydroxide	95	Schatzmayr et al. (2006) and Voss et al. (1996)
			Nixtamalization	100	
3.	Biological	Microorganisms	Bacterial consortium SAAS79	100	Deepa et al. (2022), Cavaglieri et al. (2004, 2005a,b,c), Heinl et al. (2010), Gergolet Diaz et al. (2021), Zhao et al. (2019), Heinl et al. (2010), Deepthi et al. (2016), and Jabar Ali et al. (2020)
			Strain NCB 1492	100	
			Saccharomyces cerevisiae ISI/1 SC82	22–50	
			Bacillus spp. S9, S10, S69	43–83	
			Bacillus subtilis	50–83	
			Enterococcus casseliflavus M4A	88.75	
			Azotobacter species	80–98	
			Lactobacillus plantarum	61.7	

		Essential oils	*Carway, fennel, spearmint, marigold, hazanbul, Ocimum basilicum, Cumin cyminum*	60–92	Ingok et al. (2020), Achimon et al. (2021), Houicher et al. (2018), Davari and Ezazi (2017), Sharifzadeh et al. (2016), and Lopez-Meneses et al. (2015)
		Genetic engineering	Bt Cry proteins; corn borers	>80	Hammond et al. (2004).
		Resistant varieties	Maize lipoxygenase (ZmLOX)	>50	Dowd (2001)
		Commercial products	Fumzyme, Fusaclean, Biofox C, Cedom, Cerall, T-22HB, Biofungus, Epic, Kodiak, Intercept, Mycostop, T-22G, Blue circle, Deny, Novasil, Nevalite	>70	Alberts et al. (2016) and Lanubile et al. (2014)
4.	Advanced strategy	Cold plasma	First-order kinetics at 10 min exposure	64	Murugesan et al. (2020) and Esua et al. (2022)
		Magnetic materials and nanoparticles	Maghemite, nano-gel, nanoparticles, ZON, SLN, SEN, copper	6–100	Gomez et al. (2019), Abd-Elsalam et al. (2017), and Magro et al. (2016)
		Pulsed electric field	Innovative and cost-effective		Nunes et al. (2021) and Gavahian et al. (2020)
		Polyphenols, flavonoids, plant extracts	BHA/PP THC/TT Aqueous and methanol	77 >50 50–65	Mehany et al. (2021), Deepa et al. (2012), Rawal et al. (2010), and Etcheverry et al. (2002)
		Enzymes	Carboxylesterase FumD FB1 to HFB1	100	Masching et al. (2016)
		Nutritional	Soyabean isoflavone	>70	Lu et al. (1997)

2.4.4 Irradiation

It is a feasible technique applied for removal of fumonisin among feed and food in industries. Electron beams, γ-rays, and X-rays are ionizing radiations, whereas infrared, microwave, and ultraviolet rays are non-ionizing radiations. These rays on food and feed eliminate the fumonisin inducing both biological and physiochemical effects (He and Zhou 2010). Feedstuffs on treating with γ-rays, microwave, and electron beam inactivate FB1 by 63.5–100%, 93.3%, and 58.1%, respectively (Xiao et al. 2011). Deepthi et al. (2017) reported ionizing radiation is lethal for *F. proliferatum* growth and its fumonisin B1 production at 7.5 kGy. They also reported that γ-radiation of more than 7.5 kGy effectually prohibited *F. proliferatum* growth and FB1 production by minimizing its exposure to animals and humans. Pleadin et al. (2019) stated that as per WHO-FAO-IAEA, irradiated feeds and foods less than the dose of 10 kGy are considered safe and also nutritionally adequate. Cereals such as sorghum and maize weighing 250 g on exposure to γ-radiation with 2.5, 5, 7.5, and 10 kGy for assessment of fumonisin level and its *F. verticillioides* incidence (%) at even intervals of 0, 30, 60, 90 days of storage, respectively was conducted reporting incidence of *Fusarium* species on 0 day as 48% and 38% in maize and sorghum, respectively and recorded the decrease of Fusarium incidence at 2.5 and 5 kGy after 30, 60, and 90 days of storage, respectively (Sreenivasa et al. 2009). Even though irradiations are considered to be a promising approach to decontaminating the fumonisins in feedstuffs, the issues related to its safety such as mutagenesis generate harmful microorganisms on damaging nutritional standards of feed and food stuffs (Table 2.1).

2.4.5 Adsorption

In many studies, enormous binders from many sources were reported to adsorb fumonisin and detoxify the same in feed industry. The adsorption binders with fumonisin together form a complex and avoid the mycotoxin passage into blood and other organs through the gastrointestinal tract among animals (Kabak et al. 2006; Adamovic et al. 2011). The adsorbent needs to follow certain properties such as high adsorption against mycotoxins with little hydrophobicity, high safety, palatability, and stability (Kabak et al. 2006). Aluminosilicate minerals are widely applied decontaminates of mycotoxins. Among them, illite, kaolin, hydrated sodium calcium aluminosilicate, zeolite, montmorillonite, bentonite, etc., serve as the adsorbents on degrading mycotoxins (Adamovic et al. 2011). The binding aptitude of minerals with both binders and mycotoxin structures mainly depends on charge distribution, surface area, pore size of adsorption binders along with polarity, charge distribution, and shape of mycotoxins (Kabak et al. 2006). Vila-Donat et al. (2020) stated that tri-octahedral bentonite adsorbs more than 90% of FB1 while adsorption dose was active at 0.20% (w/v). Hydrated sodium calcium aluminosilicate reports outstanding capability of FB1 adsorption in aqueous solution, ranging from 84.7–92.4% (Dakovic et al. 2007). Esterified glucomannan a broad-spectrum mycotoxin adsorbent improves adverse values of mycotoxins by immunity, performance, biochemical indices, and blood hematological values of chickens (Vila-Donat et al. 2020). It has effective binding capability for FB1 by 59% (Dakovic et al. 2007). Durian peels an agronomic waste which is widely used as an inorganic and organic pollutant adsorbent which adsorbs 86.1% FB1 by its larger superficial area and surface charge modification (Adunphatcharaphon et al. 2020) (Table 2.1).

Cross-linked chitosan polymers are used as generic adsorbents which adsorb multiple mycotoxins and reported 99% of FB1 adsorption (Zhao et al. 2015). Some bacterium adsorbs mycotoxins forming a complex and excretes with toxins reducing the hazard (Luoy et al. 2020). *Lactobacillus pentosus* X8 and *Lactobacillus plantarum* B7 detoxify 58% and 52.9% FB1, respectively (Wang et al. 2015) (Table 2.1).

Natural clay adsorbs fumonisin detoxifying the food and feed contaminants during processing stages (He et al. 2007). Natural clay adsorbents are considered generally recognized as safe (GRAS) by Food and Drug Administration (FDA), the United States (SCOGS 2015). Montmorillonite clay is substantial due to its huge superficial part and its molecular structure helps in increasing the adsorbing ability when it is wet. Montmorillonite clay, a dose of 1.5 and 3 g/day, on adsorption, successfully reduces FB1 in the aqueous solution (Robinson et al. 2012). Howes and Newman (2000) reported a combination of altered yeast cell extracts and clay improves the adsorption capability of numerous mycotoxins (Table 2.1).

2.5 Chemical Detoxification Strategies Against Fumonisin

Chemical methods destroy the fumonisin structure into non-toxic or mildly toxic products. Fumonisin is a constant molecule, but its devastation is challenging. Fumonisin decontamination primarily includes ozone treatment, alkaline treatment, and other chemical agents (Jalili and Son 2011).

2.5.1 Ozone Treatment

Many kinds of oxidizers are applied as a chemical agent that detoxifies the fumonisin by changing its molecular structure such as hydrogen peroxide, ozone, chlorine, calcium, and sodium hypochlorite. Combination of high temperature and ammonization leads to fumonisin detoxification (Sydenham et al. 1995). Scott (1998) reported application of chemical methods for destruction of fumonisin seems to be more positive than physical methods among cereals and documented 2% of ammonium hydroxide at 50 °C decreases fumonisin concentration by 89%, in comparison to treating for four days of physical method air drying by reducing the toxin to only 32% (Table 2.1).

2.5.2 Alkaline Treatment

Chemicals like ammonia, sodium carbonate, potassium, and sodium hydroxide are applied for the devastation of fumonisins among food and feed stuffs (Jalili and Son 2011). Momentous decrease of FB1 was observed up to 95% on treating maize grains with $Ca(OH)_2$, hydrogen peroxide, and sodium bicarbonate (Munkvold and Desjardins 1997). Fructose removed amine group by non-enzymatic browning causing fumonisin structural changes on disabling its ability of causing cancer in rats (Park et al. 1992). Large amounts of consumption of maize and maize-based products are at high risk of exposure to fumonisin. Certain reports stated that alkaline maize cooking using nixtamalization in production of tortillas reports hydrolyzation of fumonisins, by lowering its toxicity (Murphy et al. 1996). Complete degradation of FB1 was reported in contaminated maize products by applying a modified nixtamalization protocol (Park et al. 1996). Nixtamalization reduces FB1 levels only but not its toxicity percentage, whereas Voss et al. (1996) hence suggest that detoxification method must be capable of eliminating traces of toxin without leaving any hazardous residues in samples treated without compromising any nutritional value in the food (Schatzmayr et al. 2006) (Table 2.1).

2.6 Biological Detoxification Strategies Against Fumonisin

Even though many advanced physical and chemical decontamination techniques have been in practice to eliminate the fumonisins contaminated among food and feed complexes, certain biological strategies like biodegradation of fumonisin by microbes and enzymes have been in practice currently by many scientists (Chlebicz and Slizewska 2020; Fang et al. 2020).

2.6.1 Microorganisms as Detoxification Activity

Fumonisin biodegradation strategy involves the breaking down of fumonisin by applying intra- and extracellular enzymes or beneficial microbes' secondary metabolites producing less toxic or non-toxic degradation products. These biologically dependent degradation techniques were recognized as efficient, specific, and environmentally friendly approaches. *Bacillus subtilis* has been considered GRAS by FDA stating that the organism should be simply and genetically cultured and manipulated as it fits appropriately into industrial processes. Vertical transmission of FB1 accumulation reduced up to 50% on treatment with *B. subtilis* which shows the spreading from plant up to cob (Bacon et al. 2001). *Bacillus* species S9, S69, and S10 degraded FB1 by 43%, 48%, and 83%, respectively, whereas strain NCB 1492 and bacterial consortium SAAS79 degraded FB1 completely (Benedetti et al. 2006; Zhao et al. 2019). Combination of *Enterobacter hormaechei and Bacillus amyloliquefaciens* at absorption of 10^9 CFU/mL reduced the fumonisin production up to 82% in the soil (Pereira et al. 2011). *F. verticillioides* maize root infection reduced by treating with *B. amyloliquefaciens* and served as an active measure to prevent horizontal transmission without harming the growth of the plant (Al-Masri et al. 2011). *Bacterium* sp. (ATCC 55552), *Sphingopyxis macrogoltabida* (MTA 144) *Exophiala spinifera* (ATCC 74269) and *Rhinocladiella atrovirens* (ATCC 74270) are skilled at diminishing the FB1 production among *F. verticillioides* (Blackwell et al. 1999; Cavaglieri et al. 2005a; Heinl et al. 2010). *Enterococcus casseliflavus* M4A strain products on combination of acetic acid and diacetyl inhibited 100% *F. verticillioides* growth and 88.75% of FB1 biosynthesis (Gergolet Diaz et al. 2021) (Table 2.1).

PGPR bacteria such as *Azotobacter* and *Arthrobacter* are predominant and prevalent in the rhizoplane region and endorhizosphere of maize-growing areas (Cavaglieri et al. 2004; Chennappa et al. 2014, 2016). *Azotobacter* species were found to be the key bacteria in fumonisin degradation reporting 98% of degradation through LCMS on two hours of incubation (Deepa et al. 2022). Mixed cultures of *Microbacterium eoleovorans*, *E. cloacae*, *B. subtilis*, and *Pseudomonas solanacearum* exhibited synergistic activities on reduction of root colonization and vertical transmission by *F. verticillioides* among maize seed (Cavaglieri et al. 2005a). *Azotobacter armeniacus*, *Arthrobacter globiformis*, *P. solanacearum*, and *Bacillus* species were found to reduce FB1 production by 80% in the endorhizosphere region of maize root (Cavaglieri et al. 2004, 2005c).

Presently, application of lactic acid bacteria as safe biocontrol agent is in practice which diminishes contamination of FB1 production and its producing species.

Pediococcus pentosaceus, having GRAS status, broadly applied as biocontrol organism in ensilage quality improvement and food fermentation, and its supernatant antifungal activity exhibited FB1 production inhibition (Hermosa et al. 2012). Deepthi et al. (2016) reported *L. plantarum* MYS6 reduced 61.7% FB1 by binding mechanism. *Saccharomyces cerevisiae* IS1/1 degrades FB1 by 45% and the mixture of FB1 and FB2 by 50%. The other strain of *S. cerevisiae*, SC82 degrades FB1 and its mixture of FB1 and FB2 up to 22% and 25%, respectively (Styriak et al. 2001). Hermosa et al. (2012) have conducted *in vitro* and *in planta* in maize with GRAS status *Trichoderma viridae* and *Trichoderma harzianum* reducing effectively contamination of FB1 production and its producing species on application of antibiotics, volatile compounds, and certain extracellular enzymes (Jabar Ali et al. 2020). *S. cerevisiae* was reported to prevent FB1 production and its producing species in cereals (Cavaglieri et al. 2005b). In recent days, method of applying non-pathogenic strains as biocontrol agents suppresses the growth of FB1-producing *Fusarium* species in feed and food commodities (Luongo et al. 2005) (Table 2.1).

2.6.2 Natural Essential Oils

Natural essential oils' (NEOs') ingredients play a significant role in direct and indirect plant barricades against pathogen and serve as antimicrobial compounds (Yooussef et al. 2016; Achar et al. 2020). Essential oils extracted from thyme and anise reported 100% inhibition of *F. verticillioides*. The development of *F. verticillioides* decreased up to 79% by caraway, 86% by fennel, ˃60% by spearmint, whereas onynum, marigold, basil, hazanbul and chamomile essential oils reduced at concentration ≤ to 500 ppm (Solimana and Badeaab 2001). Certain essential oils from aromatic plants like *Aloysia polystachya*, *Mentha piperita*, *Origanum vulgane*, and *Adenophora triphylla* inhibited development and fumonisin manufacture in *F. verticillioides* (Lopez-Theumer et al. 2004). Natural oils of palmarosa, lemongrass, clove, *cinnamon* leaf, and oregano inhibited mycelial growth of FB1-producing *Fusarium* species under different temperatures (20–30 °C) and water activity (0.95–0.995) conditions (Velluti et al. 2003). Zingerone, eugenol, and geranium essential oils from *Zingiber officinale* exhibited as potential antifungal against growth of *F. verticillioides* and FB1 production (Sreenivasa et al. 2011a) (Table 2.1).

Eugenol, 2-hexanal (extracted from cinnamon, fruits, oregano, thyme, clove, and vegetables) and carvacrol effectively inhibited the conidial germination and growth of *F. verticillioides* among maize kernels (Singh et al. 2008). Certain compounds from essential oils like eugenol from *Syzygium aromaticum*, α-tumerone, β-tumerone in *Curcuma longa*, and methyl eugenol in *Pimenta dioica* repressed *F. verticillioides* growth by 88.70%, 44.20%, 53.09%, and 70.67%, respectively. Whereas *1,8-cineole* compound mined from *Rosmarinus officinalis* inhibited conidial formation in *F. verticillioides* by 53.48% (Menniti et al. 2010; Achimona et al. 2019; Achimon et al. 2021). Recently, certain essential oils mined from *Anacyclus valentinus*, *Carum carvi*, cinnamon, *Cumin cyminum*, *Thymus capitatus*, *Cymbopogon nardus*, *Ocimum basilicum*, and *Foeniculum vulgare* inhibited *F. verticillioides* growth from 75% to 92% (Zabka et al. 2009; Dambolena et al. 2010; Xing et al. 2014; Lopez-Meneses et al. 2015; Sharifzadeh et al. 2016; Davari and Ezazi 2017; Houicher et al. 2018). Application of essential oils and their components is significant because of their availability, low cost, and wide range of biological activities. Antioxidants and antibacterials of essential oils are in practice but antifungal and anti-mycotoxigenic studies are still limited (Ingok et al. 2020) (Table 2.1).

2.6.3 Detoxification by Genetic Engineering

Genetic engineering techniques improve crops which are commercially acceptable by convincing mechanisms, like fungal, natural, and insect resistance (Lanubile et al. 2014). Cry proteins isolated from *Bacillus thuringiensis* (Bt) in maize were modified genetically and also maintain GRAS status to consumers. The cry proteins are highly effective in reducing maize contamination with FB1 among non-Bt hybrids (Hammond et al. 2004). Resistant crops grown by genetic engineering were designed to avoid *Fusarium* species contamination on detoxification of FB1, and insect invasion *in planta* by gene manipulation studies (Duvick 2001; Cleveland et al. 2003; Lanubile et al. 2014). Maize lipoxygenase (ZmLOX) derived from oxylipins subsidize plant defense in contradiction of pathogens. The derivatives of lipoxygenase, upregulation of LOX genes, ZmLOX5, and ZmLOX12 are identified as precise derivatives during the host-pathogen interactions with *F. verticillioides* and maize (Dowd 2001). Certain commercial products also serve as an advanced strategy for controlling FB1 production such as Fumzyme from *S. macrogoltabida* (Heinl et al. 2010); Biofox C and Fusaclean from atoxigenic *Fusarium oxysporum*; Cerall and Cedom from *Pseudomonas chlororaphis* (Alberts et al. 2016); Mycostop from *Streptomyces griseoviridis*; Biofungus and T-22HB from *T. harzianum*; Kodiak and Epic from *B. subtilis*; Intercept from *Pseudomonas cepacia*; T-22G, Deny, and Blue circle from *Burkholderia cepacian*; and Nevalite and Novasil from clay material (Robinson et al. 2012) (Table 2.1).

2.7 Recent Advanced Detoxification Strategies Against Fumonisin

Due to increase in consumer safety awareness toward food and feed, demand for advanced strategies on controlling fumonisin contamination and its toxicity is being in practice like cold atmospheric plasma (CAP), magnetic materials and nanoparticles, polyphenols and flavonoids, and NEOs (Hamad et al. 2023).

2.7.1 Cold Plasma

Non-thermal technique serves as a novel strategy, in recent days, non-thermal technique serves as a novel strategy for removal of *Fusarium* species producing fumonisin toxin. Cold plasma is a technique with ionized gas with partially ionized atoms containing zero net charge (Misra et al. 2019). Photocatalytic detoxification seems to be another non-thermal emerging technique for removal of fumonisins among food and feed. The method involves photon absorption by solid photocatalyst which results in reduction or oxidation reaction of photocatalytic materials with free radicals interacting with FB1 and degrading it (Murugesan et al. 2020). The reduction of FB1 through this method followed first-order kinetics with exposure time of 10 minutes which ensured 64% reduction among spiked maize values with 259 ng/g. The method is measured to be the cheap and fast innovative strategy for decontaminating *Fusarium* species and fumonisin in foods, feeds, and agricultural products without any further effects on quality (Esua et al. 2022) (Table 2.1).

2.7.2 Nanoparticles and Magnetic Materials

Recently, new trends of using nanoparticles and magnetic materials have emerged to control fumonisin. Magnetic nanoparticles like surface-active maghemite; nano-gel, nano-clay; nanomaterials like selenium nanoparticles (SENs), copper nanoparticles, silver nanoparticles (SLNs), and zinc oxide nanoparticles (ZONs) were effective in removing the fumonisin associated with agricultural feed-based stuff and foods (Magro et al. 2016; Abd-Elsalam et al. 2017). FB1 was reduced by 6% on application of SEN produced from *T. harzianum* JF309 (Hu et al. 2019). SLN prevented the *Fusarium* species and FB1 production among food model systems (Gomez et al. 2019) (Table 2.1).

2.7.3 Pulsed Electric Fields

Pulsed electric fields (PEFs) are applied to food and feed-based products to inactivate the fungi and their mycotoxins, especially for the elimination of fumonisins, trichothecenes, aflatoxins, zearalenone, and ochratoxin. PEF is the most innovative and cost-effective food-processing strategy for detoxification of mycotoxins (Gavahian et al. 2020; Nunes et al. 2021). The method is measured as advanced and novel food-grade adsorbent for removal of mycotoxins in feed and food stuffs (Hamad et al. 2023).

2.7.4 Polyphenols and Flavonoids

Phytonutrients like polyphenols and flavonoids have been applied to various food and feed systems due to their biological activities like antibacterial, anti-inflammatory, antioxidant, and antiviral properties (Mehany et al. 2021). Certain antioxidants like butylated hydroxyanisole (BHA) and propylparaben (PP) are used on degrading FB1 and are considered GRAS by FDA among cosmetic and food industries and were also reported to conquer the FB1-producing *Fusarium* species growth (Etcheverry et al. 2002; Rawal et al. (2010)). Similarly, *F. verticillioides* growth reduced up to 77% for 28 days on 10–100-fold amounts of BHA/PP (500 μg/g) at water action (0.95) (Farnochi et al. 2005). Reynoso et al. (2002) documented FB1 reduction in combinational treatment of PP and BHA along with butylated hydroxytoluene (BHT) and trihydroxybutyrophenone (THBP) (Torres et al. 2003). Tetrahydrocurcuminoids (THCs) extracted from *C. longa* were found to suppress FB1 production *in vitro* (Coma et al. 2011). *Phoma moricola* product 3,6,7-trihydroxy-α-Tetralone (TT) inhibited FB1 at 200 μg/mL concentration (Roshan and Mohana 2021). Hamad et al. (2021) suggested the use of polyphenols and natural plant extracts as vital approach to inhibition of FB1 production and *Fusarium* species growth. Phenolic compounds like vanillic and caffeic acid decreased the association of *F. verticillioides* growth and its FB1 production among maize (Ferrari et al. 2003; Samapundo et al. 2007). Other compounds such as maakianin, chlorophorin, iroko, and ferulic also reported on preventing the growth of *F. verticillioides* and biosynthesis of FB1 (Beekrum et al. 2003). *Prosopis juliflora* plant extracts such as aqueous and methanol repressed the growth of *F. verticillioides* at 400 μg/mL by 50% and 65%, respectively, while alkaloid extract repressed the growth of *F. verticillioides* completely at 300 μg/mL (Deepa et al. 2012) (Table 2.1).

2.7.5 Enzymes and Nutritional as Detoxification Activity

Certain microbes are active in biodegrading fumonisins through the enzymes produced by them. The FumD (fumonisin carboxylesterase) degrades FB1 to HFB1 in GI tract, jejunum, and duodenum of pigs and turkeys (Masching et al. 2016). None of the strategies such as physiochemical or biological can completely decontaminate the fumonisin among food and feed as even low consumption of fumonisin can even cause chronic toxicity by immunosuppression in animals (Delwiche et al. 2005). Lu et al., reported (1997) soyabean isoflavone extract as a protective agent against FB1 hepatotoxicity in suppressing FB1-stimulated prostaglandin production (Table 2.1).

2.8 Summary

Fumonisins are the most dangerous and prominent toxin contaminated among food and feed as they attract attention worldwide due to their multitude effects on health of animals and humans. The chapter summarizes various strategies to eliminate or reduce fumonisin contamination followed by many detoxification methods such as physical (sorting and separation, heating, washing, adsorption, irradiation), chemical (ozone treatment, alkaline treatment), and biological (microorganism, genetic engineering) methods. Due to the cognizance of environmental safety as well as feed and food safety, more approaches are expected and need to be practiced for innovative and green technologies to prevent fumonisin. The recent innovative strategies are explained in the study like cold plasma, nanoparticles, magnetic materials, PEFs, polyphenols, enzymes, and nutrition.

2.9 Future Implications

Further future studies need to limelight on development of advanced fumonisin detoxification approaches which have commercial applications through conducting studies on toxic metabolites by novel approaches.

2.10 Study Questions

1) Synonyms for fumonisin.
2) Innovative detoxification strategies for fumonisin.
3) Molecular structure of fumonisins.
4) Effects of FB1 on humans and animals.
5) Note on acceptable limits for fumonisin among humans and animals.

Author Contributions

Conceptualization and writing D.N., Supervision, review, and editing M.Y.S., coordinating and editing A.M.V.

Acknowledgments

We wish to thank the Indian Council of Medical Research (ICMR) for providing ICMR to carry out research work on "potential antifungals from PGPR bacteria against fumonisin."

Conflict of Interest

The authors confirm that they have no conflicts of interest.

References

Abd-Elsalam, K.A., Hashim, A.F., Alghuthaymi, M.A., and Said-Galiev, E. (2017). Nanobiotechnological strategies for toXigenic fungi and mycotoXin control. In: *Food Preservation* (ed. A.M. Grumezescu), 337–364. Elsevier Academic Press.

Achar, P.N., Quyen, P., Adukwu, E.C. et al. (2020). Investigation of the antifungal and anti-aflatoxigenic potential of plant-based essential oils against *Aspergillus flavus* in peanuts. *J. Fungi* 6 (4): 383. https://doi.org/10.3390/jof6040383.

Achimon, F., Brito, V.D., Pizzolitto, R.P. et al. (2021). Chemical composition and antifungal properties of commercial essential oils against the maize pythopathogenic fungus *Fusarium verticillioides*. *Rev. Argentina De Microbiol.* 53 (4): 292–303.

Achimona, F., Brito, V.D., Pizzolittoa, R.P. et al. (2019). Chemical composition and antifungal properties of commercial essential oils against the maize phytopathogenic fungus *Fusarium verticillioides*. *J. Stored Prod. Res.* 432: 123–130.

Adamovic, M., Stojanovic, M., Grubisic, M. et al. (2011). Importance of aluminosilicte minerals in safe food production. *Macedo J. Anim. Sci.* 1: 175–180.

Adunphatcharaphon, S., Petchkongkaew, A., Greco, D. et al. (2020). The effectiveness of durian peel as a multi-mycotoxin adsorbent. *Toxins* 12 (2): 108.

Alberts, J.F., Van Zyl, W.H., and Gelderblom, W.C.A. (2016). Biologically based methods for control of fumonisin-producing *Fusarium* species and reduction of the fumonisins. *Front. Microbiol.* 7: 00548.

Alexander, N.J., Proctor, R.H., and McCormick, S.P. (2009). Genes, gene clusters, and biosynthesis of trichothecenes and fumonisins in *Fusarium*. *Toxin Rev.* 28: 198–215.

Alizadeh, A.M. (2012). Fumonisin B1 contamination of cereals and risk of esophageal cancer in a high-risk area in north eastern Iran. *Asian Pac. J. Cancer Prev.* 13 (6): 2625–2628.

Al-Masri, S.A., El-Safty, S.M.S., Nada, S.A., and Amra, H.A. (2011). *Saccharomyces cerevisiae* and probiotic bacteria potentially inhibit Fumonisin B1 production in vitro and in vivo. *J. Am. Sci.* 7: 198–205.

Anthony, S., Abeywickrama, K., Dayananda, R. et al. (2004). Fungal pathogens associated with banana fruit in Sri Lanka, and their treatment with essential oils. *Mycopathologia* 157: 91–97.

Aoyama, K., Nakajima, M., Tabata, S. et al. (2010). Four-year surveillance for ochratoxin A and fumonisins in retail foods in Japan. *J. Food Protect.* 73: 344–352.

Bacon, C.W., Yates, I.E., Hinton, D.M., and Meredith, F. (2001). Biological control of *Fusarium moniliforme* in maize. *Env. Health Persp.* 109: 325–332.

Bankole, S.A. and Adebanjo, A. (2003). Mycotoxins in food in West Africa: current situation and possibilities of controlling it. *Afr. J. Biotechnol.* 2: 254–263.

Becker-Algeri, T.A., Heidtmann-Bemvenuti, R., Hackbart, H.C.S., and Badiale-Furlong, E. (2013). Thermal tretaments and their effects on the fumonisin B1 level in rice. *Food Cont.* 34 (2): 488–493.

Beekrum, S., Govinden, R., Padayachee, T., and Odhav, B. (2003). Naturally occurring phenols: a detoxification strategy for fumonisin B1. *Food Addit. Contam.* 20: 490–493.

Ben Taheur, F., Kouidhi, B., Al Qurashi, Y.M.A. et al. (2019). Review: biotechnology of mycotoxins detoxification using microorganisms and enzymes. *Toxicon* 160: 12–22.

Benedetti, R., Nazzi, F., Locci, R., and Firrao, G. (2006). Degradation of fumonisin B1 by a bacterial strain isolated from soil. *Biodegradation* 17 (1): 31–38.

Bezuidenhout, S.C., Gelderblom, W.C.A., Gorst-Allman, C.P. et al. (1988). Structure elucidation of the fumonisins, mycotoxins from *Fusarium moniliforme*. *J. Chem. Soc. Chem. Commun.* 1476: 743–745.

Blackwell, B.A., Gilliam, J.T., Savard, M.E. et al. (1999). Oxidative deamination of hydrolysed fumonisin B1 (AP1) by cultures of *Exophiala spinifera*. *Nat. Toxins* 7: 31–38.

Boonzaaijer, G., van Osenbruggen, W.A., Kleinnijenhuis, A.J., and van Dongen, W.D. (2008). An exploratory investigation of several mycotoxins and their natural occurrence in flavour ingredients and spices, using a multi-mycotoxin LC-MS/MS method. *World Mycotoxin J.* 1: 167–174.

Braun, M.S. and Wink, M. (2018). Exposure, occurrence, and chemistry of fumonisins and their cryptic derivatives. *Compr. Rev. Food Sci. Food Saf.* 17: 769–791.

Bullerman, L.B. and Tsai, W.Y.J. (1994). Incidence and levels of *Fusarium moniliforme*, *Fusarium proliferatum*, and fumonisins in corn and corn-based foods and feeds. *J. Food Protect.* 57: 541–546.

Cavaglieri, L., Orlando, J., Rodríguez, M.I. et al. (2005a). Biocontrol of *Bacillus subtilis* against *Fusarium verticillioides* in vitro and at the maize root level. *Res. Microbiol.* 156: 748–754.

Cavaglieri, L., Orlando, J., and Etcheverry, M. (2005b). In vitro influence of bacterial mixtures on *Fusarium verticillioides* growth and fumonisin B1 production: effects of seeds treatment on maize root colonization. *Lett. Appl. Microbiol.* 41: 390–396.

Cavaglieri, L., Passone, A., and Etcheverry, M. (2004). Screening procedures for selecting rhizobacteria with biocontrol effects upon *F. vericillioides* growth and fumonisin B1 production. *Res. Microbiol.* 155: 747–754.

Cavaglieri, L.R., Andres, L., Ibáñez, M., and Etcheverry, M.G. (2005c). Rhizobacteria and their potential to control *Fusarium verticillioides*: effect of maize bacterisation and inoculum density. *Antonie van Leeuwenhoek* 87: 179–187.

Cendoya, E., Chiotta, M.L., Zachetti, V. et al. (2018). Fumonisins and fumonisin-producing *Fusarium* occurrence in wheat and wheat by products: a review. *J. Cereal Sci.* 80: 158–166.

Chennappa, G., Naik, M.K., Adkar-Purushothama, C.R. et al. (2016). PGP, abiotic stress tolerant and antifungal activity of *Azotobacter* sp. isolated from paddy soils. *Indian J. Exp. Biol.* 54 (5): 322–331.

Chennappa, G., Adkar-Purushothama, C.R., Suraj, U. et al. (2014). Impact of pesticides on PGPR activity of *Azotobacter* sp. isolated from pesticide flooded paddy soils. *Greener J. Agric. Sci.* 4 (4): 117–129.

Chlebicz, A. and Slizewska, K. (2020). In vitro detoxification of aflatoxin B1, deoxynivalenol, fumonisins, T-2 toxin and zearalenone by probiotic bacteria from genus *Lactobacillus* and *Saccharomyces cerevisiae* yeast. *Probiotics Antimicrob. Proteins* 12 (1): 289–301.

Cleveland, T.E., Dowd, P.F., Desjardins, A.E. et al. (2003). United States Department of Agriculture-Agricultural Research Service research on pre-harvest prevention of mycotoxins and mycotoxigenic fungi in US crops. *Pest Manag. Sci.* 59: 629–642.

Coma, V., Portes, E., Gardrat, C. et al. (2011). In vitro inhibitory effect of tetrahydrocurcuminoids on *Fusarium proliferatum* growth and fumonisin B1 biosynthesis. *Food Addit. Contam.* 28: 218–225.

Corpas-Hervias, C., Melero-Vara, J.M., Molinero-Ruiz, M.L. et al. (2006). Characterization of isolates of *Fusarium* spp. obtained from asparagus in Spain. *Plant Dis.* 90: 1441–1451.

Correa, J.A.F., Orso, P.B., Bordin, K. et al. (2018). Toxicological effects of fumonisin B1 in combination with other *Fusarium* toxins. *Food Chem. Toxicol.* 121: 483–494.

Dakovic, A., Tomasevic-Canovic, M., Rottinghaus, G.E. et al. (2007). Fumonisin B1 adsorption to octadecyldimethylbenzyl ammonium-modified clinoptilolitr-rich zeolitic tuff. *Microporous Mesoporous Mater.* 105: 285–290.

Dambolena, J.S., Zunino, M.P., López, A.G. et al. (2010). Essential oils composition of *Ocimum basilicum* L. and *Ocimum gratissimum* L. from Kenya and their inhibitory effects on growth and fumonisin production by *Fusarium verticillioides*. *Innov. Food Sci. Emerg. Technol.* 11: 410–414.

Damiani, T., Righetti, L., Suman, M. et al. (2019). Analytical issue related to fumonisins: a matter of sample comminution? *Food Control* 95: 1–5.

Dass, R.S., Sreenivasa, M.Y., Charith Raj, A.P., and Janardhana, G.R. (2009). PCR-based assay for the rapid detection of Fumonisin-producing *Fusarium* species in maize-based animal and poultry feeds in Karnataka, India. *Arch. Phytopathol. Plant Protect.* 42: 796–804.

Davari, M. and Ezazi, R. (2017). Chemical composition and antifungal activity of the essential oil of *Zhumeria majdae*, *Heracleum persicum* and *Eucalyptus* sp. against some important phytopathogenic fungi. *J. Mycol. Med.* 27: 463–468.

Deepa, N., Chennappa, G., Deepthi, B.V. et al. (2022). Antifungal potential of *Azotobacter* species and its metabolites against *Fusarium verticillioides* and biodegradation of fumonisin. *J. Appl. Microbiol.* 133: 2430–2444.

Deepa, N., Nagaraja, H., and Sreenivasa, M.Y. (2016a). Prevalence of fumonisin producing *Fusarium verticillioides* associated with cereals grown in Karnataka (India). *Food Sci. Human Well.* 5: 156–162.

Deepa, N., Charith Raj, A.P., and Sreenivasa, M.Y. (2016b). Multiplex PCR method for the early detection of fumonisin producing *Fusarium verticillioides*. *Food Biosci.* 13: 84–88.

Deepa, N., Nayaka, C.S., Udaya Shankar, A.C. et al. (2012). Detection and management of seed-borne toxigenic *Fusarium verticillioides* by plant alkaloids. *J. Mycol. Plant Pathol.* 42: 161–166.

Deepa, N., Achar, P., and Sreenivasa, M.Y. (2021). Current perspectives of biocontrol agents for management of *Fusarium verticillioides* and its fumonisin in cereals – a review. *J. Fungi* 7: 776.

Deepa, N. and Sreenivasa, M.Y. (2019a). Biocontrol strategies for effective management of phytopathogenic fungi associated with cereals. In: *New and Future Developments in Microbial Biotechnology and Bioengineering* (ed. J.S. Singh and D.P. Singh), 177–189. Elsevier. ISBN: 9780444641915 10.1016/B978-0-444-64191-5.00013-4.

Deepa, N. and Sreenivasa, M.Y. (2019b). Molecular methods and key genes targeted for the detection of fumonisin producing *Fusarium verticillioides* - an updated review. *Food Biosci.* 32: 100473. https://doi.org/10.1016/j.fbio.2019.100473.

Deepa, N. and Sreenivasa, M.Y. (2017a). Fumonisins: a review on its global occurrence, epidemiology, toxicity and detection. *J. Vet. Med. Res.* 4: 1093.

Deepa, N. and Sreenivasa, M.Y. (2017b). *Fusarium verticillioides*, a globally important pathogen of agriculture and livestock: a review. *J. Vet. Med. Res.* 4 (4): 1084.

Deepthi, B.V., Gnanaprakash, A.P., and Sreenivasa, M.Y. (2017). Effect of γ-irradiation on fumonisin producing *Fusarium* associated with animal and poultry feed mixtures. *3 Biotech* 7: 57.

Deepthi, B.V., Rao, K.P., Chennapa, G. et al. (2016). Antifungal attributes of *Lactobacillus plantarum* MYS6 against Fumonisin producing *Fusarium proliferatum* associated with poultry feeds. *PLoS One* 11 (6): e0155122.

Delwiche, S.R., Pearson, T.C., and Brabec, D.L. (2005). High-speed optical sorting of soft wheat for reduction of deoxynivalenol. *Plant Dis.* 89 (11): 1214–1219.

Desjardins, A.E., Busman, M., Proctor, R.H., and Stessman, R. (2007). Wheat kernel black point and fumonisin contamination by *Fusarium proliferatum*. *Food Addit. Contam.* 2007 (24): 1131–1137.

Desjardins, A.E., Manandhar, G.G., Plattner, R.D. et al. (2000). Occurrence of *Fusarium* species and mycotoxins in Nepalese maize and wheat and the effect of traditional processing methods on mycotoxin levels. *J. Agric. Food Chem.* 48: 1377–1383.

Di Mavungu, J.D., Monbaliu, S., Scippo, M.L. et al. (2009). LC-MS/MS multi-analyte method for mycotoxin determination in food supplements. *Food Addit. Contam. A* 26: 885–895.

Doko, M.B. and Visconti, A. (1994). Occurrence of fumonisin B1 and B2 in corn and corn-based human food stuff in Italy. *Food Addit. Contam.* 11: 433–439.

Domijan, A.M., Zeljezic, D., Milic, M., and Peraica, M. (2007). Fumonisin B1: oxidative status and DNA damage in rats. *Toxicology* 232: 163–169.

Dowd, P.F. (2001). Biotic and abiotic factors limiting efficacy of Bt corn in indirectly reducing mycotoxin levels in commercial fields. *J. Econ. Entomol.* 94: 1067–1074.

Duvick, J. (2001). Prospects for reducing fumonisin contamination of maize through genetic modification. *Environ. Health Persp.* 109: 337–342.

Esua, O.J., Sun, D.W., Cheng, J.H. et al. (2022). Hybridising plasma functionalized water and ultrasound pretreatment for enzymatic protein hydrolysis of *Larimichthys polyactis*: parametric screening and optimization. *Food Chem.* 132677: 385–399.

Etcheverry, M., Torres, A., Ramirez, M.L. et al. (2002). In vitro control of growth and fumonisin production by *Fusarium verticillioides* and *F. proliferatum* using antioxidants under different water availability and temperature regimes. *J. Appl. Microbiol.* 92: 624–632.

Fang, Q.A., Du, M.R., Chen, J.W. et al. (2020). Degradation and detoxification of aflatoxin b1 by tea-derived *Aspergillus niger* RAF106. *Toxins* 12 (12): 777.

Farnochi, M.C., Torres, A.M., Magan, N., and Chulze, S.N. (2005). Effect of antioxidants and competing mycoflora on *F. verticillioides* and *F. proliferatum* populations and fumonisin production on maize grain. *J. Stored Prod. Res.* 41: 211–219.

Ferrari, S., Vairo, D., Ausubel, F.M. et al. (2003). Tandemly duplicated *Arabidopsis* genes that encode polygalacturonase-inhibiting proteins are regulated coordinately by different signal transduction pathways in response to fungal infection. *Plant Cell Online* 15: 93–106.

Fransceschi, S., Bidoldi, E., Baron, A.E., and La Vecchia, C. (1990). Maize and risk of cancers of the oral cavity, pharynx, and oesophagus in Northeastern Italy. *J. Nat. Cancer Inst.* 82: 1407–1411.

Gavahian, M., Pallares, N., Al Khawli, F. et al. (2020). Recent advances in the application of innovative food processing technologies for mycotoXins and pesticide reduction in foods. *Trends Food Sci. Technol.* 106: 209–218.

Gazzotti, T., Lugoboni, B., Zironi, E. et al. (2009). Determination of fumonisin B1 in bovine milk by LC-MS/MS. *Food Control* 20: 1171–1174.

Gergolet Diaz, D.G., Pizzolitto, R.P., Vazquez, C. et al. (2021). Effects of volatile organic compounds produced by Enterococcus spp. strains isolated from maize grain silos on *Fusarium verticillioides* growth and fumonisin B1 production. *J. Stored Prod. Res.* 93: 101825.

Gomez, J.V., Tarazona, A., Mateo, F. et al. (2019). Potential impact of engineered silver nanoparticles in the control of aflatoXins, ochratoXin A and the main aflatoXigenic and ochratoXigenic species affecting foods. *Food Control* 101: 58–68.

Hamad, G.H., Mehany, T., Simal-Gandara, J. et al. (2023). A review of innovative strategies for cotrolling mycotoxins in foods. *Food Control* 144: 109350.

Hamad, G.M., Mohdaly, A.A.A., El-Nogoumy, B.A. et al. (2021). DetoXification of aflatoXin B1 and ochratoXin A using *Salvia farinacea* and *Azadirachta indica* water extract and application in meat products. *Appl. Biochem. Biotechnol.* 193 (10): 3098–3120.

Hammond, B.G., Campbell, K.W., Pilcher, C.D. et al. (2004). Lower fumonisin mycotoxin levels in the grain of Bt corn grown in the United States in 2000-2002. *J. Agric. Food Chem.* 52: 1390–1397.

He, J. and Zhou, T. (2010). Patented techniques for detoxification of mycotoxins in feeds and food matrices. *Rec. Pat. Food Nutr. Agric.* 2: 96–104.

Heinl, S., Hartinger, D., Thamhesl, M. et al. (2010). Degradation of fumonisin B1 by the consecutive action of two bacterial enzymes. *J. Biotechnol.* 145: 120–129.

Hermosa, R., Viterbo, A., Chet, I., and Monte, E. (2012). Plant-beneficial effects of *Trichoderma* and of its genes. *Microbiology* 158: 17–25.

Houicher, A., Hamdi, M., Hechachna, H., and Özogul, F. (2018). Chemical composition and antifungal activity of *Anacyclus valentinus* essential oil from Algeria. *Food Biosci.* 25: 28–31.

Howes, A.D. and Newman, K.E. (2000). Compositions and methods for removal of mycotoxins from animal feed. U.S. Patent 6,045,834. Washington, DC: U.S. Patent and Trademark Office (accessed 4 April 2000).

Hu, D. and Wu, A. (2019). Chemical and physical treatments for reducing mycotoxin contaminantions. In: *Food Safety and Mycotoxins* (ed. A. Wu), 145–162. Singapore: Springer.

Hu, D., Yu, S., Yu, D. et al. (2019). Biogenic *Trichoderma harzianum*-derived selenium nanoparticles with control functionalities originating from diverse recognition metabolites against phytopathogens and mycotoXins. *Food Control* 106: 106748.

Ingok, A.M., Devoglu, D., Dikmetas, N. et al. (2020). Antibacterial, antifungal, antimycotoxigenic, antioxidant activities of essential oils: an updated review. *Molecules* 25: 4711.

International Agency for Research on Cancer (IARC) and World Health Organisation (WHO) (2002). Fumonisin B1. In: *IARC Monographs on the Evaluation of Carcinogenic Risks to Humans, Some Traditional Herbal Medicines, Some Mycotoxins, Naphthalene and Styrene*, vol. 82, 301–366. Lyon: IARC Press.

Jabar Ali, A., Faraj Jubair, A., and Talib Mohammadali, M. (2020). Antifungal activity of *Tagetes erecta* extract and *Trichoderma harzianum* on the pathogenic fungus *Fusarium verticillioides*. *Plant Arch.* 20: 185–188.

Jackson Di, L.S., DeVries, J.W., and Bullerman, L.B. (1996). Fumonisin in food. In: *Advances in Experimental Medicine and Biology* (ed. L.S. Jackson, J.W. DeVries, and L.B. Bullerman), 392. New York: Plenum Press.

Jalili, M. and Son, S. (2011). The effect of chemical treatment on resuction of aflatoxins and ochratoxin A in black and white pepper during washing. *Food Addit. Contam. Part A Chem. Anal. Control Expo. Risk Assess.* 28 (4): 485–493.

Jindal, N., Mahipal, S.K., and Rottinghaus, G.E. (1999). Occurrence of fumonisin B1 in maize and poultry feeds in Haryana, India. *Mycopathologia* 148: 37–40.

Joint FAO/WHO Expert Committee on Food Additives. Meeting (74th: 2011: Rome, Italy) & World Health Organization. (2012). Safety evaluation of certain food additives and contaminants: prepared by the seventy fourth meeting of the Joint FAO/WHO expert committee on food additives (JECFA). World Health Organization.

Kabak, B., Dobson, A., and Var, I. (2006). Strategies to prevent mycotoxin contamination of food and animal feed: a review. *Crit. Rev. Food Sci. Nutr.* 46 (8): 593–619.

Karbancioglu-Guler, F. and Heperkan, D. (2009). Natural occurrence of fumonisin B1 in dried figs as an unexpected hazard. *Food Chem. Toxicol.* 47: 289–292.

Karlovsky, P., Suman, M., Berthiller, F. et al. (2016). Impact of food processing and detoxification treatments on mycotoxin contamination. *Mycotoxin Res.* 32 (4): 179–205.

Kovacic, S., Pepeljnjak, S., Petrinec, Z., and Klaric, M.S. (2009). Fumonisin B1 neurotoxicity in young carp (*Cyprinus carpio* L.). *Arh. Hig. Rada Toksikol.* 60: 419–426.

Kumar, P., Mahato, D.K., Kamle, M. et al. (2017). Aflatoxins: a global concern for food safety, human health and their management. *Front. Microbiol.* 7: 2170.

Lanubile, A., Ferrarini, A., Maschietto, V. et al. (2014). Functional genomic analysis of constitutive and inducible defense responses to *Fusarium verticillioides* infection in maize genotypes with contrasting ear rot resistance. *BMC Genom.* 15: 710.

Liu, Y., Yamdeu, J.H., Gong, Y.Y., and Orfila, C. (2020). A review of post-harvest approaches to reduce fungal and mycotoxin contamination of foods. *Compr. Rev. Food Sci. Food Saf.* 1521–1560.

Logrieco, A., Ferracane, R., Haidukowsky, M. et al. (2009). Fumonisin B2 production by *Aspergillus niger* from grapes and natural occurrence in must. *Food Addit. Contam. A* 26: 1495–1500.

Logrieco, A., Ferracane, R., Visconti, A., and Ritieni, A. (2010). Natural occurrence of fumonisin B2 in red wine from Italy. *Food Addit. Contam. A* 27: 1136–1141.

Lopez-Meneses, A.K., Plascencia-Jatomea, M., Lizardi-Mendoza, J. et al. (2015). Antifungal and antimycotoxigenic activity of essential oils from *Eucalyptus globulus, Thymus capitatus* and *Schinus molle*. *Food Sci. Technol.* 35: 664–671.

Lopez-Theumer, M.G., Zygadlo, J.A., and Rubinstein, H.R. (2004). Aromatic plants essential oils activity on *F. verticillioides* fumonsin B1 production in corn grains. *Mycopathologia* 158: 343–349.

Lu, Z., Dantler, R.W., Hopsman, E.C. et al. (1997). Reaction with fructose detoxifies fumonisin B1 while stimulating liver-associated natural killer cell activity in rats. *J. Agric. Food Chem.* 45: 803–809.

Luongo, L., Galli, M., Corazza, L. et al. (2005). Potential of fungal antagonists for bio-control of *Fusarium* spp. in wheat and maize through competition in crop debris. *Biocon. Sci. Technol.* 15: 229–242.

Luoy, L.X., Yuan, L., and Li, J. (2020). Complicated interactions between bio-adsorbents and mycotoxins during mycotoxin adsorption. Current research and future prospects. *Trends Food Sci. Tech.* 96: 127–134.

Magro, M., Moritz, D.E., Bonaiuto, E. et al. (2016). Citrinin mycotoXin recognition and removal by naked magnetic nanoparticles. *Food Chem.* 203: 505–512.

Manjula, K., Hell, K., Fandohan, P. et al. (2009). Aflatoxin and fumonisin contamination of cassava products and maize grain from markets in Tanzania and republic of the Congo. *Toxin Rev.* 28: 63–69.

Martins, M.L., Martins, H.M., and Bernardo, F. (2001). Fumonisins B1 and B2 in black tea and medicinal plants. *J. Food Protect.* 2001 (64): 1268–1270.

Masching, S., Naehrer, K., Karin, N. et al. (2016). Gastrointestinal degradation of Fumonisin B1 by carboxylesterase FumD pevents fumonisin induced alteration of sphingolipid metabolism in turkey and swine. *Toxins* 8 (3): 84.

Matumba, L., Poucke, C.V., Ediage, E.N. et al. (2015). Effectiveness of hand sorting, flotation/ washing, dehulling and combinations thereof on the decontamination of mycotoxin-contaminated white maize. *Food Addit. Contam. Part A Chem. Anal. Control Expo. Risk Assess.* 32 (6): 960–969.

Mehany, T., Khalifa, I., Barakat, H. et al. (2021). Polyphenols as promising biologically active substances for preventing SARS-CoV-2: a review with research evidence and underlying mechanisms. *Food Biosci.* 40: 100891.

Menniti, A.M., Gregori, R., and Neri, F. (2010). Activity of natural compounds on *Fusarium verticillioides* and fumonisin production in stored maize kernels. *Int. J. Food Microbiol.* 136: 304–309.

Misra, N.N., Yadav, B., and Roopesh, M.S. (2019). Cold plasma for effective fungal and mycotoxin control in foods: mechanisms, inactivation effects, and applications. *Compr. Rev. Food Sci. Food Saf.* 18: 106–120.

Mohammadi, A., Nejad, R.F., and Mofrad, N.N. (2012). *F. verticillioides* from sugarcane, vegetative compatability groups and pathogenecity. *Plant Protect. Sci.* 48: 80–84.

Munkvold, G.P. and Desjardins, A.E. (1997). Fumonisin in maize, can we reduce their occurrence? *Plant Dis.* 81: 556–565.

Murphy, P.A., Hendrich, S., Hopmans, E.C. et al. (1996). Effect of processing on fumonisin content of corn. In: *Fumonisin in Food* (ed. L.S. Jackson, J.W. Devries, and L.B. Bullerman), 323–334. New York: Plenum Press.

Murugesan, P., Brunda, D.K., and Moses, J.A. (2020). Photolytic and photocatalytic detoxification of mycotoxins in foods. *Food Control* 123: 107748.

Mutungi, C., Muthoni, F., Bekunda, M. et al. (2019). Physical quality of mize grain harvested and stored by small holder farmers in the northern highlands of Tanzania: effects of harvesting and pre-storage handling practices in two marginally contrasting agro-locations. *J. Stored Prod. Res.* 84: 101517.

Nagaraja, H., Gurikar, C., Deepa, N. et al. (2022). Antifungal potential of *Azotobacter salinestris* strain Azt 31 against phytopathogenic *Fusarium* spp. associated with cereals. *J. Fungi* 8: 473.

Njobeh, P.B., Dutton, M.F., Koch, S.H. et al. (2010). Simultaneous occurrence of mycotoxins in human food commodities from Cameroon. *Mycotoxin Res.* 26: 47–57.

Nunes, V.M., Moosavi, M., Khaneghah, A.M., and Oliveira, C.A. (2021). Innovative modifcations in food processing to reduce the levels of mycotoxins. *Curr. Opin. Food Sci.* 38: 155–161.

Omurtag, G.Z. and Yazicioglu, D. (2004). Determination of fumonisins B1 and B2 in herbal tea and medicinal plants in Turkey by high-performance liquid chromatography. *J. Food Protect.* 67: 1782–1786.

Pankaj, S.K., Shi, H., and keenara, K.M. (2018). A review of novel physical and chemical decontamination technologies for aflatoxin in food. *Trends Food Sci. Tech.* 71: 73–83.

Park, D.L., Lopez-Garcia, R., Trujillo-Preciado, S., and Price, R.L. (1996). Reduction of risk associated with fumonisin contamination in corn. In: *Fumonisin in Food* (ed. L.S. Jackson, J.W. Devries, and L.B. Bullerman), 335–344. New York: Plenum Press.

Park, D.L., Rua, S.M., Mirocha, C.J. et al. (1992). Mutagenic potential of fumonisin contaminated corn following ammonia decontamination procedure. *Mycopathologia* 117: 105–108.

Pereira, P., Sabrina, G.I., Agostini, E., and Etcheverry, M. (2011). Effects of maize inoculation with *Fusarium verticillioides* and with 2 bacterial biocontrol agents on seedlings growth and antioxidative enzymatic activities. *Appl. Soil Ecol.* 51: 52–59.

Pitt, J.I., Wild, C.P., Baan, R. et al. (2012). *Improving Public Health Through Mycotoxin Control.* Scientific Publication no. 2012, 158. Lyon: IARC Press; International Agency for Res on Cancer (IARC).

Pleadin, J., Frece, J., and Markov, K. (2019). Mycotoxins in food and feed. *Adv. Food Nutr. Res.* 89: 297–345.

Prelusky, D.B., Miller, J.D., and Trenholm, H.L. (1996). Disposition of ^{14}C-derived residues in tissues of pigs fed radiolabelled fumonisin B1. *Food Addit. Contam.* 13: 155–162.

Rawal, S., Kim, J.E., and Coulombe, R. Jr. (2010). Aflatoxin B1 in poultry: toxicology, metabolism and prevention. *Res. Vet. Sci.* 89: 325–331.

Reddy, K.R., Reddy, C.S., Abbas, H.K. et al. (2008). Mycotoxigenic fungi, mycotoxins and management of rice grains. *Toxin Rev.* 27: 287–317.

Reynoso, M.M., Torres, A.M., Ramirez, M.L. et al. (2002). Efficacy of antioxidant mixtures on growth, fumonisin production and hydrolytic enzyme production by *Fusarium verticillioides* and *F. proliferatum* in vitro on maize-based media. *Mycol. Res.* 106: 1093–1099.

Rheeder, J.P., Marasas, W.F.O., and Vismer, H.F. (2002). Production of fumonisin analogs by *Fusarium* species. *Appl. Environ. Microbiol.* 68: 2101–2105.

Robinson, A., Johnson, N.M., Strey, A. et al. (2012). Calcium montmorillonite clay reduces urinary biomarkers of fumonisin B_1 exposure in rats and humans. *Food Addit. Contam. Part A Chem. Anal. Control Expo. Risk Assess.* 29 (5): 809–818.

Rocha, L.O., Reis, G.M., Silva, V.N., and Braghini, R. (2011). Molecular characterization and fumonisin production by *F. verticillioides* isolated from corn grains of different geographic origins in Brazil. *Int. J. Food Microbiol.* 145: 9–12.

Roshan, A.B. and Mohana, D.C. (2021). Antimicrobial and antimycotoxigenic activities of (3s)-3,6,7-trihydroxy-α-tetralone isolated from endophytic *Phoma moricola*. *Pharma Innov. J.* 10 (7): 852–860.

Samapundo, S., De Meulenaer, B., Osei-Nimoh, D. et al. (2007). Can phenolic compounds be used for the protection of corn from fungal invasion and mycotoxin contamination during storage? *Food Microbiol.* 24: 465–473.

Santos, L., Marın, S., Sanchis, V., and Ramos, A.J. (2009). Screening of mycotoxin multicontamination in medicinal and aromatic herbs sampled in Spain. *J. Sci. Food Agric.* 89: 1802–1807.

Schatzmayr, G., Zehner, F., Taubel, M. et al. (2006). Microbiologicals for deactivating mycotoxins. *Mol. Nutr. Food Res.* 50: 543–551.

Scott, P.M. (1998). Industrial and farm detoxfication process for mycotoxins. *Rev. Med. Vet. Fr.* 146 (6): 543–548.

Scott, P.M. (2012). Recent research on fumonisins: a review. *Food Addit. Contam.* 23 (2): 242–248.

Seefelder, W., Gossmann, M., and Humpf, H.U. (2002). Analysis of fumonisin B1 in *Fusarium proliferatum*-infected asparagus spears and garlic bulbs from Germany by liquid chromatography-electrospray ionization mass spectrometry. *J. Agric. Food. Chem.* 50: 2778–2281.

Senyuva, H.Z. and Gilbert, J. (2008). Identification of fumonisin B2, HT-2 toxin, patulin, and zearalenone in dried figs by liquid chromatography-time-of-flight mass spectrometry and liquid chromatography-mass spectrometry. *J. Food Protect.* 71: 1500–1504.

Shapira, R. and Paster, N. (2004). Control of mycotoxins in storage and techniques for their decontamination. In: *Mycotoxins in Food - Detection Control* (ed. N. Magan and M. Olsen), 190–213. Boca Raton Boston New York Washington, DC: CRC Woodhead publishing Limited.

Sharifzadeh, A., Javan, A.J., Shokri, H. et al. (2016). Evaluation of antioxidant and antifungal properties of the traditional plants against foodborne fungal pathogens. *J. Mycol. Med.* 26: e11–e17.

Shephard, G.S., Vander-Westhuizen, L., Gatyeni, P.M. et al. (2005). Fumonisin mycotoxins in traditional Xhosa maize beer in South Africa. *J. Agric. Food Chem.* 53: 9634–9637.

Shi, H.T., Li, S.L., Bai, Y.Y. et al. (2018). Mycotoxin contamination of food and feed in China: occurrence, detection techniques, toxicological effects and advances in mitigation technologies. *Food Control* 91: 202–215.

Singh, G., Kapoor, I.P.S., Singh, P. et al. (2008). Chemistry, antioxidant and antimicrobial investigations on essential oil and oleoresins of *Zingiber officinale*. *Food Chem. Toxicol.* 46: 3295–3302.

Smith, E.R. and Merrill, A.H. (1995). Differential roles of de novo sphingolipid biosynthesis and turnover in the "burst" of free sphingosine and sphinganine, and their 1-phosphates and n-acyl-derivates, that occurs upon changing the medium of cells in culture. *J. Biol. Chem.* 270: 18749–18758.

Solimana, K.M. and Badeaab, R.I. (2001). Effect of oil extracted from some medicinal plants on different mycotoxigenic fungi. *Food Chem. Toxicol.* 40: 1669–1675.

Sreenivasa, M.Y., Dass, R.S., Charithraj, A.P., and Janardhana, G.R. (2007). PCR method for the detection of genus *Fusarium* and fuonisin producing isolates from freshly harvested sorghum grains grown in Karnataka, India. *J. Food Saf.* 28: 236–247.

Sreenivasa, M.Y., Dass, R.S., Charithraj, A.P. et al. (2011a). Assessment of the growth inhibiting effect of some plant essential growth inhibiting effect of some plant essential oils on different *Fusarium* species isolated from Sorghum and maize grains. *J. Plant Dis Protect.* 118: 208–213.

Sreenivasa, M.Y., Diwakar, B.T., Charith Raj, A.P. et al. (2012). Determination of toxigenic potential of *Fusarium* species occurring on sorghum and maize grains produced in Karnataka, India by using thin layer chromatography. *Int. J. Life Sci.* 6: 31–36.

Sreenivasa, M.Y., Gonzalez Jaen, M.T., Dass, R.S. et al. (2008a). A PCR based assay for the detetction and differentiation of potential fumonisin producing *Fusarium verticillioides* isolated from maize kernels. *Food Biotechnol.* 22: 160–170.

Sreenivasa, M.Y., Dass, R.S., Charith Raj, A.P., and Janardhana, G.R. (2008b). PCR-based detection of genus *Fusarium* and Fumonisin-producing isolates from freshly harvested Sorghum grains grown in Karnataka, India. *J. Food Saf.* 28: 236–237.

Sreenivasa, M.Y., Maheshwar, P.K., Sanjay, S.R. et al. (2009). Effect of gamma irradiation on the incidence and fumonisin production by *Fusarium* species occurring on maize and sorghum grains. *J. Agric. Technol.* 5: 325–335.

Sreenivasa, M.Y., Dass, R.S., Charith Raj, A.P., and Janardhana, G.R. (2011b). Mycological evaluation of maize grains produced in Karnataka (India) for the post-harvest fungal contamination. *World Appl. Sci. J.* 13 (4): 688–692.

Styriak, I., Conkova, E., Kmec, V. et al. (2001). The use of yeast for microbial degradation of some selected mycotoxins. *Mycotoxin Res.* 17 (1): 24–27.

Sydenham, E.W., Stockenstrom, S., Thiel, P.G. et al. (1995). Potential of alkaline hydrolysis for the removal of fumonisin from contaminated corn. *J. Agric. Food Chem.* 43: 1198–1201.

Tesso, T., Claflin, L.E., and Tuinstra, M.R. (2004). Estimation of combining ability for resistance to *Fusarium* stalk rot in grain sorghum. *Crop Sci.* 44: 1195–1199.

Thiel, P.G., Marasas, W.F.O., Sydenham, E.W. et al. (1992). The implications of naturally occurring levels of fumonisins in corn for human and animal health. *Mycopathologia* 117: 3–9.

Torres, A.M., Ramirez, M.L., Arroyo, M. et al. (2003). Potential use of antioxidants for control of growth and fumonisin production by *Fusarium verticillioides* and *Fusarium proliferatum* on whole maize grain. *Int. J. Food Microbiol.* 83: 319–324.

Trucksess, M.W., Stack, M.E., Allen, S., and Barrion, N. (1995). Immunoaffinity column coupled with liquid chromatography for the determination of fumonisin B1 in canned and frozen sweet corn. *J. Assoc. Off. Anal. Chem. Int.* 78: 705–710.

Velluti, A., Sanchis, V., Ramos, A.J. et al. (2003). Inhibitory effect of cinnamon, clove, lemongrass, oregano and palmarose essential oils on growth and fumonisin B1 production by *Fusarium proliferatum* in maize grain. *Int. J. Food Microbiol.* 2003 (89): 145–154.

Vila-Donat, P., Marin, S., Sanchis, V., and Ramos, A.J. (2020). Tri-octahedral bentonites as potential technological feed additive for *Fusarium* mycotoxin reduction. *Food Addit. Contam. Part A Chem. Anal. Control Expo. Risk Assess.* 37 (8): 1374–1387.

Voss, K.A., Bacon, C.W., Meredith, F.I., and Norred, W.P. (1996). Comparative subchronic toxicity studies of nixtamalized and water-extracted *Fusarium moniliforme* culture material. *Food Chem. Toxicol.* 34: 623–632.

Voss, K.A., Riley, R.T., Snook, M.E., and Waes, J.G. (2009). Reproductive and sphingolipid metabolic effects of fumonisin B1 and its alkaline hydrolysis product in LM/Bc mice: hydrolyzed fumonisin B1 did not cause neural tube defects. *Toxicol. Sci.* 112: 459–467.

Vudathala, D.K., Prelusky, D.B., Ayround, M. et al. (1994). Pharmacokinetic fate and pathological effects of ^{14}C-fumonisin B1 in laying hens. *Nat. Toxins* 2: 81–88.

Wang, J., Zhou, Y., Liu, W. et al. (2008). Fumonisin level in corn-based food and feed from Linxian country, a high-risk area for esophageal cancer in China. *Food Chem.* 106: 241–246.

Wang, X., Zheng, J.Y., Peng, X.L. et al. (2015). Study on the removal of fumonisins by *Lactobacillus* strains. *Sci. Technol. Food Ind.* 101 (4): 849–856.

Westhuizen, L., Shephard, G.S., Rheeder, J.P. et al. (2011). Optimising sorting and washing of home-grown maize to reduce fumonisin contamination under laboratory-controlled conditions. *Food Control* 22: 396–400.

Xiao, L.X., Wang, F., Yu, H.T. et al. (2011). Detoxification of aflatoxin B1 and fumonisin B1 in purple corn. *Food Sci.* 32 (9): 114–117.

Xing, F., Hua, H., Selvaraj, J.N. et al. (2014). Growth inhibition and morphological alterations of *Fusarium verticillioides* by cinnamon oil and cinnamaldehyde. *Food Control* 46: 343–350.

Yooussef, M.M., Pham, Q., Achar, P.N., and Sreenivasa, M.Y. (2016). Antifungal activity of essential oils on *Aspergillus parasiticus* isolated from peanuts. *J. Plant Protect. Res.* 56 (2): 139–142. https://doi.org/10.1515/jppr-2016-0021.

Zabka, M., Pavela, R., and Slezakova, L. (2009). Antifungal effect of *Pimenta dioica* essential oil against dangerous pathogenic and toxinogenic fungi. *Ind. Crops Prod.* 30: 250–253.

Zhao, Z.Y., Liu, N., Yang, L.C. et al. (2015). Cross-linked chitosan polymers as generic adsorbents for simultaneous adsorption of multiple mycotoxins. *Food Cont.* 57: 362–369.

Zhao, Z.Y., Zhang, Y.M., Gong, A.D. et al. (2019). Biodegradation of mycotoxin fumonisin B1 by a novel bacterial consortium SAAS79. *Appl. Microbiol. Biotechnol.* 103 (17): 7129–7140.

Further Reading

Agriopoulou, A., Stamatelopoulou, E., and Varzakas, T. (2020). Advances in occurrence, importance and mycotoxin control strategies: prevention and detoxification in foods. *Foods* 9: 137.

Hamad, G.M., Mehany, T., Simal-Gandara, J. et al. (2023). A review of recent innovative strategies for controlling mycotoxins in foods. *Food Control.* 144: 144–155.

Kamle, M., Mahato, D.K., Devi, S. et al. (2019). Fumonisins: impact on agriculture, food and human health and their management strategies. *Toxins* 11: 328.

Liu, M., Zhao, L., Gong, G. et al. (2022). Invited review: remediation strategies for mycotoxin control in feed. *J. Anim. Sci. Biotechnol.* 13: 19.

3

Innovative Strategies to Decontaminate Ochratoxin A in Food and Feed

Priyanthi Chandravarnan[1,2,3]*, Dominic Agyei*[1]*, and Azam Ali*[2]

[1] *Department of Food Science, Division of Sciences, University of Otago, Dunedin, New Zealand*
[2] *Center for Bioengineering and Nanomedicine, Faculty of Dentistry, Division of Health Sciences, University of Otago, Dunedin, New Zealand*
[3] *Department of Biosystems Technology, University of Jaffna, Jaffna, Sri Lanka*

CONTENTS

Abstract

Ochratoxins (OTs) are mainly produced by species of *Aspergillus* and *Penicillium*. Ochratoxin A (OTA) is most abundant and toxic to humans and animals, with significant economic losses. This primary concern occurred due to commonly contaminated food and feed commodities. Pre-harvest approaches can prevent the growth of toxigenic fungi and mycotoxin production. However, avoiding fungal infection and growth in food and feed is difficult. Therefore, different strategies are practiced to decontaminate OTA. Conventional methods practiced so far are

Anti-Mycotoxin Strategies for Food and Feed, First Edition. Edited by Deepa Nagaraju, Sreenivasa Marikunte Yanjarappa, Premila N. Achar, and Angel Medina Vaya.

ineffective, time-consuming, laborious, and may alter the sensory quality of the commodity. Therefore, new strategies, approaches, and technologies are essential to control, reduce, eliminate, or degrade OTA, and ensure food safety. This chapter provides insights into the use of several technologies for OTA decontamination. Technologies including irradiation, cold plasma, pulsed light, ultrasound, physical adsorption, ozone, and microbiological methods have been discussed.

Keywords *Ochratoxin A, decontamination technologies, food, feedstuffs*

Graphical Representation

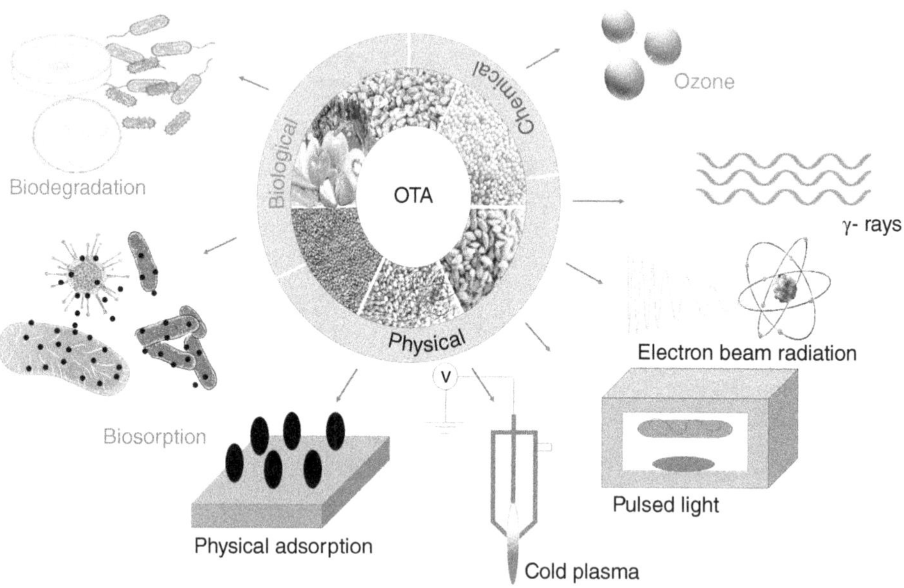

3.1 Introduction

Ochratoxins (OTs) are common mycotoxins in various food and feed, such as cereals, pulses, coffee beans, grapes, cocoa beans, nuts, spices, and animal-based foods. OTs are secondary metabolites produced by *Aspergillus* and *Penicillium* species. There are three classes of OTs, namely Ochratoxin A (OTA), Ochratoxin B (OTB), and Ochratoxin C (OTC), according to their molecular structure (Figure 3.1). Amongst these, OTA is the most prevalent and also risky to both humans and animals (Denli and Perez 2010). Studies on animals have revealed that OTA is immunotoxic, teratogenic, neurotoxic, hepatotoxic, and nephrotoxic, causing eventual death in animals (Klimke and Wu 2015; Kumar et al. 2020).

The research studies on OTA in food or feed have increased over the years but peaked in 2021 (Figure 3.2). It was estimated that the global incidence of OTA in raw cereals was 29% from the data published between 2007 and 2017 (Lee and Ryu 2017). The prevalence of OTA contamination between 2013 and 2022 was around 11–23% for finished feed samples, corn, and cereals collected worldwide (Biomin 2022). The prevalence of OTA contamination in Asia was 32%, in the Middle East and North Africa was 23%, and in Europe, 12% in 2022, according to Biomin World Mycotoxin Survey (Biomin 2022).

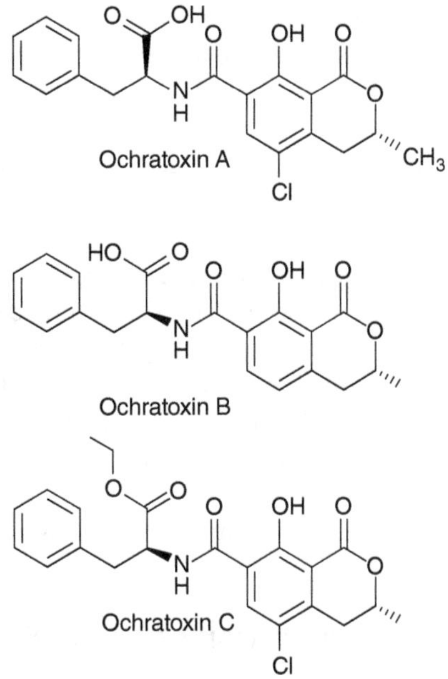

Figure 3.1 Molecular structures of OTA, OTB, and OTC (*Source:* Samuel et al. 2021).

Factors that affect the OTA-producing fungi and OTA contamination in food and feed are geographical locations, soil and climate conditions, agronomic measures (such as crop varieties, fertilizers, crop protection, cultivation, pests, and diseases), climatic conditions during harvesting, postharvest practices such cleaning and drying, storage conditions, processing methods, and transport conditions. Moreover, contamination of these mycotoxins can cause postharvest quality losses in food and feed. Contaminated food and feeds are rejected in the international market due to mycotoxin regulations. The OTA may interact with phytochemicals in the food and reduce their availability for absorption (Prakash et al. 2015). The color, sensory, and nutritional quality of the commodities can be reduced, which could result in economic losses. Likewise, contamination of animal feed can reduce the available feed nutrients, nutrient digestibility, uptake, absorption, and production. Finally, OTA bioaccumulates in animal tissues (muscle, liver, kidney), eggs, and milk due to its high affinity for protein (e.g. serum albumin) (Kumar et al. 2020; Li et al. 2021).

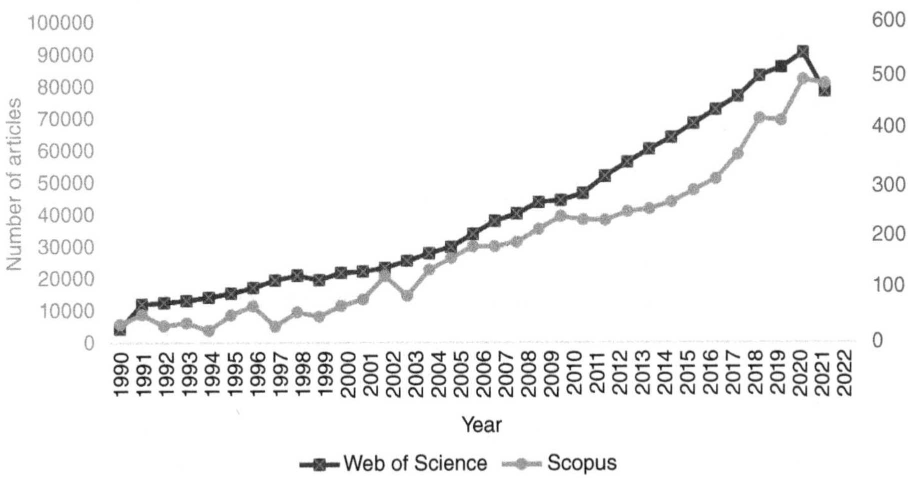

Figure 3.2 Number of published articles on OT (Scopus and Web of Science databases from 1900 to 2022 using the search term "Ochratoxin or OTA and feed OR food" in article titles, abstracts, and keywords [accessed 17 February 2023]).

Hence, there is a necessity for eliminating and reducing the OTA contamination in foods and feedstuff. There are conventional OTA decontamination techniques such as washing, dehulling, steeping, milling, density segregation, and manual sorting, but these have been shown to be inefficient and time-consuming (Wang et al. 2022a; Deepa and Sreenivasa 2019a, b; Deepa et al. 2021). A number of patents (e.g. US 8,496.984 B2, US 2012/0027747 A1, US 2012/0082759 A1, US2017/0156372 A1) have been filed that describe techniques for the decontamination of OTA in food and feed. Further, approaches like high heat processing and fungicide application may alter and reduce the color, flavor, texture, and nutritional content of food and feed through processes such as lipid oxidation, breakdown of vitamins, and depolymerization and repolymerization of polysaccharides (Zhang et al. 2019b). Further, the release of chemical residuals can harm the environment. Consequently, there is growing demand for innovative strategies that will decontaminate OTA, have little or no undesirable effects, or perhaps improve the organoleptic quality of food and feed (Sreenivasa et al. 2011a, b). This chapter discusses recent innovative strategies to decontaminate OTA in foods and feedstuffs.

3.2 Production of OTA in Fungi

OTA is mainly produced by toxigenic fungi *Aspergillus* and *Penicillium*. Among *Aspergillus* species, *Aspergillus alliaceus*, *Aspergillus carbonarius*, *Aspergillus ochraceus*, *Aspergillus steynii*, *Aspergillus niger*, and *Aspergillus westerdijkiae* are the major producers of OTA in food and feed (Copetti et al. 2010; Taniwaki et al. 2019). Among *Penicillium* species, *Penicillium verrucosum*, *Penicillium nordicum*, and *Penicillium thymicola* are the significant producers of OTA in foods and feedstuffs. *A. ochraceus* grows at 12–37 °C temperature, and optimum OTA production occurs at 25–30 °C and 0.98–0.99 a_w (Zhihong et al. 2015). *Aspergillus niger*, the optimum growth temperature was 35–41 °C, and the optimum OTA producing temperature was 20–25 °C. The optimal temperature condition for *A. carbonarius* is 32–35 °C, and the optimal a_w for spore germination is 0.83 a_w at 30 °C (Zhihong et al. 2015). *Philodendron verrucosum* and *Penicillium nordicum* produce OTA in 0.99–0.90 a_w and 15–25 °C (Sanchez-Montero et al. 2019).

OTA has an isocoumarin core bonded via an amide bond to the amino acid phenylalanine. The chemical name of OTA is L-phenylalanine-N-[(5-chloro-3,4-dihydro-8-hydroxy-3methyl-1oxo-1H-2-benzopyrane-7-yl) carbonyl]-(R)-isocoumarin. Acetyl CoA and malonyl CoA are the precursors of OTA biosynthesis. The biosynthesis pathway of OTA is explained in Figure 3.3. Identification of chemical compounds such as OTB, OTC, Ochratoxin β (OTβ), and Ochratoxin α (OTα) in the OTA – producing fungi culture clears up the order of the OTA biosynthesis pathway (Gallo et al. 2017). First, the isocoumarin group is synthesized through polyketide synthase. Then the ligation of the isocoumarin moiety with phenylalanine by a peptide synthetase generates OTB, and the dihydroisocoumarin-based structure of OTB is then chlorinated to form OTA. Phenylalanine was formed through the shikimic acid pathway (Sreenivasa et al. 2008; Gallo et al. 2012; Gallo et al. 2017). Here, OTα may be a product of the hydrolysis of OTA. OTα may be phosphorylated and linked to the ethyl ester of phenylalanine to produce OTC.

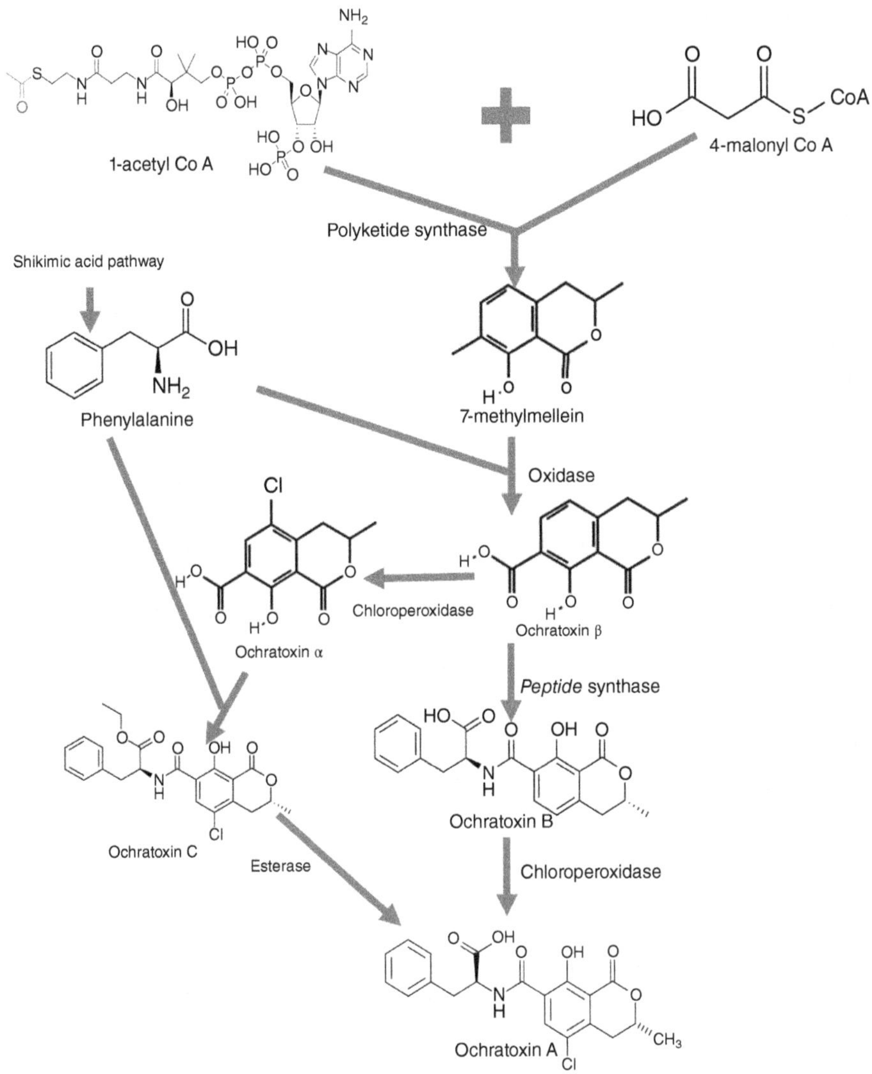

Figure 3.3 Biosynthesis pathway of OTA.

3.3 Occurrence and Distribution

OTA commonly occurs in various foods and feeds such as wheat and wheat products, corn and corn products, sorghum, rice and rice products, barely, rye, millet, sesame, wine, tea, coffee, cocoa, herbs, milk and milk products, poultry, beef, fish, pork and eggs, fruits and vegetables, beans, dried products, infant foods and poultry, and other animal feeds (Taniwaki et al. 2019; Kumar et al. 2020; Ganesan et al. 2022). OTA contamination initiates during pre-harvesting, harvesting or post-harvesting processes such as processing, transportation, packaging, and storage (Deepa et al. 2016; Deepa and Sreenivasa 2017).

Table 3.1 Maximum permitted OTA levels in some common foods.

Food/feed	Maximum limit (μg/kg)	References
Unprocessed cereals	5	
Cereals and cereal products	3	
Dried vine fruit (currants, raisins, and sultanas)	10	
Roasted coffee beans and ground roasted coffee	5	European Commission (2006a,b)
Soluble coffee (instant coffee)	10	
Wine, grape juice	2	
Processed cereal-based foods and baby foods for infants and young children	0.5	
Wheat, barley, rye	5	Codex-Alimentarius (2013)
Spices (*Capsicum* spp., *Piper* spp., Nutmeg, ginger, and turmeric)	15	European Commission (2006a,b)
Liquorice root, an ingredient for herbal infusion	20	European Commission (2010)
Liquorice extract	80	
Complementary and complete poultry feed	100	
Feed (cereal and cereal products)	250	Europen Commission (2012)
Complementary and complete pig feed	50	

OTA-producing fungi can infect foods and feed in both fields and storage, and these fungi grow in the commodity when favorable factors such as high humidity and temperatures and nutrients are available and finally produce toxins. Joint FAO/WHO Expert Committee on Food Additives (JECFA) consults governments and the Codex Alimentarius Commission (the inter-governmental standards-setting body for food) to establish the highest concentration of mycotoxins in food and help control or prevent mycotoxin contamination. The maximum permitted limits of OTs in several foods are given in Table 3.1.

3.4 OTA Toxicity and Its Effects on Humans and Animals

OTA is a group 2B carcinogens. Studies have indicated that OTA is toxic and carcinogenic to humans and animals. OTA mainly targets the kidney and causes nephrotoxic. Further, it causes tumors in the urinary tract, renal failure, and human Balkan endemic nephropathy, even in low amounts. OTA damages the cells by causing physiological oxidative stress, damages DNA and protein synthesis, and results in mutations (Ganesan et al. 2022). It is more likely to be absorbed because of its affinity to plasma proteins and subsequently reach its target organs via blood. OTA has also been reported to be hepatotoxic, neurotoxic, teratogenic, immunotoxic, and genotoxic (Kumar et al. 2020).

3.5 Recent Strategies Used in OTA Decontamination

3.5.1 Physical Methods

3.5.1.1 Gamma Radiation

Gamma (γ) rays are electromagnetic radiation diffused from the radioactive isotope (e.g. ^{60}Co, ^{192}Ir, ^{139}Cs, and ^{70}Tm). γ radiation is typically a physical and/or chemical means that interacts directly with the double bonds in the aromatic or heterocyclic rings of mycotoxin molecules and destroys the molecular structure through highly reactive free radicals produced by radiolysis of water, oxidation, and ionization reaction (Wang et al. 2022a). Generation of positively charged water radicals (H_2O^+) and negative free solvated electrons (e^-) lead to the production of the reactive species hydrogen radical ($H^•$), hydroxyl radical ($HO^•$), $HO_2^•$ (hydroperoxyl radical), OH^- (hydroxide), H_3O^+ (hydronium), H_2, and H_2O_2, which play an essential role in the destruction of the structure of OTA. No adverse effects on humans or animals were observed at the irradiation dose of 10 kGy and considered safe for food without nutritional losses (WHO 1999) (Table 3.2).

In sorghum, a 32% reduction was achieved at a 10 kGy radiation (Ben Amara et al. 2022). The same study observed that the effects of γ irradiation on mycotoxin reduction depend significantly on initial concentration and irradiation dose. γ irradiation treatment at 8 kGy reduced 47.2% of OTA contamination (Mehrez et al. 2016). Increasing the moisture content of the sample further increased the degradation rate (Mehrez et al. 2016). Calado et al. (2018) observed the highest OTA reduction of 24%, 11%, and 19% in wheat flour, grape juice, and wine at 30 kGy radiation. These findings show that irradiation has a limited effect on OTA in food matrices. The scavengers in the food can react with free radicals or absorb the radiation energy and reduce the number of free radicals produced through water hydrolysis. Dissolved solids and total solids can act as protective layers for OTA from radiation. Furthermore, the water solution of OTA was degraded entirely (98%) by γ radiation at 8.6 kGy, and only 12% of degradation was achieved in dry OTA. The results showed that γ radiation is effective in water due to water radiolysis (Table 3.2).

OTA reduction rate was 61.1% at 20 kGy in maize (Khalil et al. 2021). OTA was reactive to the highest irradiation exposures (10 and 20 kGy) compared to aflatoxin B1 and aflatoxin B2. The study recommended irradiating the grain at least by 6.0 kGy dose to inactive mycotoxin-producing molds before they produce mycotoxin to avoid the application of high radiation doses for mycotoxin degradation. OTA was effectively reduced by 62% in contaminated millet flour by irradiation at 4 kGy, and the reduction rate is dose-dependent (Maatouk et al. 2019). γ irradiation reduced the initial levels of OTA at 5 kGy dose, and γ irradiated mycotoxins showed lower toxicity than non-irradiated OTA (Domijan et al. 2019). There are several contradictory statements about the impact of γ rays on the detoxification of OTA in naturally occurring foods and feeds. Some studies have summarized

Table 3.2 Summary of physical and chemical degradation of Ochratoxin A in food and feed.

Treated sample	Treatment conditions	OTA concentration	Decontamination rate	References
Physical methods				
Gamma radiation				
Sorghum	10 kGy	30 μg/g	32%	Ben Amara et al. (2022)
Wheat	8 kGy	5000 μg/kg	47.2%	Mehrez et al. (2016)
Wheat	30.5 kGy	93.7 μg/kg	24%	Calado et al. (2018)
Grape juice	30 kGy	20 μg/L	11%	
Wine	30 kGy	20 μg/L	19%	
Maize	20 kGy	Not mentioned	61.1%	Khalil et al. (2021)
Millet flour	4 kGy	9 μg/kg	62%	Maatouk et al. (2019)
Chicken products	10 kGy	0.3–0.92 mg/kg	73.44%	Abd El-Tawaab et al. (2019)
Electron beamed radiation				
Pure solution	10 kGy	0.5 μg/mL	75.2%	Luo et al. (2017)
Corn	50 kGy	60.18 μg/kg	67.9%	
Methanol solution	16 kGy	1 μg/mL	84.16%	Yang et al. (2020)
Acetonitrile solution			91.56%	
UV radiation				
Poultry feed	0.1 mW/cm^2 at 254 nm for 40 min	150 μg/kg	100%	Ameer Sumbal et al. (2016)
Red rice	2.06 kJ/cm^2 at 254 nm	12.3 μg/kg	92%	Ferreira et al. (2021)
Black rice		12.1 μg/kg	55%	
Pure solution	25 W at 295 nm for 15 days	10 μg/mL	96.5%	Yang et al. (2020)
Pulsed light				
Grape juice	39 J/cm^2, 40 pulses	50 μg/L	95.18%	Wang et al. (2022b)
Red pepper	9.1 J/cm^2, 61 pulses, 20 s	239.5 μg/kg	36.9%	Woldemariam et al. (2021)
Cold plasma technology				
Roasted coffee	Cold plasma, 30 W, 850 V, gas helium, gas flow rate 1.5 L/min, for 30 min	Not given	0%	Casas-Junco et al. (2019)

Table 3.2 (Continued)

Treated sample	Treatment conditions	OTA concentration	Decontamination rate	References
Rice grain	Dielectric barrier discharge 25 kV, 8 min	Not given	55.64%	Guo et al. (2023)
Barley	Diffuse coplanar surface barrier discharge (DCSBD) plasma 350 W, Gas: dry air, CO_2 or 80% CO_2 + 20% O_2 gas flow rate: 10 L/min, for 1 or 3 min	49 ng/g 56.9 ng/g	$CO_2 + O_2$–43.9% in 1 min and 51.4% in 3 min Air – 54.8% in 1 min and 64.5% in 3 min	Durek et al. (2018)
Physical adsorption				
Solution	Surfactant-modified zeolites (natural zeolite with 5 mmol/100 g benzalkonium chloride) 2 mg/mL – pH = 3	2 mg/L	92.6%	Markovic et al. (2017)
Animal feed	Bentonite 0.02% W/V	1 mg/L	20.3%	Vila-Donat et al. (2019)
Palm kernel cake-feed	Chitosan pH = 4, for 8 h, at 35 °C	5, 25, 100 ng/g	87.96%	Pirouz et al. (2020)
Palm kernel cake-feed	Magnetic graphene oxide nanocomposite – pH = 5	100 ng/g	59.96%	Pirouz et al. (2021)
Wine	Nano-MgO microporous ceramic membrane	20 ng/mL	90%	Nan et al. (2022)
Chemical methods				
Ozone				
Corn	O_3-concentration 10 mg/L, 120 s	67.6 μg/kg	65.4%	Qi et al. (2016)
Corn	O_3-concentration 40 mg/L, 180 min	18 μg/kg	70.3%	
Sultanas	O_3-concentration 12.8 mg/L, 120 s	16.7 μg/kg	60.2%	Krstovic et al. (2020)
Acetonitrile solution	O_3-concentration 50 mg/L, 180 s	5 μg/mL	34%	
Corn	O_3-concentration 10 mg/L, 120 s	67.6 μg/kg	65.4%	

that γ radiation is an effective technology for detoxifying OTA, while others have reported low or no efficacy on the food matrices. This may be due to various irradiation factors such as dosage, mycotoxin level, type of food or feed, moisture content, sampling, and environmental conditions that affect irradiation efficiency (Table 3.2).

3.5.1.2 Electron Beam Radiation

Electron beam irradiation is a sterilization method where the electron is generated by commercial electricity in a vacuum condition. Then a beam of the electron is formed by the electron gun in sequence. The detoxification mechanisms of mycotoxins can be explained by the direct contact of electrons with mycotoxins, resulting in the straight destruction of their structure and the indirect degradation caused by reactive species such as $H^•$, $OH^•$, active oxygen, and $e^-(aq)$ produced during the radiolysis of water molecules in the solution of mycotoxins or the matrix of food and feed (Khaneghah et al. 2020).

A study by Yang et al. (2020) explained that the degradation rate of OTA in methanol was 84.16% and acetonitrile was 91.56% by electron beam radiation. The degradation rate is reduced in methanol compared to acetonitrile due to the free radical-scavenging effect of methanol. A significant reduction of OTA (67.9%) at 50 kGy dose was observed in corn kernels and flour (Luo et al. 2017). Amylose content, essential and total amino acid contents in corn reduced considerably with increasing irradiation dose (Luo et al. 2020a). The degradation pathway of OTA is studied in (Figure 3.4). Peng et al. (2015) explained the OTA pathway by electron beam radiation in three pathways. First is the production of OTB, and the second is the production of hydrogenated and oxidated compounds of OTA ($C_{22}H_{26}ClNO_8$). Finally, the amide bond breaks down and produces phenylalanine and OTα. OTα is further oxidized and forms $C_{13}H_{11}ClNO_5$. Finally, $C_{13}H_{16}O_7$ is produced by chlorine removal.

Irradiation can initiate fat oxidation and lead to rancidity and odor or color changes. The free fatty acid values were increased due to the decomposition of fat by high-dose irradiation (Luo et al. 2017). A higher level of moisture content, high radiation dose, and lower level of initial mycotoxins enhanced the degradation rate of OTA. In addition to these factors, the food matrix also affects the degradation rate of OTA. The toxicity of the OTA was

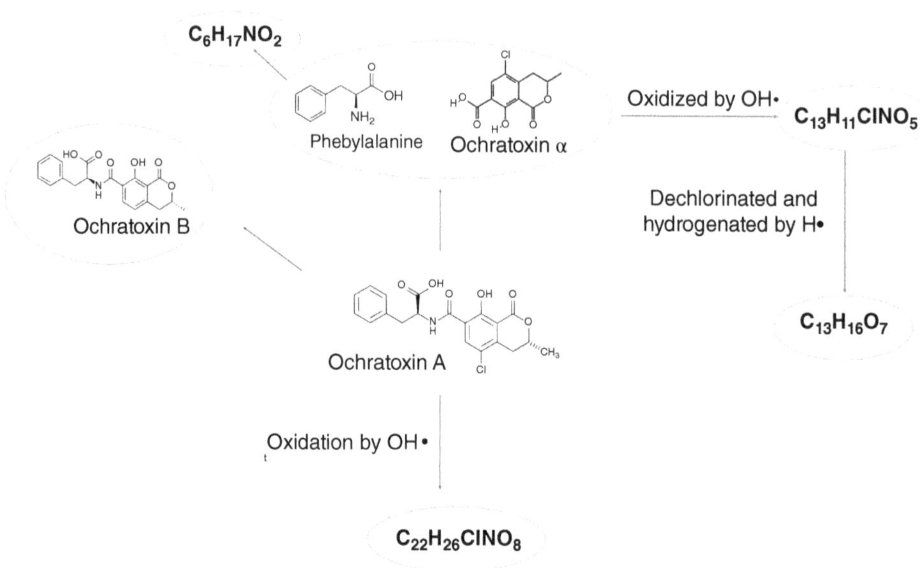

Figure 3.4 Degradation pathway of OTA by electron beam radiation.

reduced by electron beam irradiation (Luo et al. 2020a), but the results in OTA by-products were unknown (Table 3.2).

UV Radiation UV irradiations effectively removed OTA from the contaminated poultry feed samples. Poultry feeds naturally contaminated 150 μg/kg OTA might be lowered to 100 μg/kg (the highest permissible limit of OTA in feeds) after 20 minutes of UV treatment and completely decontaminated after 40 minutes of UV irradiation. However, it took six hours to reduce the OTA to 100 μg/kg with sunlight treatment (Ameer Sumbal et al. 2016). Ferreira et al. (2021) showed that the dosage of 2.06 kJ/cm^2 UV-C irradiation treatment when exposed to one hour, is effective in OTA decontaminating when subjected to one hour without changing the cooking and color properties of rice. A higher dosage of 6.18 kJ/cm^2, when exposed for three hours, removed OTA 100% and 92% in red and black rice, respectively, but reduced the total content of phenolic compounds (Table 3.2).

Zhang et al. (2021) concluded that short-wavelength lights could inhibit OTA release by *A. ochraceus* and *A. carbonarius*, and UV-B had the most apparent inhibition. The degradation rate was 75.89% in 15 days for 1 μg/mL pure OTA solution, whereas the degradation rate was increased to 96.5% when the concentration of OTA solution was increased to 10 μg/mL. So, the UV radiation technique could be used on an industrial scale as a cost-effective approach to control OTA in poultry feeds (Ameer Sumbal et al. 2016).

Pulsed Light Technology Pulsed light treatment involves a short-time, highly intense, broad spectrum of pulsed energy. The decontamination mechanisms of pulsed light are photochemical, photothermal, and photophysical (Kaya et al. 2020; Chen et al. 2021; Preetha et al. 2021). Photochemical breakdown of mycotoxin is due to intense short-duration flashes with high peak power of the UV-C spectrum. Though pulsed light is known as non-thermal technology, short-time heating of mycotoxins causes photothermal destruction of mycotoxin, which is explained as photochemical mechanisms (Yousefi et al. 2021).

The maximum fluence (9.1 J/cm^2, 61 pulses, 20 seconds) reduced the 36.9% OTA in red pepper (Woldemariam et al. 2021). The treatment intensity and the broad spectrum of pulsed light wavelength, exposure time, thickness, and composition of the food substrate, mycotoxin concentration increase the degradation rate of OTA (Woldemariam et al. 2021; Yousefi et al. 2021; Wang et al. 2022c). Pulsed light degrades OTA to less toxic phenylalanine and OTα. Pulsed light treatment slightly differed in the carotenoid content, total antioxidant activity, organic acid content, and color of the red pepper and grape juice (Woldemariam et al. 2021; Wang et al. 2022b). Interestingly, the total phenolic content increased in the pulsed light-treated sample may be due to improved extraction caused by the photothermal impact that improved the dry weight within the sample and the increase in phenolic compounds. The aroma of the grape juice was reduced following pulsed light application (Wang et al. 2022b) due to losses in volatile compounds such as alcohols, esters, and aldehydes (Table 3.2).

Cold Plasma Technology Few studies have concluded the effectiveness of cold plasma in the degradation of OTA. Cold plasma decreases 50% of OTA in coffee following 30 minutes of treatment and reduces the toxicity of OTA compared to untreated samples (Casas-Junco et al. 2019). In another study by Guo et al. (2023), a 55.64% reduction of OTA in rice grains was observed at 25 kV of cold plasma for eight minutes. Air plasma reduced OTA production. In contrast, using only CO_2 as a plasma gas increased OTA production by 48.8% insignificantly (Durek et al. 2018).

The cold plasma on OTA detoxification has resulted in reactive species, including ions, electrons, radicals, UV photons, and free radicals. Free radicals include reactive oxygen species, such as atomic oxygen (O), singlet oxygen ($^1O_2$), superoxide anion (O_2^-), and ozone (O_3), OH^- anion, $^{\bullet}OH$ radical or H_2O_2, reactive nitrogen species, such as atomic nitrogen N, excited nitrogen, nitric oxide ($NO^{\bullet}$), as well as UV irradiation and etching (Deng et al. 2020). These species could break the amide bond and produce OTα and L-phenylalanine. The oxidation of the chlorinated ring in OTA may produce free chlorine and phenylalanine (Table 3.2).

Cold plasma has been demonstrated as feasible for commercial usage in food industries for safety and shelf-life extension. The cold plasma influences the nutritional and sensory attributes of food, increasing the oxidation of unsaturated fatty acids and functional quality (Sarangapani et al. 2018; Rao et al. 2023). Cold plasma technology is confined to food surface treatment even though cold plasma is highly effective in degrading toxins with less effect on food quality (Wang et al. 2022c).

Physical Adsorption Physical adsorbents such as active carbon, natural zeolite, bentonite, nano-MgO microporous ceramic membrane, and chitosan are recently used to adsorb the OTA from food and feed (Markovic et al. 2017; Vila-Donat et al. 2019; Pirouz et al. 2020; Pirouz et al. 2021; Nan et al. 2022). The mycotoxins adsorb through electrostatic attraction forces, hydrogen bonding, and valency forces between the adsorbent and the adsorbate.

Pirouz et al. (2020) showed the removal of OTA in animal feed using chitosan. Chitosan is more attractive as an adsorbent because of its hydrophilicity, biodegradability, non-toxic nature, and anti-bacterial properties. The application of magnetic graphene oxide nanocomposite for OTA adsorption in animal feed was investigated by Pirouz et al. (2021). The positively charged nano-magnesium oxide microporous ceramic membrane provided an inexpensive method for removing OTA from drinks by electrostatic adsorption (Nan et al. 2022). Furthermore, the adsorption process was spontaneous, exothermic, and monolayer adsorption, which is dependent on the electrical charge of the adsorbate. During filtration, wine components smaller than the membrane pore size pass through smoothly, absorbent, and OTA complex, which are larger than the membrane remains. Absorbents can be removed easily from the liquid food (Table 3.2).

3.5.2 Chemical Methods

3.5.2.1 Ozone

Ozonation has been used in the degradation of OTA in corn, coffee, and sultanas. Qi et al. (2016) observed a 65.4% degradation rate in 5 μg/mL of OTA solution after 120 seconds of treatment with 10 mg/L of ozone. According to Qi et al. (2016), the initial OTA level in contaminated corn with 14.1% moisture content was decreased by 64.2% after treatment with 100 mg/L ozone for 180 minutes. The degradation rate was increased to 90.7% when the moisture of the corn was 19.5%. Another study by Krstovic et al. (2020) reported 70.3% degradation of OTA in corn with 40 mg/L ozone in 180 minutes. Sultanas were ozonated (12.8 mg/L) for 120 minutes to degrade the OTA to 60.2%, and the degradation rate was further increased to 82.5% when treated for 240 minutes (Torlak 2019). OTA degradation in acetonitrile solution peaked (34%) at 180 seconds (Yang et al. 2020).

The OTA in the solution is more easily degraded than the dry OTA because the ozone solubilizes in the water, increases the reaction area, and rapidly decomposes into atomic oxygen and hydroxyl ions in water. In addition to ozone, hydroxyl radicals formed in the solutions can further trigger OTA degradation. The ozonation process depends on the exposure time, ozone concentration, temperature, moisture content, and product composition. The degradation rates improved with ozone concentration, treatment time, and moisture content. Reactive oxygen species can react with the organic substances in the food. Ozone may oxidize the double bonds and hydroxyl groups on an aromatic ring of OTA. Thus, the breakdown of OTA can be due to ozone-induced oxidation of double bonds and the hydroxyl group in the structure of the molecule. The ozonolysis of OTA may result in phenylalanine and OTα (Table 3.2).

The changes in the nutritional and sensory properties of food after ozone treatment should be considered. No significant changes in the concentration of phenolic substances in sultanas were reported after the ozonation (Torlak 2019). The color of the corn was reduced due to the bleaching effect of ozone. Oxidizing properties of ozone stimulated the oxidation reactions of fat components and increased the fatty acid value of the corn with the ozone application. However, optimizing ozone conditions can minimize detrimental effects on the quality due to ozone treatment.

3.5.3 Biological Methods

Recently, many studies have been done on the biological degradation of OTA because of efficiency, cost-effectiveness, specificity, less nutritional and organoleptic losses, and eco-friendly (Luo et al. 2020b). Microorganisms such as lactic acid bacteria, actinobacteria, filamentous fungi, yeast, and enzymes secreted by these microorganisms degrade or detoxify the OTA or adsorb the mycotoxin (Table 3.3).

3.5.3.1 Biosorption

The most effective mechanism to remove OTA by microorganisms is binding with the cell wall. The bacterial cell wall has peptidoglycan matrices, polysaccharides, teichoic and lipoteichoic acid, and a protein S-layer. The cell wall of the microorganism binds with the OTA, and no by-products are produced. In the study of Fouad et al. (2021), *Lactococcus rhamnosus*, *Lactococcus plantarum*, and *Lactococcus reuteri* reduced 59.3, 52.0, and 50.2% of OTA after incubation for six hours, respectively, in phosphate buffer saline. When increasing the incubation period to 12 and 36 hours, the removal rate was increased to 68.1 and 81.4% of OTA in *L. rhamnosus*, respectively. The binding efficiency of lactic acid bacteria cells with OTA increased with incubation time.

Furthermore, thermally inactivated cells bind more than viable cells due to structural changes in the cell surface. Heat treatment could reduce the thickness of the peptidoglycan or increase the pore size in the cell wall. Heat treatment might also cause protein denaturation or the Maillard reaction between polysaccharides and peptides, increasing the OTA-binding sites on the bacterial cell surface. The binding of toxin by bacterial cells is also affected by electron donor–acceptor and Lewis' acid–base interactions; this may be because the cells of

Table 3.3 Summary of biological decontamination of Ochratoxin A.

Microorganisms	Source	Conditions	OTA concentration	Reduction (%)	Source
Adsorption by microorganisms					
Acetobacter syzygii	Kefir grain	25 °C for 24 h in milk	1 μg/mL	50	Ben Taheur et al. (2017)
Lactobacillus kefiri	Kefir milk	25 °C for 24 h in milk	1 μg/mL	81	Ben Taheur et al. (2017)
Kazachstania servazzii	Kefir milk	25 °C for 24 h in milk	1 μg/mL	62	Ben Taheur et al. (2017)
Lactococcus rhamnosus	Dairy products	37 °C for 6 h in phosphate buffer	10 μg/L	59.3	Fouad et al. (2021)
Lactococcus plantarum	Dairy products	37 °C for 6 h in phosphate buffer	10 μg/L	52.0	Fouad et al. (2021)
Lactococcus reuteri	Dairy products	37 °C for 6 h in phosphate buffer	10 μg/L	50	Fouad et al. (2021)
Streptococcus thermophilus	Dairy products	37 °C for 36 h in phosphate buffer	10 μg/L	80.3	Fouad et al. (2021)
Bifidobacterium bifidum	Dairy products	37 °C for 36 h in phosphate buffer	10 μg/L	80.4	Fouad et al. (2021)
Bacillus megaterium	Soil	30 °C for 72 h in a liquid medium	2.5 μg/mL	80.3	Shang et al. (2019)
Saccharomyces cerevisiae	Wine	25 °C for 28 days in a liquid medium	5 μg/L	34.52–48.96	Pulvirenti et al. (2020)
Lactobacillus kefiranofaciens	Tibetan kefir grains	25 °C for 24 h in dairy products	1 μg/mL	90	(Du et al. 2021)
Kazachstania turicensis					
Candida intermedia	Pure solution	25 °C for 48 h in grape juice	20 μg/kg	70	Farbo et al. (2016)
Bacillus subtilis	Fermented food	2 h in wine	20 μg/L	85.33	Shukla et al. (2020)
Biodegradation by microorganism					
Streptomyces sp.	Compost	25 °C for 12 days	280 ng/mL	99	Campos-Avelar et al. (2020)
Trichoderma afroharzianum-peroxidase	Pure culture	8 days	0.01 mg/L	46	Dini et al. (2022)
Trichoderma koningii	Pure culture	10 days at 30 °C	5 μg/mL	100	Ismaiel et al. (2022)
Aspergillus niger	Wheat bran	5 days, 30 °C	1 μg/g	59.84	Zou et al. (2022)
Yarrowia lipolytica	Grape	28 °C for 48 h	1 μg/mL	88	Yang et al. (2016)

lactic acid bacteria consider strong electron donors and weak electron acceptors, which is supported by the hydrophilic nature of their surface. The hydrophobic characteristics of the cell wall and cell wall components (polysaccharides, peptidoglycan, lipoteichoic acids, and teichoic), as well as electron donor–acceptor and Lewis' acid–base interactions, also contribute to the binding of toxins by bacterial cells (Piotrowska 2014; Shukla et al. 2018). *Saccharomyces* strains adsorb OTA from musts and wines during fermentation (Petruzzi et al. 2015; Pulvirenti et al. 2020). The cell wall component (e.g. β-glucan) interacts with the functional groups of OTA through non-covalent interaction, hydrogen bond, and ionic or hydrophobic interaction. This interaction mechanism is affected by the charge of the cell wall surface and the polarity, solubility, and charge distribution of the toxin (Piotrowska and Masek 2015). A study by Farbo et al. (2016) suggested that the encapsulation of yeast cells in alginate beads does not alter the OTA adsorption. However, autoclaving of the yeast cells improves the adsorption capacity by increasing the adsorption cell sites. *Bacillus subtilis* was immobilized onto alginate beads, which showed no significant difference from free *B. subtilis* in removing OTA from wine by Shukla et al. (2020). However, encapsulated microorganisms can be easily removed from the aqueous solution with a magnet, cleaned, and reused (Table 3.3).

3.5.3.2 Biodegradation

The microorganism and the microbial enzymes degrade the OTA into less/non-toxic products. The degradation of OTA by microorganisms is mainly by enzymes produced by them. Carboxypeptidase A was the first identified enzyme which degrades the amide bond in the OTA and produces OTA-α and L-β-phenylalanine (Chen et al. 2018). Another hypothesized biodegradation mechanism of degradation by the enzyme is hydrolysis in the lactone ring of the OTA, which produces opened lactone form of OTA, as shown in Figure 3.5. The breakdown process can be affected by the microorganism type and concentration, OTA concentration, temperature, and pH (Yang et al. 2016).

Yang et al. (2014) have explained that the OTA degradation using *Yarrowia lipolytica* was the most effective at 28 °C and a pH of 4. Moreover, a high yeast concentration, low initial concentration of OTA, acidic environment, and optimal temperature (28 °C) increase the OTA degradation efficiency. Environmental pH affects the ionization state of OTA by changing the charges of the carboxyl and hydroxyl groups in OTA. Carboxypeptidase was involved in this process (Zhang et al. 2018). Another study by Campos-Avelar et al. (2020) showed that 33 strains of *Actinobacteria* could degrade OTA almost entirely in a liquid medium, while only five decreased it in a solid medium, and two of them reduced OTA to a lower limit. However, no by-products of OTA (i.e. OTα, OTβ, L-β-phenylalanine) were identified by HPLC-MS/MS, which might be due to a different detoxification mechanism or breakdown of OTA into unknown products by enzymes and secondary metabolites of microorganisms (Nagaraja et al. 2016; Achar et al. 2020).

Extracellular enzymes (carboxypeptidases, hydrolases, amidases, and lactamase) produced by *B. subtilis* were able to degrade OTA. However, carboxypeptidase genes were expressed in *Escherichia coli* through the recombinant protein, and the detoxification of OTA was effective (Xu et al. 2021). A recombinant carboxypeptidase expressed from *Lysobacter* sp. degraded OTA. However, the degradation activity of the host strain was much more efficient than that of the expressed protein (Wei et al. 2020). *Alcaligenes faecalis* produce an enzyme that hydrolyses the amide bond in OTA to Otα (Zhang et al. 2017).

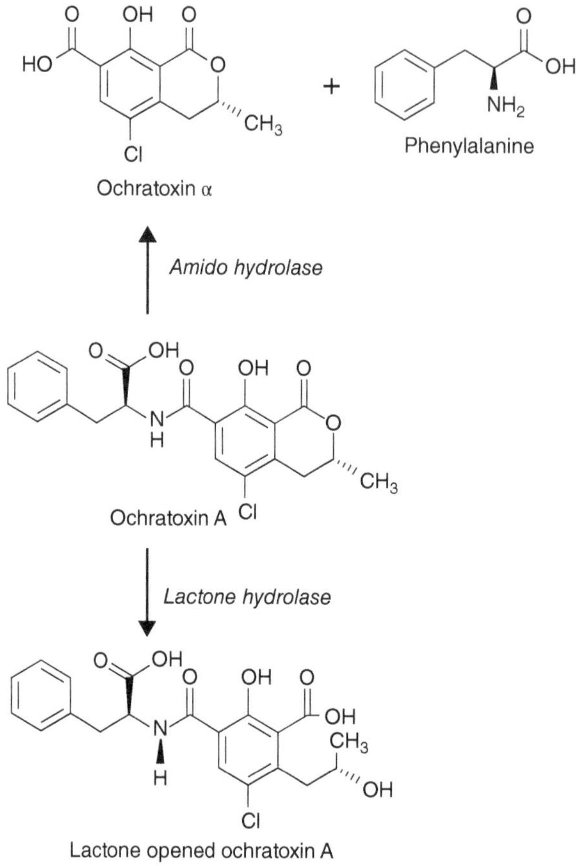

Figure 3.5 Biodegradation of OTA.

Later, a newly expressed enzyme N-acyl-L-amino acid amidohydrolase from *A. faecalis* efficiently degraded OTA and had broad thermal and pH stability while food and feed processing (Zhang et al. 2019a). Leitao and Enguita (2021) showed that ochratoxinase produced by OT-producing fungi (*A. niger*) had more catalytic properties to break the OTA.

Recombinant DNA technology can produce these microbial enzymes on a commercial scale. These enzymes are easy to handle as optimum conditions for the growth of microorganisms are not needed, and they are effective. The advantages and disadvantages of each method are discussed in Table 3.4.

3.6 Summary

OTA contamination in food and feedstuffs is a global problem for the food and feed industry due to its toxicity to both human and animal, quality and the economic losses of products. Once the mycotoxin is produced in the product, preventive measures are ineffective and need decontamination techniques. Limitations such as labor and time-consuming in the conventional methods hasten the research to novel decontamination

Table 3.4 Advantages and disadvantages of various decontamination methods.

Decontamination methods	Advantages	Disadvantages
Gamma radiation	Deep penetration into food Little loss of food quality Environmentally friendly approach Applicable for large-scale production since	The initial cost is high Unsuitable for high-lipid foods Use of radioactive materials
Electron beam radiation	Environmentally friendly approach Use of electricity rather than radioactive materials	Surface decontamination approach
UV radiation	Large-scale application	Limited penetration depth
Cold plasma technology	Negligible loss of nutritional and sensory attributes Does not alter the physical structure of foods No risk of chemical contamination Non-toxic byproducts	High set-up cost Not applicable for high-lipid food
Physical adsorption	Specific	Can bind with micronutrients
Ozone	Does not leave any residues in the environment	Unstable and quick decomposition High oxidation/reduction potential
Biological method	Specific Low cost No toxic residuals	Efficiency can be affected by food matrix Effective under specific conditions (pH, temperature) Possible partial adsorption of toxins

strategies. Until now, gamma radiation, electron beam radiation, pulsed light technology, UV radiation, cold plasma technology, physical adsorption, ozone, biosorption, and biodegradation have been used in OTA degradation. These methods are environmentally friendly and effective in OTA inactivation, having little or no effect on the nutritional and sensory quality of commodities. The effectiveness of these techniques may be further increased by combining these technologies. Further commercialization of these strategies should be done.

3.7 Future Implications

The detailed degradation mechanism of the techniques mentioned above, and the toxicity of the resulting products could be studied. The effect of decontamination techniques with different doses and treatment times on the physical characteristics of different food and feedstuffs could be further explored. The combined effect of decontamination technology on OTA deactivation and their effect on the physical and functional characteristics of food and feedstuffs should be studied.

3.8 Study Questions

1) What is the rationale for use of novel techniques in decontaminating OTA in food and feedstuffs?
2) Give examples and explain the mechanism behind physical, chemical, and biological methods of OTA decontamination.
3) Discuss the advantages and disadvantages of biological detoxification techniques.

Acknowledgments

Priyanthi Chandravarnan acknowledges the support of the Accelerating Higher Education Expansion and Development (AHEAD) Program in her PhD studies.

Conflict of Interest

The authors declare no conflict of interest.

Author Contributions

Priyanthi Chandravarnan; Writing the original draft. Dominic Agyei; Supervision, reviewing, editing; Azam Ali; Supervision, conception, and design, reviewing.

References

Achar, P.N., Quyen, P., Adukwu, E.C. et al. (2020). Investigation of the antifungal and anti-aflatoxigenic potential of plant-based essential oils against *Aspergillus flavus* in peanuts. *J. Fungi* 6 (4): 383. https://doi.org/10.3390/jof6040383.

Ameer Sumbal, G., Hussain Shar, Z., Hussain Sherazi, S.T. et al. (2016). Decontamination of poultry feed from ochratoxin A by UV and sunlight radiations. *J. Sci. Food Agric.* 96: 2668–2673.

Abd El-Tawaab, A.A., El-Hofy, F.I., Mahmoud, A.H., and Rashed, D.M. (2019). Mycotoxin residues in different chicken products by HPLC and their inactivation using Gamma radiation. *Int. J. Pharm. Res. Allied Sci.* 8 (4): 71–81.

Ben Amara, A., Mehrez, A., Ragoubi, C. et al. (2022). Fungal mycotoxins reduction by gamma irradiation in naturally contaminated sorghum. *J. Food Process. Preserv.* 46: 16345–16362.

Ben Taheur, F., Fedhila, K., Chaieb, K. et al. (2017). Adsorption of aflatoxin B1, zearalenone and ochratoxin A by microorganisms isolated from *Kefir* grains. *Int. J. Food Microbiol.* 251: 1–7.

Biomin. (2022). Biomin world mycotoxin survey 2022. https://www.dsm.com/anh/products-andservices/products/mycotoxindeactivators.html (accessed 20 January 2023).

Calado, T., Fernandez-Cruz, M.L., Cabo Verde, S. et al. (2018). Gamma irradiation effects on ochratoxin A: degradation, cytotoxicity and application in food. *Food Chem.* 240: 463–471.

Campos-Avelar, I., Colas De La Noue, A., Durand, N. et al. (2020). Minimising ochratoxin A contamination through the use of actinobacteria and their active molecules. *Toxins* 12: 296–306.

Casas-Junco, P.P., Solis-Pacheco, J.R., Ragazzo-Sanchez, J.A. et al. (2019). Cold plasma treatment as an alternative for ochratoxin A detoxification and inhibition of mycotoxigenic fungi in roasted coffee. *Toxins* 11: 337–345.

Chen, D., Mosher, W., Wiertzema, J. et al. (2021). Effects of intense pulsed light and gamma irradiation on *Bacillus cereus* spores in mesquite pod flour. *Food Chem.* 344: 128675–128683.

Chen, W., Li, C., Zhang, B. et al. (2018). Advances in biodetoxification of ochratoxin A-a review of the past five decades. *Front. Microbiol.* 9: 1386–1397.

Codex-Alimentarius. (2013). General standard for contaminatnts and toxins in food and feed. Codex Alimentarius Commission: procedural manual. https://www.cabdirect.org/cabdirect/abstract/20133318613 (accessed 15 December 2022).

Copetti, M.V., Pereira, J.L., Iamanaka, B.T. et al. (2010). *Ochratoxigenic* fungi and ochratoxin A in cocoa during farm processing. *Int. J. Food Microbiol.* 143: 67–70.

Deng, L.-Z., Tao, Y., Mujumdar, A.S. et al. (2020). Recent advances in non-thermal decontamination technologies for microorganisms and mycotoxins in low-moisture foods. *Trends Food Sci. Technol.* 106: 104–112.

Denli, M. and Perez, J.F. (2010). Ochratoxins in feed, a risk for animal and human health: control strategies. *Toxins* 2: 1065–1077.

Deepa, N. and Sreenivasa, M.Y. (2017). Fumonisins: a review on its global occurrence, epidemiology, toxicity and detection. *J. Vet. Med. Res.* 4 (6): 1093.

Deepa, N., Achar, P.N., and Sreenivasa, M.Y. (2021). Current perspectives of biocontrol agents for management of *Fusarium verticillioides* and its Fumonisin in cereals—a review. *J. Fungi* 7: 776. https://doi.org/10.3390/jof7090776.

Deepa, N., Charith Raj, A.P., and Sreenivasa, M.Y. (2016). Multiplex PCR method for the early detection of fumonisin producing *fusarium verticillioides*. *Food Biosci.* 13: 84–88.

Deepa, N. and Sreenivasa, M.Y. (2019a). Biocontrol strategies for effective Management of Phytopathogenic Fungi Associated with cereals. In: *New and Future Developments in Microbial Biotechnology and Bioengineering* (ed. J.S. Singh and D.P. Singh), 177–189. Elsevier. ISBN: 9780444641915 10.1016/B978-0-444-64191-5.00013-4.

Deepa, N. and Sreenivasa, M.Y. (2019b). Molecular methods and key genes targeted for the detection of fumonisin producing *Fusarium verticillioides* - an updated review. *Food Biosci.* 32: 100473. https://doi.org/10.1016/j.fbio.2019.100473.

Dini, I., Alborino, V., Lanzuise, S. et al. (2022). *Trichoderma* enzymes for degradation of aflatoxin B1 and ochratoxin A. *Molecules* 27: 3959–3971.

Domijan, A.M., Marjanovic Cermak, A.M., Vulic, A. et al. (2019). Cytotoxicity of gamma irradiated aflatoxin B(1) and ochratoxin A. *J. Environ. Sci. Health B* 54: 155–162.

Du, G., Liu, L., Guo, Q. et al. (2021). Microbial community diversity associated with *Tibetan kefir* grains and its detoxification of ochratoxin A during fermentation. *Food Microbiol.* 99: 103803–103813. https://doi.org/10.1016/j.fm.2021.103803.

Durek, J., Schluter, O., Roscher, A. et al. (2018). Inhibition or stimulation of ochratoxin A synthesis on inoculated barley triggered by diffuse coplanar surface barrier discharge plasma. *Front. Microbiol.* 9: 2782–2791.

Europen-Commission. (2012). Commission Regulation (EU) No 594/2012 of 5th July 2012 amending Regulation (EC) 1881/2006 as regards the maximum levels of the contaminants ochratoxin A, non dioxin-like PCBs and melamine in foodstuffs. https://eur-lex.europa.eu/legal-content/EN/TXT/PDF/?uri=CELEX:32012R0594 (accessed 10 December 2022).

Europian-Commission. (2010). Commission Regulation (EU) No 105/2010 of 5th February 2010 amending Regulation (EC) No 1881/2006 setting maximum levels for certain contaminants in foodstuffs as regards ochratoxin A. https://eur-lex.europa.eu/legal-content/EN/ALL/?uri=celex:32010R0105 (accessed 10 December 2022).

European-Commission. (2006a). Commiossion Regulation (EC) No 1881/2006 of 19th December 2006 setting maximum levels for certain contaminants in foodstuffs. https://eur-lex.europa.eu/LexUriServ/LexUriServ.do?uri=OJ:L:2006:364:0005:0024:EN:PDF (accessed 10 December 2022).

European-Commission. (2006b). Commission Recommendation of 17th August 2006 on the presence of deoxynivalenol, zearalenone, ochratoxin A, T-2 and HT-2 and fumonisins in products intended for animal feeding,§ 229. https://eurlex.europa.eu/LexUriServ/LexUriServ.do?uri=OJ:L:2006:229:0007:0009:EN:PDF (10 December 2022).

Farbo, M.G., Urgeghe, P.P., Fiori, S. et al. (2016). Adsorption of ochratoxin A from grape juice by yeast cells immobilised in calcium alginate beads. *Int. J. Food Microbiol.* 217: 29–34.

Ferreira, C.D., Lang, G.H., Lindemann, I.D.S. et al. (2021). Postharvest UV-C irradiation for fungal control and reduction of mycotoxins in brown, black, and red rice during long-term storage. *Food Chem.* 339: 127810–127820.

Fouad, M.T., El-Shenawy, M., and El-Desouky, T.A. (2021). Efficiency of selected lactic acid bacteria isolated from some dairy products on aflatoxin B1 and ochratoxin. *J. Pure Appl. Microbiol.* 15: 312–319.

Gallo, A., Bruno, K.S., Solfrizzo, M. et al. (2012). New insight into the ochratoxin A biosynthetic pathway through deletion of a nonribosomal peptide synthetase gene in *Aspergillus carbonarius*. *Appl. Environ. Microbiol.* 78: 8208–8226.

Gallo, A., Ferrara, M., and Perrone, G. (2017). Recent advances on the molecular aspects of ochratoxin A biosynthesis. *Curr. Opin. Food Sci.* 17: 49–56.

Ganesan, A.R., Mohan, K., Karthick Rajan, D. et al. (2022). Distribution, toxicity, interactive effects, and detection of ochratoxin and deoxynivalenol in food: a review. *Food Chem.* 378: 131978–131990.

Guo, J., He, Z., Ma, C. et al. (2023). Evaluation of cold plasma for decontamination of molds and mycotoxins in rice grain. *Food Chem.* 402: 134159–134168.

Ismaiel, A.A., Mohamed, H.H., and El-Sayed, M.T. (2022). Biodegradation of ochratoxin A by endophytic *Trichoderma koningii* strains. *World J. Microbiol. Biotechnol.* 39 (2): 53–66.

Kaya, Z., Unluturk, S., Martin-Belloso, O., and Soliva-Fortuny, R. (2020). Effectiveness of pulsed light treatments assisted by mild heat on *Saccharomyces cerevisiae* inactivation in verjuice and evaluation of its quality during storage. *Innov. Food Sci. Emerg. Technol.* 66: 102517–102529.

Khalil, O.A.A., Hammad, A.A., and Sebaei, A.S. (2021). *Aspergillus flavus* and *Aspergillus ochraceus* inhibition and reduction of aflatoxins and ochratoxin A in smaise by irradiation. *Toxicon* 198: 111–120.

Khaneghah, A., Hashemi Moosavi, M., Oliveira, C.A.F. et al. (2020). Electron beam irradiation to reduce the mycotoxin and microbial contaminations of cereal-based products: an overview. *Food Chem. Toxicol.* 143: 111557–111565.

Klimke, T.R. and Wu, F. (2015). Ochratoxin A and human health risk: a review of the evidence. *Crit. Rev. Food Sci. Nutr.* 55: 1860–1869.

Krstovic, S., Krulj, J., Jaksic, S. et al. (2020). Ozone as decontaminating agent for ground corn containing deoxynivalenol, zearalenone, and ochratoxin A. *Cereal Chem.* 98: 135–143.

Kumar, P., Mahato, D.K., Sharma, B. et al. (2020). Ochratoxins in food and feed: occurrence and its impact on human health and management strategies. *Toxicon* 187: 151–162.

Lee, H.J. and Ryu, D. (2017). Worldwide occurrence of mycotoxins in cereals and cereal-derived food products: public health perspectives of their co-occurrence. *J. Agric. Food Chem.* 65: 7034–7051.

Leitao, A.L. and Enguita, F.J. (2021). Systematic structure-based search for ochratoxin-degrading enzymes in proteomes from *Filamentous* fungi. *Biomolecules* 11: 1040–1057.

Li, X., Ma, W., Ma, Z. et al. (2021). The occurrence and contamination level of ochratoxin A in plant and animal-derived food commodities. *Molecules* 26: 6928–6942.

Luo, X., Qi, L., Liu, Y. et al. (2017). Effects of electron beam irradiation on zearalenone and ochratoxin A in naturally contaminated corn and corn quality parameters. *Toxins* 9: 84–101.

Luo, X., Zhai, Y., Qi, L. et al. (2020a). Influences of electron beam irradiation on the physical and chemical properties of zearalenone- and ochratoxin A-contaminated corn and in vivo toxicity assessment. *Foods* 9: 1–14.

Luo, Y., Liu, X., Yuan, L., and Li, J. (2020b). Complicated interactions between bio-adsorbents and mycotoxins during mycotoxin adsorption: current research and future prospects. *Trends Food Sci. Technol.* 96: 127–134.

Maatouk, I., Mehrez, A., Amara, A.B. et al. (2019). Effects of gamma irradiation on ochratoxin A stability and cytotoxicity in methanolic solutions and potential application in Tunisian millet samples. *J. Food Protect.* 82: 1433–1439.

Markovic, M., Dakovic, A., Rottinghaus, G.E. et al. (2017). Ochratoxin A and zearalenone adsorption by the natural zeolite treated with benzalkonium chloride. *Colloids Surf. A* 529: 7–17.

Mehrez, A., Maatouk, I., Romero-González, R. et al. (2016). Assessment of ochratoxin A stability following gamma irradiation: experimental approaches for feed detoxification perspectives. *World Mycotoxin J.* 9 (2): 289–298.

Nan, M.N., Bi, Y., Qiang, Y. et al. (2022). Electrostatic adsorption and removal mechanism of ochratoxin A in wine via a positively charged nano-MgO microporous ceramic membrane. *Food Chem.* 371: 131157–1311165.

Nagaraja, H., Chennappa, G., Rao, P.C.R.K. et al. (2016). Diversity of toxic and phytopathogenic fusarium species occurring on cereals grown in Karnataka state, India. *3 Biotech* 6: 57.

Peng, C., Ding, Y., An, F. et al. (2015). Degradation of ochratoxin A in aqueous solutions by electron beam irradiation. *J. Radioanal. Nucl. Chem.* 306: 39–46.

Petruzzi, L., Corbo, M.R., Baiano, A. et al. (2015). In vivo stability of the complex ochratoxin A – *Saccharomyces cerevisiae* starter strains. *Food Control* 50: 516–520.

Piotrowska, M. and Masek, A. (2015). Saccharomyces cerevisiae cell wall components as tools for ochratoxin A decontamination. *Toxins* 7: 1151–1162.

Piotrowska, M. (2014). The adsorption of ochratoxin A by *Lactobacillus* species. *Toxins* 6: 2826–2839.

Pirouz, A., Selamat, J., Sukor, R., and Noorahya Jambari, N. (2021). Effective detoxification of aflatoxin B1 and ochratoxin A using magnetic graphene oxide nanocomposite: isotherm and kinetic study. *Coatings* 11: 1346–1351.

Pirouz, A., Selamat, J., Zafar Iqbal, S., and Iskandar Putra Samsudin, N. (2020). Efficient and simultaneous chitosan-mediated removal of 11 mycotoxins from palm kernel cake. *Toxins* 12: 115–129.

Prakash, B., Kedia, A., Mishra, P.K., and Dubey, N.K. (2015). Plant essential oils as food preservatives to control moulds, mycotoxin contamination and oxidative deterioration of agri-food commodities – potentials and challenges. *Food Control* 47: 381–391.

Preetha, P., Pandiselvam, R., Varadharaju, N. et al. (2021). Effect of pulsed light treatment on inactivation kinetics of *Escherichia coli* (MTCC 433) in fruit juices. *Food Control* 121: 107547–107558.

Pulvirenti, A., De Vero, L., Blaiotta, G. et al. (2020). Selection of wine *Saccharomyces cerevisiae* strains and their screening for the adsorption activity of pigments, phenolics and ochratoxin A. *Fermentation* 6: 80–93.

Qi, L., Li, Y., Luo, X. et al. (2016). Detoxification of zearalenone and ochratoxin A by ozone and quality evaluation of ozonised corn. *Food Addit. Contam. Part A Chem. Anal. Control Expo. Risk Assess.* 33: 1700–1710.

Rao, W., Li, Y., Dhaliwal, H. et al. (2023). The application of Cold Plasma Technology in low-moisture foods. *Food Eng. Rev.* 15: 86–112.

Samuel, M.S., Jeyaram, K., Datta, S. et al. (2021). Detection, contamination, toxicity, and prevention methods of ochratoxins: an update review. *J. Agric. Food Chem.* 69: 13974–13989.

Sanchez-Montero, L., Cordoba, J.J., Peromingo, B. et al. (2019). Effects of environmental conditions and substrate on growth and ochratoxin A production by *Penicillium verrucosum* and *Penicillium nordicum*: relative risk assessment of OTA in dry-cured meat products. *Food Res. Int.* 121: 604–611.

Sarangapani, C., Patange, A., Bourke, P. et al. (2018). Recent advances in the application of Cold Plasma Technology in foods. *Annu. Rev. Food Sci. Technol.* 9: 609–629.

Shang, L., Bai, X., Chen, C. et al. (2019). Isolation and identification of a *Bacillus megaterium* strain with ochratoxin A removal ability and antifungal activity. *Food Control* 106: 106743–106751.

Shukla, S., Park, J.H., and Kim, M. (2020). Efficient, safe, renewable, and industrially feasible strategy employing *Bacillus subtilis* with alginate bead composite for the reduction of ochratoxin A from wine. *J. Cleaner Prod.* 242: 118344–118354.

Shukla, S., Park, J.H., Chung, S.H., and Kim, M. (2018). Ochratoxin A reduction ability of biocontrol agent *Bacillus subtilis* isolated from Korean traditional fermented food Kimchi. *Sci. Rep.* 8: 8039–8049.

Sreenivasa, M.Y., Dass, R.S., Adkar-Purushothama, C.R. et al. (2011a). Assessment of the growth inhibiting effect of some plant essential oils on different *Fusarium* species isolated from sorghum and maize grains. *J. Plant Dis. Protect.* 118 (6): 208–213.

Sreenivasa, M.Y., Dass, R.S., Charith Raj, A.P., and Janardhana, G.R. (2008). PCR-based detection of genus *Fusarium* and Fumonisin-producing isolates from freshly harvested sorghum grains grown in Karnataka, India. *J. Food Saf.* 28: 236–237.

Sreenivasa, M.Y., Dass, R.S., Charith Raj, A.P., and Janardhana, G.R. (2011b). Mycological evaluation of maize grains produced in Karnataka (India) for the post harvest fungal contamination. *World Appl. Sci. J.* 13 (4): 688–692.

Taniwaki, M.H., Pitt, J.I., Copetti, M.V. et al. (2019). Understanding mycotoxin contamination across the food chain in Brazil: challenges and opportunities. *Toxins* 11: 411–428.

Torlak, E. (2019). Use of gaseous ozone for reduction of ochratoxin A and fungal populations on sultanas. *Aust. J. Grape Wine Res.* 25: 25–29.

Vila-Donat, P., Marín, S., Sanchis, V., and Ramos, A.J. (2019). New mycotoxin adsorbents based on tri-octahedral bentonites for animal feed. *Anim. Feed Sci. Technol.* 255: 114228–114241.

Wang, L., Hua, X., Shi, J. et al. (2022a). Ochratoxin A: occurrence and recent advances in detoxification. *Toxicon* 210: 11–18.

Wang, L., Liu, X., Cai, R. et al. (2022b). Detoxification of ochratoxin A by pulsed light in grape juice and evaluation of its degradation products and safety. *Innov. Food Sci. Emerg. Technol.* 78: 103024–103032.

Wang, Y., Shang, J., Cai, M. et al. (2022c). Detoxification of mycotoxins in agricultural products by non-thermal physical technologies: a review of the past five years. *Crit. Rev. Food Sci. Nutr.* 62: 1–12.

Wei, W., Qian, Y., Wu, Y. et al. (2020). Detoxification of ochratoxin A by *Lysobacter* sp. CW239 and characteristics of a novel degrading gene carboxypeptidase cp4. *Environ. Pollut.* 258: 113677–113687.

WHO (1999). *High- Dose Irradiation: Wholesomeness of Food Irradiated with Doses above 10 KGy*. Joint FAO/IAEA/WHO Study Group.

Woldemariam, H.W., Harmeling, H., Emire, S.A. et al. (2021). Pulsed light treatment reduces microorganisms and mycotoxins naturally present in red pepper (*Capsicum annuum* L.) powder. *J. Food Process Eng.* 45: 13948–13959.

Xu, X., Pang, M., Liu, J. et al. (2021). Genome mining reveals the genes of carboxypeptidase for OTA-detoxification in *Bacillus subtilis* CW14. *Int. J. Biol. Macromol.* 186: 800–810.

Yang, J., Li, J., Jiang, Y. et al. (2014). Natural occurrence, analysis, and prevention of mycotoxins in fruits and their processed products. *Crit. Rev. Food Sci. Nutr.* 54: 64–83.

Yang, K., Li, K., Pan, L. et al. (2020). Effect of ozone and electron beam irradiation on degradation of zearalenone and ochratoxin A. *Toxins* 12: 138–148.

Yang, Q., Wang, J., Zhang, H. et al. (2016). Ochratoxin A is degraded by *Yarrowia lipolytica* and generates non-toxic degradation products. *World Mycotoxin J.* 9: 269–278.

Yousefi, M., Mohammadi, M.A., Khajavi, M.Z. et al. (2021). Application of novel non-thermal physical technologies to degrade mycotoxins. *J. Fungi* 7: 395–413.

Zhang, H.H., Wang, Y., Zhao, C. et al. (2017). Biodegradation of ochratoxin A by *Alcaligenes faecalis* isolated from soil. *J. Appl. Microbiol.* 123: 661–668.

Zhang, H., Wang, G., Yang, Q. et al. (2021). Effects of light on the ochratoxigenic fungi *Aspergillus ochraceus* and *A. carbonarius*. *Toxins* 13: 251–262.

Zhang, H., Zhang, Y., Yin, T. et al. (2019a). Heterologous expression and characterization of A novel ochratoxin A degrading enzyme, N-acyl-L-amino acid Amidohydrolase, from *Alcaligenes faecalis*. *Toxins* 11: 518–537.

Zhang, X., Yang, H., Apaliya, M.T. et al. (2018). The mechanisms involved in ochratoxin A elimination by *Yarrowia lipolytica* Y-2. *Ann. Appl. Biol.* 173: 164–174.

Zhang, Z.-H., Wang, L.-H., Zeng, X.-A. et al. (2019b). Non-thermal technologies and its current and future application in the food industry: a review. *Int. J. Food Sci. Technol.* 54: 1–13.

Zhihong, L., Kunlunt, H., and Yunbo, L. (2015). Ochratoxin A and ochratoxin-producing fungi on cereal grain in China: a journal article. *Food Addit. Contam. Part A Chem. Anal. Control Exposure Risk Assess.* 32: 461–470.

Zou, D., Ji, J., Ye, Y. et al. (2022). Degradation of Ochratoxin A by a UV-mutated *Aspergillus niger* strain. *Toxins (Basel)* 14: 343–358.

Further Reading

Klimke, T.R. and Wu, F. (2015). Ochratoxin A and human health risk: a review of the evidence. *Crit. Rev. Food Sci. Nutr.* 55: 1860–1869.

4

Patulin-Effective Mitigation Strategies in Food and Feed

S. Divyashree[1], G. Adithi[1], B. Shruthi[1], and M.Y. Sreenivasa[2]

[1] *Applied Mycology Laboratory, Department of Studies in Microbiology, University of Mysore, Mysuru, India*
[2] *Molecular Mycotoxicology Laboratory, Department of Studies in Microbiology, University of Mysore, Mysuru, Karnataka, India*

CONTENTS

Abstract

Patulin is a toxic metabolite ensuing from enzymatic pathway cascades, often produced by molds, and is a food safety concern and economic menace. Patulin is produced predominantly by 22 *Penicillium* spp., 3 *Aspergillus* spp., 3 *Paecilomyces* spp., and 1 *Xylaria* spp. The occurrence of patulin in food/products as a natural contaminant poses a worldwide human health problem related to immunological, gastrointestinal, and neurological outcomes. Therefore, effective detoxification and mitigation strategies are necessary to extend the product life. This book

Anti-Mycotoxin Strategies for Food and Feed, First Edition. Edited by Deepa Nagaraju, Sreenivasa Marikunte Yanjarappa, Premila N. Achar, and Angel Medina Vaya.

chapter presents an outline of patulin distribution, sources of occurrence in various foods, and effects of patulin in pre- and post-harvest stages. Moreover, patulin mitigation strategies are uniformly important using various physical, chemical, and biological methods and their disadvantages. This book chapter also summarizes the detoxification, binding methods, and degradation products, and their safety from patulin.

Keywords *Patulin, binding, degradation, fruits,* Penicillium *spp.*

Graphical Representation

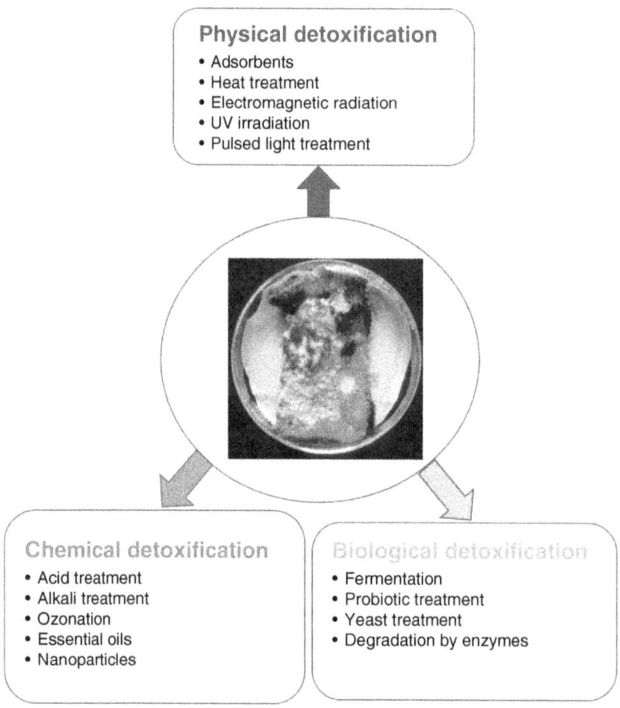

4.1 Introduction

Patulin (4-hydroxy-4H-furo-[3,2-c] pyran-2(6H)-one) is one of the most important secondary metabolites produced by numerous species of *Penicillium*, *Aspergillus*, and *Byssochlamys* (Steiman et al. 1989). Among *Aspergillus*, patulin-producing species include: *Aspergillus giganteus*, *Aspergillus clavatus*, and *Aspergillus longivesica* (Varga et al. 2007). In the *Penicillium* genera, there are 13 Patulin (PAT)-producing species such as *Penicillium clavigerum*, *Penicillium carneum*, *Penicillium concentricum*, *Penicillium dipodomyicola*, *Penicillium coprobium*, *Penicillium glandicola*, *Penicillium expansum*, *Penicillium gladioli*, *Penicillium marinum*, *Penicillium griseofulvum*, *Penicillium sclerotigenum*, *Penicillium paneum*, and *Penicillium vulpinum* (Frisvad and Samson 2004; Sreenivasa et al. 2008). Among them, *P. expansum* produces bulky amounts of PAT.

Compiling multiple researches has shown now PAT to take place naturally in fruit and vegetable products as apple, apple-acerola, pear, grape, sour cherry, orange, blackcurrant, pineapple and passion fruit juices, corn, blackcurrant and blueberry jams, strawberry, red raspberry, cranberry, and some types of baby food along with certain cereals (Larsen et al. 1998; Nagaraja et al. 2016). In addition, PAT has also been isolated from grain products such as wheat, malts, barley, feed silages, bread, and related dough products as well as cereal stubbles and cheddar cheese (Lopez-Diaz and Flannigan 1997; Pittet and Harbarth 1998).

Numerous researchers around the globe have investigated the degree and extension of food product contamination by PAT. Tyllinen et al. (1977) conducted research on PAT production in bread samples and found 27–160 g/kg and PAT attributed to death of 100 cows through feeding malt (Ciegler 1977). PAT have been documented as life-threatening substances identified from a variety of food products from various countries; India-Mysore (Jayashree and Farhath 2015), England (Sommer et al. 1974), China (Ji et al. 2017), Canada (Harwig et al. 1973), United States (Reid and Ware 1974), New Zealand (Walker 1969), and South Africa (Leggott and Shephard 2001). In addition, PAT has also been found in apple juices from Belgium (Tangni et al. 2010), Iran (Azizi and Rouhi 2013), Italy (Ritieni 2003), Austria (Romero-steiner et al. 1999), and France (Sommer et al. 1974).

In vivo studies on consumption of contaminated foods with PAT reported ulceration and hemorrhage, and gastrointestinal effects such as distension, agitation, edema, convulsions, intestinal inflammation as well as vomiting (Magan 2014). Current studies have also confirmed that patulin in humans alters the function of gastrointestinal barrier. Moreover, PAT cause immunotoxicity, neurotoxicity, teratogenicity, and genotoxicity (Moake et al. 2005). In this book chapter, we widely summarize effective detoxification and mitigation strategies to extend the product life and present an outline of PAT distribution, sources of occurrence in various foods, and effects of patulin in pre- and post-harvest stages. Moreover, PAT mitigation strategies are uniformly important using various physical, chemical, and biological methods with their disadvantages (Figure 4.1). This book chapter also summarizes the detoxification, binding methods, and degradation products and their safety from PAT.

4.2 Occurrence and Distribution of Patulin

Patulin is a secondary metabolite that occurs in various food products such as apples, apricots, kiwis, plums, peaches, and cereal-based food formed by numerous filamentous fungi within several genera, for instance, *Bysochlamys*, *Eupenicillium*, *Penicillium*, *Aspergillus*, and *Paecilomyces* (Reddy et al. 2010). Currently, *P. expansum*, also called the blue mold, which causes soft rot of apples, pears, cherries, and other fruits, is largely documented as a common offender in patulin contamination (Zbyňovská et al. 2016). PAT is one of the most

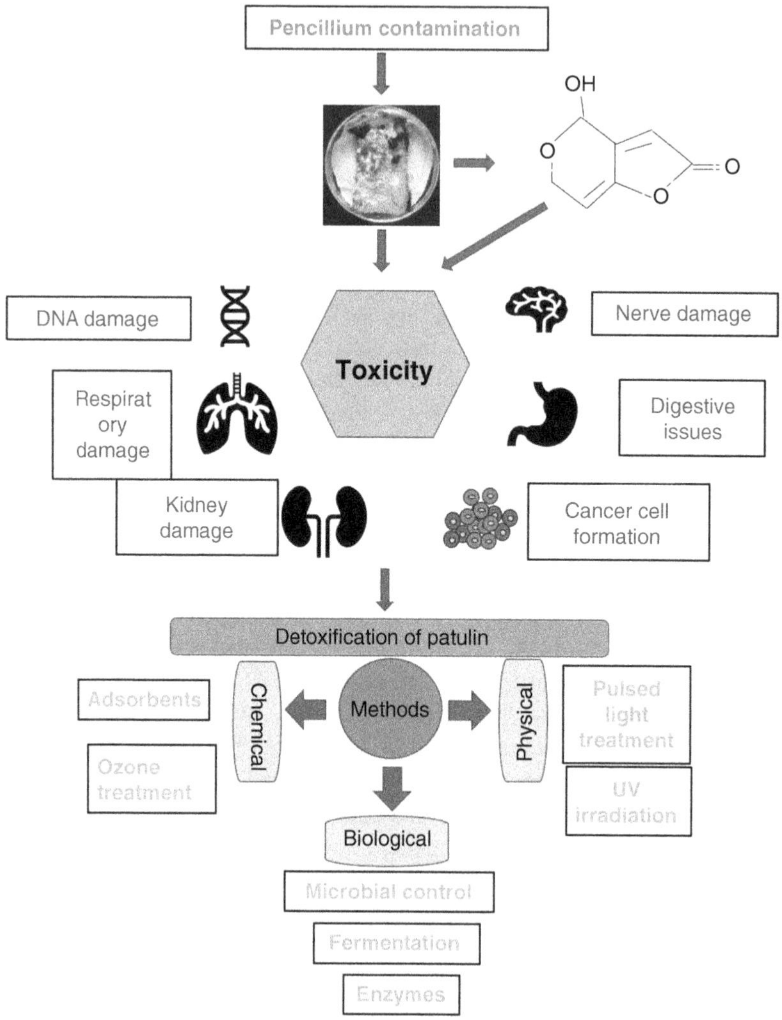

Figure 4.1 Mitigation strategies for the degradation of patulin.

dangerous mycotoxins produced by some of the fungal species amongst all toxic metabolites. PAT toxin incidence in food products, fruits, and vegetables is mentioned in Table 4.1.

4.3 Effect of both Pre- and Post-harvest Stages

Apple and its commercial foodstuffs can contain PAT, the mycotoxin produced by various fungi of the Penicillium genus. Among the species of these genera, *P. expansum* is the foremost producer of PAT in addition to also being considered a significant pre- and post-harvest pollutant of apples all over the world (Riachy et al. 2021). *P. expansum* is probably the most associated with apples and is the cause of the so-called blue rot. Even though PAT occurs frequently in damaged fruit, the mold may not be externally visible, which does not

Table 4.1 Contamination of patulin in various food products.

Products	Country	Patulin concentration	References
Apple and apple juice	Brazil	757 μg/kg in apples and 1298 μg/L in apple juice	Díaz et al. (2020)
Dried apricot	South Brazil	40 μg/kg	Hartwig et al. (2020)
Commercial pineapple juice and fruit juices	Malaysia	19.4 mg/L	Ping et al. (2014)
Apple products	China	>50 μg/kg	Yuan et al. (2010)
Homogenized fruits and tomato products	Italy	4.05 ng/mL in tomato sauce 5.23 ng/mL in baby foods 0.85 ng/mL in homogenized apple of 0.79 ng/mL in homogenized pear	Sarubbi et al. (2016)
Apple juice	India	191 mg/L	Saxena et al. (2009)
Chilgoza (pine nuts)	India	4.556 ± 2.219 ng/g	Sharma et al. (2015)
Dried figs, dried longans (seedless), and dried hawthorn products	China	87.6, 68.4, and 5.1 mg/kg, respectively	Ji et al. (2017)
Grape juice	Pakistan	53.9 μg/kg	Hussain et al. (2020)
Strawberries	Poland	5–100 μg/kg	Sadok et al. (2017)

mean the absence of mycotoxin, but the mold growth is not constantly superficially visible. Internal fungal growth may arise sometimes, through insect incursion or from other sorts of damage, resulting in incidence of PAT in the unharmed fruit. However, the spores of several PAT-producing fungi are present on the fruits; the growth of molds will not be seen during harvesting. But the mold's growth and PAT production can arise post-harvest due to being affected by disease or else insect injury or through the fruits which fell into the ground were used in processing (Deepa and Sreenivasa 2017b; Deepa et al. 2021). This demonstrates the importance of applying good agricultural practices in the stages involved in the pre-harvest of the fruits. During the processing of juice, the grade of apples used must be assured, and many pre-harvest procedures must be taken, such as the exclusion and obliteration of fruits which are rotten, the trees must be spaced adequately to let for continuous air and light penetration between them, the control of pests and diseases that could cause fruit rot or denote a point of entrance for PAT-producing molds, the application of fungicides to prevent mold germination and growth during and after harvest, the use of fertilizers based on calcium and phosphorus for the plantation to improve cell structure and reduce the susceptibility to fruit rot, do not store fruit with poor mineral composition for long periods of time (more than three to four months) due to their greater susceptibility to physiological disorders and rots such as those caused by *Gloeosporium* and *Penicillium* spp. maintain registers of the rot indexes for each orchard since, to this date, the history of an orchard is the best indication of the need to apply fungicides and of the fruit storage potential (Sant'Ana et al. 2008). Moreover, the epiphytic microbiome of fruits consists of a large number of microorganisms that play more or less an important role in maintaining health; during pre- and post-harvest steps, quality and disease resistance of fruit will also be maintained by epiphytic microbiomes. Consequently, most microbiome studies related to apples have mostly been attentive to the assessment of microbial diversity by post-harvest point (Deepa et al. 2016a, b; Riachy et al. 2021).

4.4 Mitigation Strategies Against Patulin Mycotoxin

4.4.1 Physical Control

Physical treatment strategies involve strengthening the selection and cleaning of the raw resources, physical adsorption, and clarification (Figure 4.2). The selection of prime raw materials is the primary step in the way to reduce or avoid contamination by PAT. Grinding, skin mutilation, and any other damage that occurred physically could easily encourage the growth and progress of PAT toxin-producing fungi and production of patulin toxin. The better-quality cleaning of raw materials can also successfully reduce the PAT contents in food products (Baert et al. 2012).

Presently, adsorbent is broadly used in the physical treatment for elimination of PAT in fruit juice, among them; magnetic chitosan, resin, and activated carbon are frequently preferred for the absorption of PAT in the food industry. Luo et al. (2016) used a loftier magnetic chitosan in combination with Fe_3O_4 particles by the technique called water-in-oil micro-emulsion encapsulation, that is binding the PAT (200 μg/L, 10 mL) in kiwi fruit juice. The PAT-binding capability up to 19.4 μg/g by 100 mg magnetic chitosan in the nine hours at 35 °C is observed. Langmuir isotherm model was fitted with this PAT-biding behavior. In the meantime, the quality and flavor of kiwi juice remained same, and the color and luster were also enhanced (Luo et al. 2016). Adsorption by resin is the usually used method for eradicating PAT during the production of apple juice in industries. Investigation has proven that cross-linked xanthate chitosan resin had an adsorption competence of 130 mg/g for PAT removal at pH 4.0, 30 °C for 18 hours from the apple juice, and it shadowed the pseudo-second-order model and Freundlich isotherm model (Peng et al. 2016).

Electromagnetic radiation has been shown in initial studies to decrease the content of PAT and other mycotoxins within juice. In an investigation, juice treated with 0.35-kGy ionizing radiation instigated a 50% of reduction in PAT content without acceleration of nonenzymatic browning of the juice (Moake et al. 2005).

Further, UV radiation detoxification of PAT is still a research hot spot currently. The UV exposure treatments of apple juice (14.2–99.4 mJ/cm^2) lessened the PAT content by 5.2–72.6%. This reaction followed first-order kinetic modeling (Assatarakul et al. 2012). Several studies have proposed that pH value, turbidity, and chromophores remained as important aspects in the UV decontamination of PAT from fruit juice (Chandra et al. 2017; Ibarz et al. 2017). Furthermore, conferring the previous study, microwave, high hydrostatic pressure (HHP), and ultrasonic have been revealed as a virtuous method for the removal of PAT in fruit products (Avsaroglu et al. 2015). The UV light sensitivity of aflatoxins has been

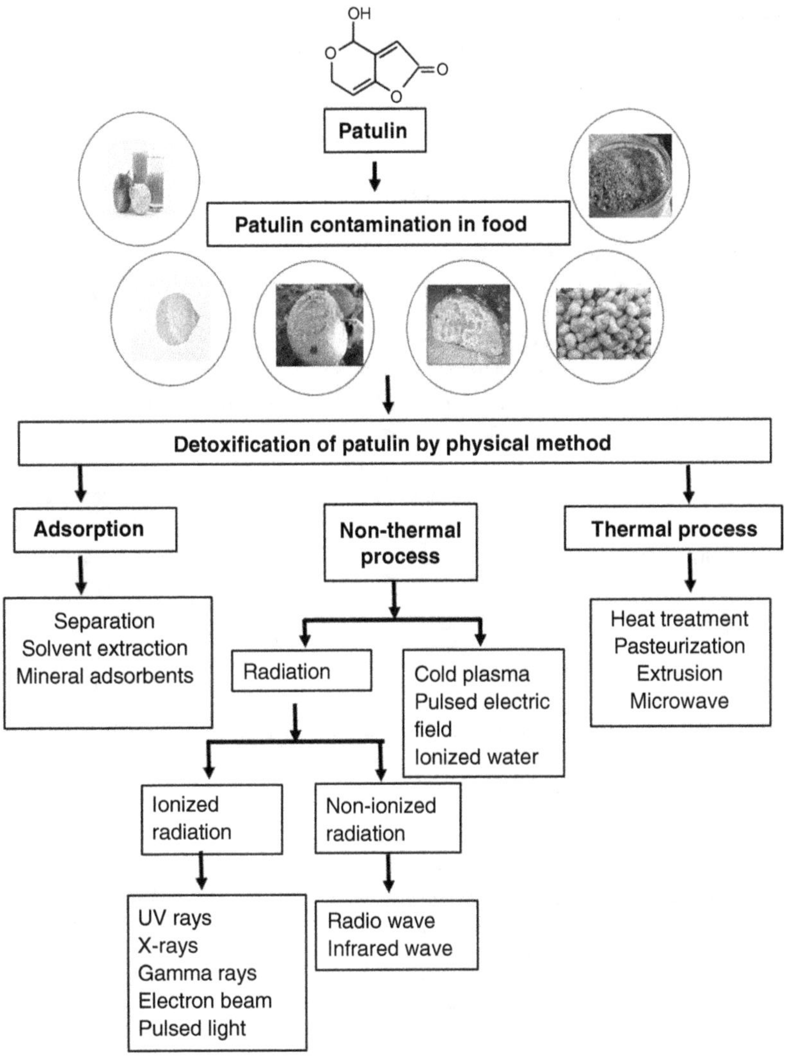

Figure 4.2 Physical method for the patulin degradation.

demonstrated on several accounts, but no studies have been performed specifically on PAT (Moake et al. 2005) (Figure 4.2).

Additionally, use of pulsed light is an alternative processing method that has been projected for the decrease of PAT content in the food products (Funes et al. 2013). Pulsed light is a non-thermal food preservation strategy that includes the use of short (1 μs–0.1 s) bursts of broad-spectrum light with wavelengths ranging from 200 to 1100 nm (Gómez et al. 2012). PAT toxin was reduced by using pulsed light in Mcllvaine buffer (composed of citric acid and disodium hydrogen phosphate, also known as a citrate-phosphate buffer), apple juice, and apple puree (Funes et al. 2013). Action with pulsed light was capable to reduce PAT by 85–95% in Mcllvaine buffer, 22% in apple juice, and 51% in apple puree (Table 4.2).

Table 4.2 Anti-patulin strategies in food and feed.

S. No.	Anti-patulin strategy		Methodology	Percent of reduction (%)	References
1.	Physical	irradiation	UV rays, high hydrostatic pressure, ultrasonic rays, microwave, pulsed light	52–72.6	Chandra et al. (2017), Avsaroglu et al. (2015), and Gómez et al. 2012
		Storage	Harvest, transportation, and sorting	70	Baert et al. (2012)
		Heat treatment	Pasteurization and high temperature	18.81–50.6	Kadakal and Nas (2003)
		Adsorbent	Magnetic chitosan, resin, activated carbon	65–72	Luo et al. (2016) and Peng et al. (2016)
2.	Chemical	ozone	Gaseous ozone detoxification equipment	35.22–93.9	Appell et al. (2011)
		Chemical additives	Sulfur dioxide, ammonia, ascorbic acid, acidic potassium permanganate, potassium sorbate, sodium benzoate, ozone, pyridoxine hydrochloride, calcium-d-pantothenate, and thiamine hydrochloride	60–90	Yazici and Velioglu (2002) and Appell et al. (2011)
3.	Biological	microorganisms	*Candida tropicalis*, *Rhodosporidium paludigenum*, *Lactobacillus rhamnosus*, *Pichia caribbica*, *Saccharomyces cerevisiae*, *Gluconobacter oxydans*, *Candida guilliermondii*, and *Kodameae ohmeri*	58.9–85.1	Luo et al. (2015), Zhu et al. (2015), and Fu et al. (2021)
		Essential oils	White vinegar, acetic acid, cymbopogon citrates, decanal	44–68	Caldwell et al. (2016), Opez et al. (2018), and Zhou et al. (2018)
		Nanoparticles	Multiwalled carbon nanotube, magnetic oxide, chitosan oxide, SeNPs, gold nanoparticles	62–90	Ge et al. (2017), Luo et al. (2017), and Silici and Karaman (2013)

Table 4.2 (Continued)

S. No.	Anti-patulin strategy		Methodology	Percent of reduction (%)	References
4.	Advanced strategy	Binding of PAT to heat-treated cells	Cell wall of heat-treated yeast strain and LAB cells, C—O, OH, and NH groups, polysaccharides, proteins	20.5–48.6	Guo et al. (2012) and Wang et al. (2015)
		DNA aptamers	ssDNA	83.3–99.8	Tang et al. (2022)
		Enzymes	Porcine pancreatic lipase	80–90	Liu et al. (2018)
		Fermentation	Yeast	90–99	Moss et al. (2010)

4.4.2 Chemical Control of Patulin and Its Producers

Chemical degradation methods to detoxify PAT have great potential and are liable as the most suitable in food industry for commercial application presently. Several of these include novel compounds and others are chemical additives. Sulfur dioxide, ammonia, ascorbic acid, acidic potassium permanganate, potassium sorbate, sodium benzoate, ozone, pyridoxine hydrochloride, calcium-d-pantothenate, and thiamine hydrochloride have been widely studied to effectively degrade PAT (Yazici and Velioglu 2002; Appell et al. 2011).

Ozone is the most effective chemical oxidant used to detoxify PAT in food products. According to the reported literature, treatment of ozonization is worned due to their food safety, low cost, and eco-friendly without any patulin toxin residues (Miller and Silva 2013). In addition, PAT releases its end product into oxalic acid, carbon dioxide, water, and diglycolic acid after degradation at high ozone concentration and depending on the time of ozonation (Cataldo and Cataldo 2008; Appell et al. 2011). Diao et al. (2018) applied ozone concentration of 7 mg/L for 10 minutes using gaseous ozone to apple juice and reduced 35.22% of original PAT concentration. Cataldo and Cataldo (2008) reduced PAT in water to 8% and apple juice to 0% from the original PAT concentration. In another study with one minute of ozonation time, PAT was reduced to 4.5 ppb from 250, with a 98% reduction of PAT. Therefore, ozone treatment methods have significant consequences on quality of food products.

Some other chemical treatments are also effectively responsible for the degradation of PAT in food processing. Similar to the ozone treatment, in the presence of ascorbic acid after 34 days of storage, PAT was reduced to 70% (Drusch et al. 2007) and between 25 and 85 °C of thermal detoxification process, the PAT concentration was significantly decreased (Kokkinidou et al. 2014). In addition, sulfur-containing compounds such as sulfur dioxide, cysteine, glutathione, β-aminobutyric acid, gamma-aminobutyric acid, boric acid (Lai et al. 2016), sodium hypochlorite (Cerioni et al. 2013), potassium sorbate, and sodium propionate and N-acetylcysteine has been successfully studied for the reduction of PAT in food products. A study conducted by Loi et al. (2017) found a 12% and 90% reduction of PAT after 24 and 48 hours of incubation since amino, NH_2, and thiol groups as well as sulfhydryl groups covalently bind to PAT structure. Similarly, other chemical compounds such as potassium permanganate degrade PAT by about 99.9% in aqueous solution (Loi et al. 2017) and calcium D-pantothenate brings about 94.3% of PAT degradation (Yazici and Velioglu 2002). The chemical treatments proved to be most effective in PAT degradation, but it ends with an unidentified residue and leads to irreversible changes, hence needing further effective studies (Table 4.2).

4.4.3 Biological Control of Patulin-Producing Fungi

Fruits and fruit-oriented products are supposed to be majorly affected by PAT contamination and it has become a foremost task for food industries (Zhong et al. 2018). Biological methods meant for control of PAT have become a significant part to increase their efficiency and safety. The yeast *Pichia caribbica* is identified as an efficient PAT-degrading isolate (Zheng et al. 2018; Deepa and Sreenivasa 2019a, b). Biological methods have shown great potential, with high efficiency and no effect on product quality, several microorganisms including *Lactobacillus rhamnosus*, *P. caribbica*, *Saccharomyces cerevisiae*, *Gluconobacter oxydans*, *Candida guilliermondii*, *Kodamaea ohmeri* are effective at PAT degradation (Ricelli et al. 2007; Hatab et al. 2012; Guo et al. 2012; Fu et al. 2021). 85.1% of PAT-adsorbing efficiency can be seen by *Candida tropicalis* N-10 (Luo et al. 2015). *P. expansum* can be effectively inhibited by *Lactobacillus plantarum* by preventing its germination and growth in addition to possessing the ability to degrade PAT to E-/Z-ascladiol and hydroascladiol, a novel biomarker, *in vitro* (Reddy et al. 2010; Ren et al. 2021). Food quality and safety of commodities can be increased by the use of LAB as biocontrol agents for PAT treatment (Hawar et al. 2013). Zheng et al. (2020) showed that LAB strain *Lactobacillus casei* YZU01 can effectively degrade PAT by extracellular enzymes and its cell wall can absorb PAT. The degradation of PAT in the contaminated fruit juice can be done by *L. casei* YZU01. Hence *L. casei* YZU01 can be used in food products as a biocontrol agent for the degradation of PAT.

Zhong et al. (2020) demonstrated that *S. cerevisiae* S288C could effectively reduce PAT during fermentation and showed that projected glutathione and intracellular enzymes are liable for decrease in PAT during the fermentation of *S. cerevisiae* S288C. Cao et al. (2013) experiment results showed that the application of *P. caribbica* significantly reduced the postharvest blue mold decay of apples caused by *P. expansum*. This indicates that the extensive variety of pathogens which grow and survive in diverse conditions can be controlled by *P. caribbica*. To maintain freshness of fruits and vegetables, they must be stored at a low temperature (Zhang et al. 2007). The biocontrol capability of the antagonist under common shelf-life conditions (low temperature and ambient storage) suggests that the combination of low temperature with *P. caribbica* can be used to enhance the storage and disease control ability. These results showed that *P. caribbica* treatment did not impair quality parameters of apples during storage, including weight loss, fruit firmness, toxic shock syndrome (TSS), titratable acidity, browning, and ascorbic acid. These outcomes illustrate that *P. caribbica* can be used as a potent biocontrol agent to minimize the post-harvest diseases caused by apples.

Tolaini et al. (2010) demonstrated the use of culture filtrates from the edible mushroom *Lentinula edodes* (LF23) can greatly improve the biocontrol activity exerted by *Cryptococcus laurentii* (LS28) and can also contribute directly to controlling the patulin contamination.

Moreover, LF23 extracts are not only nontoxic for human health but better still, they can have a positive effect on health. The edible mushroom *L. edodes* could have a useful role in the formulation of a commercial product for rot disease and PAT control in apple fruits.

Lima et al. (2011) concluded that the integration of the selected biocontrol yeasts isolates *Rhodosporidium kratochvilovae* LS11 and *C. laurentii* LS28 with low dosages of the recently developed fungicides boscalid (BOSC) and cyprodinil (CYPR) appears to be a very promising method to control blue mold and maintain both fungicide residues and PAT accumulation low in apples. Díaz et al. (2020) reported that efficient protection was achieved after short exposure to a low concentration of yeast cells, *Clavispora lusitaniae* which is known as a wide-range biocontrol agent as it has the capacity to degrade PAT content present in citrus fruits. The fruit odor will not be affected by yeast treatment. Hence, *C. lusitaniae* is used in formulation to control PAT contamination present in citrus fruits.

L. plantarum 13M5 reduces PAT levels by degrading PAT into ascladiol which has lower toxicity than PAT, whereas results suggest that 13M5 can positively remove PAT from apple juice. Additionally, *L. plantarum* 13M5 improved PAT-induced cytotoxicity and oxidative stress and reversed the expression of apoptosis and TJ protein-related genes in Caco-2 cells. These results show that *L. plantarum* 13M5 has ability to decrease or eradicate PAT contamination exist in fermented fruit juice and also can be used as a supplement in diet to decrease PAT toxicity (Wei et al. 2020). The mixture of two antagonists, *C. laurentii* and *Kosakonia radicincitans*, with varied requirements and different antagonistic capacities, leads to a combination which acts as potent antifungal agents against *P. expansum* and with the capability to decrease the PAT concentration (Lambrese et al. 2021). Numerous studies on lactobacillus and plant growth promoting rhizobacteria as biocontrol agent has been recorded (Chennappa et al. 2012, 2014, 2016; Yooussef et al. 2016; Rao et al. 2017).

Lai et al. (2022) aimed to assess the PAT detoxification ability of LAB strains and provide a promising biological detoxification idea during apple juice fermentation and *in vitro* digestion model. The result exhibited that Lpe-4 (*L. pentosus*) can show fermentation ability and also can eradicate 53.15% of PAT present in fermented apple juice in 24 hours. The LAB strains are used in the degradation and decrease of PAT content. The decontamination of PAT was moderately constant and after washing, minor amount of PAT residue was released. Moreover, the degradation of PAT was enhanced and improved by different factors. Through 5% inoculation and shaking incubation of Lpe-4, PAT in spiked apple juice could be efficiently degraded. These results indicated that PAT content in apple juice fermentation can be decreased by means of *L. pentosus* (DSM 20314) and it provided a new method to decrease PAT contamination (Table 4.2).

Tang et al. (2019) explored orotate phosphoribosyltransferase isolated from *Rhodotorula mucilaginosa* helps in the reduction of PAT in apple juice. PAT degradation in apple juice and its degradation conditions and characteristic changes were estimated. The research exhibited 25 °C for 18 hours is the optimum degradation condition, and adding about 0.15 g/L of orotate phosphoribosyltransferase helped in degradation of 1 mg/L of PAT. In addition, there were observed no significant changes in the apple juice quality. Eighty percent (1 mg/L) of PAT degradation effect was observed. Yeast *Rhodosporidium paludigenum* was also used for the degradation of PAT. This yeast converted patulin into desoxypatulinic acid (DPA); the product produced after degradation was less noxious to *Arabidopsis thaliana* and also to human liver cells than PAT and it was also not toxic to *Escherichia coli* at the maximum concentration checked. The PAT contamination in food and feeds can be minimized by *R. paludigenum* and can be entitled as a promising tool (Zhu et al. 2015).

Zhang et al. (2016) isolated a new wild-type microorganism FF1-2 strain for biodegradation of high concentrations of PAT. The fungus FF1-2 was identified as *Byssochlamys nivea* (CCTCC M2013547), which was isolated from the fermented liquor pit mud. Different conditions such as culture media, pH, and temperature were used to study the degradation of PAT by FF1-2 strain. The strain FF1-2 grew and reduced PAT at 20–46 °C, and pH at 3.0–5.0. This study presented that PAT degradation was affected by temperature than a change in pH. 37 °C was the ideal temperature for the degradation of PAT, and 500 mg/mL of PAT level in culture media was degraded to a practically unnoticeable range in five days. About 97.1% of the PAT degradation was observed in apple puree at 30 °C after nine days. This was the first study which found that filamentous fungi have the capability to degrade PAT. Biodegradation of PAT using *Pichia ohmeri* 158 and *S. cerevisiae* indicated the promising application of innocuous yeasts isolated from natural ecosystems. The combined biodegradation/adsorption/antifungal activities of such yeasts exhibit a productive and effectual choice of biological control to avoid undesirable post-harvest fungi through storage. The use of antagonistic yeasts with wide activity and the ability to degrade PAT should be continued with additional studies on the mode of action and toxicity prior to *in vivo* application (Coelho et al. 2008). Mitigation strategies using biological methods were shown in (Figure 4.3).

4.5 Detoxification of Patulin

4.5.1 Storage

During harvest and transportation, there are chances of physical damage and wounds that gave way for *P. expansum* penetration and infection. Decreasing wound incidence lessens PAT concentration, for instance, about 99% of damage control is caused by a 70% PAT reduction (Baert et al. 2012). Henceforth, it is important to reduce wounds and physical damage by taking maximum precautions throughout transportation and harvesting. Other factors considered while harvesting are picking the fruit in dry conditions, keeping them in clean bins, transporting directly to stores and storing them in cold storage at 1.5–4.0 °C within 18 hours after harvest to minimize the occurrence of the fungal infection (Kabak and Dobson 2007). According to Baert et al. (2012), sorting the fruits in an accurate atmosphere by eliminating the diseased apples with lesions is very effective in decreasing PAT concentration since the PAT may contaminate further non-infected fruits.

4.5.2 Heat Treatment

The use of thermal treatments to decrease the risk of PAT has been questioned due to its resistance to heat (Lovett et al. 1975). Pasteurization has factually shown differing and distinct fallouts with regard to PAT reduction. About 50% of reduction is found by the pasteurization for about 20 minutes at 80 °C for apple juice contaminated with PAT (Scott and Somers 1968). However, further investigation reported that PAT content was constant at 80 °C for 30 minutes in apple juice, and an extensive treatment of 120 °C for 30 minutes was

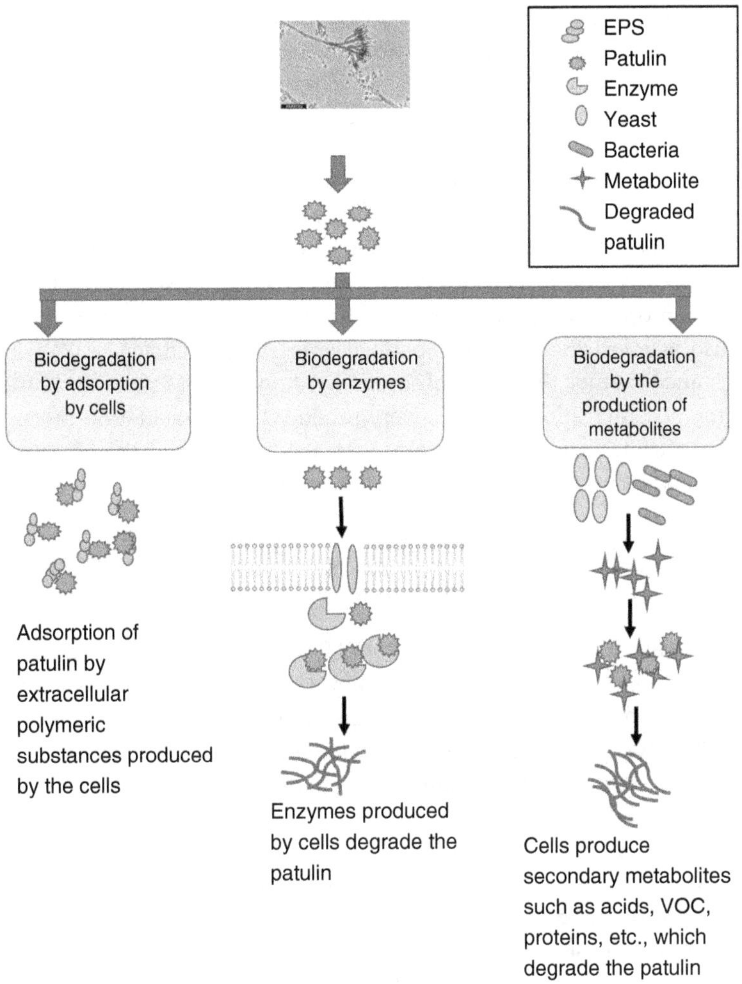

Figure 4.3 Biological strategies for patulin detoxification.

vital to attain PAT content reduction (Wheeler et al. 1987). High-temperature short-time (HTST) system remained to cause effective reduction in PAT (18.8% decrease at 90 °C) compared to the batch pasteurization. It is observed that reassessment of two approaches with extensive pasteurization of 20 minutes at 90 and 100 °C led to the reduction of about 18.81% and 25.99% PAT, respectively. Contradictory outcomes continue to be engendered by various investigators when comparing HTST and batch pasteurization (Kadakal and Nas 2003).

4.5.3 Fermentation

Fermentation is one of the processes where yeast sugars are converted into alcohols, gases, and/or acids. Several studies have been reported on unfermented apple juice contamination by the PAT, though few surveys have reported PAT contamination in alcoholic cider (Moss et al. 2010). It was observed that fermentation with yeast isolates has the potential to reduce PAT up to 90% (Burroughs 2000; Divyashree et al. 2021). In another study, eight yeast strains were used and various methods of fermentation processes were carried out to evaluate the effectivity of PAT toxin in apple juice spiked with 15 mg/L PAT content and observed that all conducted methods were capable to degrade the PAT by 99% after two weeks of fermentation period (Stinson et al. 1978). Correspondingly, in an investigation of the capability of three dissimilar strains of *S. cerevisiae* to reduce PAT content in apple juice, it was observed that all three strains were substantial at decreasing the PAT content during the fermentation process but were unsuccessful during aerobic growth period (Moss et al. 2010). This recommends that the decrease of PAT observed is a consequence of deprivation by fermentation process as opposed to adsorbing to the cells of yeast strains themselves. This study also assessed the products obtained after the breakdown of PAT by fermentation process and whether they were absorbed by the yeasts (Moss et al. 2010). They found that many decomposition products were produced by fermentation process and remained in juice after fermentation. Of note, E-ascabiol was one of the products, which is also mycotoxin by itself, however considered toxic than the PAT (Suzuki et al. 1971).

4.5.4 Nanoparticles

A novel magnetic multi-walled carbon nanotube (MWCNT) adsorbent was effectively synthesized, and its adsorption features for the effective removal of PAT from aqueous solution were examined. The maximum adsorption capability of the as-prepared magnetic MWCNTs reached 640.2 μg/g, which was more than biological material-based absorbents ($p < 0.05$), and the adsorption equilibrium time was significantly shortened to one hour ($p < 0.05$) (Zheng et al. 2018).

Magnetic Fe_3O_4@CTS nanoparticles were layered with the inactivated *Candida utilis* CICC1769 cells and was used as a novel biosorbent for the elimination of PAT in fruit juice. This new biosorbent was found to decrease PAT content by over 90% in orange juice deprived of any substantial undesirable impressions on the quality parameters like Brix, Vitamin C, and titratable acidity (Ge et al. 2017). Chitosan-coated Fe_3O_4 elements were synthesized as the magnetic adsorbents by reverse oil-in-water microemulsion system by means of Triton X-100. Chitosan-coated Fe_3O_4 adsorbent was revealed to be a significant absorbent for PAT toxin adsorption with a determined adsorption capability of 6.67 mg/g within five hours by the addition of 300 lg adsorbents into 10 mL 200 lg/L PAT aqueous. Furthermore, the retrieval rate of chitosan-coated Fe_3O_4 adsorbent grasped to 99.95% within 60 minutes, exhibited its outstanding recoverable performance (Luo et al. 2017). Selenium nanoparticles (SeNPs) were synthesized based on cross-linked Se-chitosan/L-cysteine nanoparticles and used for the effectual elimination of PAT from an aqueous solution (Paimard et al. 2021). Different concentrations of propolis (0.1, 1, and 2 mg/mL) and sodium benzoate (0.35 mg/mL) were supplemented into apple juice after *P. expansum* inoculation. Apple juice samples were later assorted with propolis, and the PAT toxin content was investigated in 1st, 24th, and 48th hour. Substantial PAT reduction was attained with the addition of propolis in the apple juice. The best outcome was attained at 2 mg/mL propolis-supplemented group for about 48 hours of incubation (Silici and Karaman 2013). SeNPs were synthesized by decreasing the sodium selenite with the chitosan as stabilizer and cast off for averting PAT-induced gastro intestine, liver, and kidney damage. Assessment of serum biochemical parameters, histopathology, oxidative stress biomarkers, and activities of antioxidant enzymes in a mouse model presented that pre-treatment with SeNPs (2 mg Se/kg body weight) could reduce PAT-induced oxidative damage to the kidney and liver of mice (Deepa and Sreenivasa 2017a; Divyashree et al. 2022).

4.5.5 Essential Oils

Treatment of apples with slight heat or fumigating them with vaporized peracetic acid or white vinegar enhanced the capability of the *Pseudomonas* biocontrol agents to prevent the growth of fungi in wounds and injuries, during a short storage period of two to three weeks. Several studies have proven essential oils (EOs) as one of the prevention strategies for fungi (Prasad et al. 2010; Sreenivasa et al. 2011a, b; Achar et al. 2020). White vinegar was immensely remarkable in its capacity to reduce populations of both existing fungi and inoculated *P. expansum* (Caldwell et al. 2016). The antagonistic effect of vapor phase lemongrass (*Cymbopogon citratus*) EO on the growth of *P. expansum* inoculated on the bread was assessed. Thirteen compounds were the chief compounds in the EO, with the presence of citral as the key compound. The fungi *P. expansum* was repressed for 21 days at 20 °C with 750 μL of EO/L_{air}, and its decrease in growth increased with increasing the EO concentrations (Opez et al. 2018). The effects of exogenic EO decanal on the development and synthesis of PAT by *P. expansum* were determined. Outcomes showed that 0.12 g/L decanal could efficiently inhibit the development of *P. expansum* mycelium *in vitro*. About 0.24 g/L decanal presented a good inhibitory activity against the blue mold rot on apple and pear fruit (Zhou et al. 2018) (Table 4.2).

4.6 Degradation Products of Patulin

PAT in foods and their commodities are one of the high-risk factors to human health as well as for animals. The PAT toxicity mostly depends on its structure hemiacetal as well as lactone ring. Therefore, damage to its structure would effectively reduce PAT toxicity (Wallen et al. 1839). The physical treatments such as pH, heating at 80 °C for 40 minutes, and UV detoxification strategies effectively degraded the PAT to its end products glyoxylic acid and 3-keto-5-hydroxypentanal, which gives opportunity for PAT hemiacetal moiety followed by lactone hydrolysis and retroaldolization. However, these degraded products have not been studied. Similarly, the strongest oxidant ozone which could completely degrade PAT had also not been evaluated, though it significantly decreased the PAT. On the other side, chemical treatment such as ascorbic acid and sulfur dioxide neutralizes toxicity of PAT by forming adducts during the breaking of lactone ring and interacting with thiols (Appell et al. 2011). Moreover, numerous studies have been investigated with bacteria and yeast as biocontrol agents for the degradation of PAT toxicity in food products. A study conducted by Hawar et al. (2013) reported PAT degradation into ascladiol-(E), ascladiol-(Z), and hydroascladiol at 4 °C in the presence of *L. plantarum* cell-free incubation for four weeks. Yeast strains were also investigated on PAT degradation to its products, same as *Lactobacillus* through fermentation followed by enzymolysis (Castoria et al. 2011). In addition, some yeast strains have also been reported to produce DPA (Zhu et al. 2015). Therefore the use of microorganisms significantly degraded PAT products and their toxicity in humans derived from study conducted on kidney, liver, intestinal tract, and immune system (Tannous et al. 2017).

4.7 Binding Methods

4.7.1 Binding Mechanism of Patulin to Heat-Treated Cells

Guo et al. (2012) investigated that cell wall of the heat-treated yeast strain plays a role in PAT binding, and cell wall integrity is important in binding process and also showed that proteins and polysaccharides are significant components of cell walls of heat-treated cells that could be associated with removal of PAT. Hydrophobic interactions participate as chief role in binding PAT to heat-treated strains of yeast. Wang et al. (2015) reported that the heat-inactivated LAB cells, which had higher specific surface area and surface hydrophobicity, were more likely to have a higher capacity to absorb PAT from the aqueous solution. Additionally, adsorption of PAT was also supposed to be done by C—O group and OH, NH groups which were linked to carbohydrate and protein components.

4.7.2 DNA Aptamers as Capture Probes

A high-affinity ssDNA aptamer that specifically binds to PAT was generated using the systemic evolution of ligands by exponential enrichment (SELEX) procedure assisted by graphene oxide (GO). The colorimetric aptasensor exhibited a linear range from 50 to 2500 pg/mL and the detection limit was found to be 48 pg/mL. The results indicated that GO-SELEX technology was suitable for screening of aptamers in contradiction of small-molecule toxins, presenting as capable application aimed at aptamer-based biosensors (Wu et al. 2016). To detect the PAT toxin using gold nanoparticles functionalized by Streptavidin Tang et al. (2022) introduced sensitive aptamer-involved lateral flow assay (LFA). The detection limit was found about 0.19 ng/mL in buffer and in real sample, it was found 0.36 ng/mL. The retrievals were 83.3% up to 107.1%, with an acceptable RSD rate of 6.5–7.5%. Therefore, the established FLA might be used as swift, simple, on-the-spot screening tool used for the determination of PAT in apple juice.

4.7.3 Binding Mechanism of Patulin Using Enzymes

Xing et al. (2021) exhibited that the yeast, *C. guilliermondii* was cloned with short-chain dehydrogenase/reductase (SDR) gene, CgSDR which is indicated in *E. coli*. Expression of CgSDR gene deliberated durable PAT tolerance and also eradication capability toward *E. coli*, then purified CgSDR possibly will transfigure PAT in *in vitro* condition into E-ascladiol by using NADPH as coenzyme. In addition, adding CgSDR by 150 μg/mL might decrease 80% of PAT content in apple juice. Similarly, biodegradation method did not impact the quality of apple juice. Liu et al. (2018) studied biodegradation of PAT using porcine pancreatic lipase (PPL). The high-performance liquid chromatography (HPLC) method was used to examine the PAT concentration. Ideal deprivation conditions of PPL aimed at PAT were detected at pH 7.5, 40 °C by 48 hours. Above 90% of degradation was reached. It showed that PPL was efficient in reducing PAT in vegetables and fruit juices.

4.8 Future Implications

Currently, to facilitate the commercial application of biological detoxification approaches, further future studies should spotlight on development of detailed PAT degradation mechanisms by conducting studies on toxic metabolites through investigating novel analytical methods.

4.9 Summary

Patulin contamination in food products is a risk factor for humans. Deeply understanding the detoxification methods such as physical, chemical, and biological lead to the investigation of ideal methods since these methods are capable of decreasing the PAT amount to a certain extent. However, based on the reported literature, PAT irradiation is very difficult in processing stages. Physical, chemical, and biological methods are also explored to detoxify PAT, but their efficacy is compromised due to their residues which are hazardous to environment in one or the other way. Hence, for commercial application, an alternative method for the progress of advanced degradation methods as well as equipment is necessary in the future.

4.10 Study Questions

1) Mitigation strategies against patulin mycotoxin
2) Detoxification treatments of patulin
3) Degradation products of patulin

Acknowledgments

We are grateful to the Institution of Excellence, Manasagangotri, and University of Mysore for supporting us to carry out the research. S. Divyashree and B. Shruthi were supported by the Indian Council for Medical Research (ICMR; New Delhi) for a Senior Research Fellowship (FBO/Fell/1/2022-ECD-II) and (Myco/Fell/8/2022-ECD-II), respectively. Adithi G was supported as SRF by DST/SERB (REF.CRG/2021/008325).

Conflict of Interest

The authors declare no competing interests.

Author Contributions

The author contributions are as follows: S. Divyashree, Adithi G, B. Shruthi, and M.Y. Sreenivasa designed the book chapter. SD, AG, and BS for writing book chapter preparation and software handling. M. Y. Sreenivasa edited and submitted the final version of the book chapter. M.Y. Sreenivasa – Supervision. All authors read and approved for publication.

References

Achar, P.N., Quyen, P., Adukwu, E.C. et al. (2020). Investigation of the antifungal and anti-aflatoxigenic potential of plant-based essential oils against *Aspergillus flavus* in peanuts. *J. Fungi* 6 (4): 383. https://doi.org/10.3390/jof6040383.

Appell, M., Jackson, M.A., and Dombrink-kurtzman, M.A. (2011). Removal of patulin from aqueous solutions by propylthiol functionalized SBA-15. *J. Hazard. Mater.* 187: 150–156. https://doi.org/10.1016/j.jhazmat.2011.01.002.

Assatarakul, K., Churey, J.J., Manns, D.C., and Worobo, R.W. (2012). Patulin reduction in apple juice from concentrate by UV radiation and comparison of kinetic degradation models between apple juice and apple cider. *J. Food Protect.* 75 (4): 717–724. https://doi.org/10.4315/0362-028X.JFP-11-429.

Avsaroglu, M.D., Bozoglu, F., Alpas, H. et al. (2015). Use of pulsed-high hydrostatic pressure treatment to decrease patulin in apple juice. *High Press. Res.* 35 (2): 214–222. https://doi.org/10.1080/08957959.2015.1027700.

Azizi, I.G. and Rouhi, S. (2013). Determination of patulin in fruit juices and compote of apple and pear. *J. Toxicol. Toxin Rev.* 32 (3): 39–42. https://doi.org/10.3109/15569543.2013.801354.

Baert, K., Devlieghere, F., Amiri, A., and De Meulenaer, B. (2012). Evaluation of strategies for reducing patulin contamination of apple juice using a farm to fork risk assessment model. *Int. J. Food Microbiol.* 154: 119–129. https://doi.org/10.1016/j.ijfoodmicro.2011.12.015.

Burroughs, L.F. (2000). Stability of patulin to sulfur dioxide and to yeast fermentation. *J. AOAC* 60: 100–103.

Caldwell, L. (2016). The use of vinegar vapor and post-harvest biological control to reduce patulin in apple cider. Electronic thesis and dessertations. Four Peaks Environmental Science & Data Solutions.

Cao, J., Zhang, H., Yang, Q., and Ren, R. (2013). Efficacy of *Pichia caribbica* in controlling blue mold rot and patulin degradation in apples. *Int. J. Food Microbiol.* 162: 167–173. https://doi.org/10.1016/j.ijfoodmicro.2013.01.007.

Castoria, R., Mannina, L., Durán-Patrón, R. et al. (2011). Conversion of the mycotoxin patulin to the less toxic desoxypatulinic acid by the biocontrol yeast *Rhodosporidium kratochvilovae* strain LS11. *J. Agric. Food Chem.* 59 (21): 11571–11578. https://doi.org/10.1021/jf203098v.

Cataldo, F. and Cataldo, F. (2008). Ozone decomposition of patulin — a micotoxin and food contaminant. *Ozone Sci. Eng.* 30: 9512. 10.1080/01919510801925930.

Cerioni, L., Lazarte, M.D.L.Á., Rodríguez-montelongo, L., and Volentini, S.I. (2013). Inhibition of *Penicillium expansum* by an oxidative treatment. *Food Microbiol.* 33: 298–301. https://doi.org/10.1016/j.fm.2012.09.011.

Chandra, S., Patras, A., Begum, A., and Sasges, M. (2017). Patulin degradation and cytotoxicity evaluation of UV irradiated apple juice using human peripheral blood mononuclear cells. *J. Food Process Eng* 1–9. https://doi.org/10.1111/jfpe.12586.

Chennappa, G., Adkar-Purushothama, C.R., Naik, M.K. et al. (2012). Impact of pesticides on pgpr activity of *Azotobacter* sp. isolated from pesticide flooded paddy soils. *Greener J. Agric. Sci.* 4 (4): 117–129. https://doi.org/10.15580/GJAS.2014.4.010314003.

Chennappa, G., Adkar-Purushothama, C.R., Suraj, U. et al. (2014). Impact of pesticides on PGPR activity of *Azotobacter* sp. isolated from pesticide flooded paddy soils. *Greener J. Agric. Sci.* 4 (4): 117–129.

Chennappa, G., Naik, M.K., Adkar-Purushothama, C.R. et al. (2016). PGP, abiotic stress tolerant and antifungal activity of *Azotobacter* sp. isolated from paddy soils. *Indian J. Exp. Biol.* 54 (5): 322–331.

Ciegler, A. (1977). Patulin. In: *Mycotoxins in Human and Animal Health* (ed. J.V. Rodricks, C.W. Hesseltine, and M.A. Mehlman), 609–624. Park Forest South, IL: Pathotox Publishers.

Coelho, A., Celli, M., Sataque Ono, E. et al. (2008). Patulin biodegradation using *Pichia ohmeri* and *Saccharomyces cerevisiae*. *World Mycotoxin J.* 1: 325–331. https://doi.org/10.3920/wmj2008.1040.

Deepa, N. and Sreenivasa, M.Y. (2017a). *Fusarium verticillioides*, a globally important pathogen of agriculture and livestock: a review. *J. Vet. Med. Res.* 4 (4): 1084.

Deepa, N. and Sreenivasa, M.Y. (2017b). Fumonisins: a review on its global occurrence, epidemiology, toxicity and detection. *J. Vet. Med. Res.* 4 (6): 1093.

Deepa, N. and Sreenivasa, M.Y. (2019a). Biocontrol strategies for effective management of phytopathogenic fungi associated with cereals. In: *New and Future Developments in Microbial Biotechnology and Bioengineering* (ed. J.S. Singh and D.P. Singh), 177–189. Elsevier. ISBN: 9780444641915 https://doi.org/10.1016/B978-0-444-64191-5.00013-4.

Deepa, N. and Sreenivasa, M.Y. (2019b). Molecular methods and key genes targeted for the detection of fumonisin producing *Fusarium verticillioides* – an updated review. *Food Biosci.* 32: 100473. https://doi.org/10.1016/j.fbio.2019.100473.

Deepa, N., Charith Raj, A.P., and Sreenivasa, M.Y. (2016a). Multiplex PCR method for the early detection of fumonisin producing *Fusarium verticillioides*. *Food Biosci.* 13: 84–88.

Deepa, N., Nagaraja, H., and Sreenivasa, M.Y. (2016b). Prevalence of fumonisin producing *Fusarium verticillioides* associated with cereals grown in Karnataka (India). *Food Sci. Human Well.* 5: 156–162. https://doi.org/10.1016/j.fshw.2016.07.001.

Deepa, N., Achar, P.N., and Sreenivasa, M.Y. (2021). Current perspectives of biocontrol agents for management of *Fusarium verticillioides* and its Fumonisin in cereals—a review. *J. Fungi* 7: 776. https://doi.org/10.3390/jof7090776.

Diao, E., Wang, J., Li, X. et al. (2018). Patulin degradation in apple juice using ozone detoxification equipment and its effects on quality. *J. Food Process. Preserv.* 1–7: https://doi.org/10.1111/jfpp.13645.

Díaz, M.A., Pereyra, M.M., Santander, F.F.S. et al. (2020). Protection of citrus fruits from postharvest infection with *Penicillium digitatum* and degradation of patulin by biocontrol yeast *Clavispora lusitaniae* 146. *Microorganisms* 8: 1–12. https://doi.org/10.3390/microorganisms8101477.

Divyashree, S., Anjali P.G., Rakesh Somashekaraiah, & Sreenivasa M.Y., 2021. Probiotic properties of *Lactobacillus Casei* – MYSRD 108 and *Lactobacillus Plantarum*-MYSRD

71 with potential antimicrobial activity against Salmonella Paratyphi. *Biotechnol. Rep.* 32. Elsevier B.V.:e00672. doi:https://doi.org/10.1016/j.btre.2021.e00672.

Divyashree, S., Anjali P.G., Deepthi B.V., Rakesh Somashekaraiah, Walid Mottawea, Riadh Hammami, & Sreenivasa, M.Y., 2022. Black cherry fruit as a source of probiotic candidates with antimicrobial and antibiofilm activities against *Salmonella*. *S. Afr. J. Bot.* 150. Elsevier B.V.:861–872. doi:https://doi.org/10.1016/j.sajb.2022.08.045.

Drusch, S., Kopka, S., and Kaeding, J. (2007). Food chemistry stability of patulin in a juice-like aqueous model system in the presence of ascorbic acid. *Food Chem.* 100: 192–197. https://doi.org/10.1016/j.foodchem.2005.09.043.

Frisvad, J.C. and Samson, R.A. (2004). Polyphasic taxonomy of *Penicillium* subgenus *Penicillium* a guide to identification of food and air-borne terverticillate Penicillia and their mycotoxins. *J. Stud. Mycol.* 49: 1–174.

Fu, Y., Yang, Q., Solairaj, D. et al. (2021). Biodegradation of mycotoxin patulin by the yeast *Meyerozyma guilliermondii. Biol. Control* 160: https://doi.org/10.1016/j.biocontrol.2021.104692.

Funes, G.J., Gómez, P.L., Resnik, S.L., and Alzamora, S.M. (2013). Application of pulsed light to patulin reduction in mcilvaine buffer and apple products. *Food Control* 30: 405–410. https://doi.org/10.1016/j.foodcont.2012.09.001.

Ge, N., Xu, J., Li, F. et al. (2017). Immobilization of inactivated microbial cells on magnetic Fe3O4 @ CTS nanoparticles for constructing a new biosorbent for removal of patulin in fruit juice. *Food Control* 82: 83–90. https://doi.org/10.1016/j.foodcont.2017.06.027.

Gómez, P.L., Salvatori, D.M., García-loredo, A., and Alzamora, S.M. (2012). Pulsed light treatment of cut apple: dose effect on color, structure, and microbiological stability. *Food Bioprocess Technol.* 5: 2311–2322. https://doi.org/10.1007/s11947-011-0598-3.

Guo, C., Yuan, Y., Yue, T. et al. (2012). Binding mechanism of patulin to heat-treated yeast cell. *Lett. Appl. Microbiol.* 55: 453–459. https://doi.org/10.1111/j.1472-765x.2012.03314.x.

Hartwig, N., Fetter, C., Ferreira, J. et al. (2020). Dry fruit as source of fungal contaminants or functional compounds. *Food Sci. Technol.* 40: 76–83. https://doi.org/10.1590/fst.32118.

Harwig, J., Chen, Y., Kennedy, B.P.C., and Scott, P.M. (1973). Occurrence of patulin and patulin-producing strains of *Penicillium expansum* in natural rots of apple in Canada. *Cancer Inst. Food Sci. Technol.* 6: 22–25. https://doi.org/10.1016/S0315-5463(73)73959-6.

Hatab, S., Yue, T., and Mohamad, O. (2012). Removal of patulin from apple juice using inactivated lactic acid bacteria. *J. Appl. Microbiol.* 112 (5): 892–899. https://doi.org/10.1111/j.1365-2672.2012.05279.x.

Hawar, S., Vevers, W., Karieb, S. et al. (2013). Biotransformation of patulin to hydroascladiol by *Lactobacillus plantarum*. *Food Control* 34: 502–508. https://doi.org/10.1016/j.foodcont.2013.05.023.

Hussain, S., Asi, M.R., Iqbal, M. et al. (2020). Surveillance of patulin in apple, grapes juices and value-added products for sale in Pakistan. *Foods* 9: 1–12.

Ibarz, R., Garvín, A., and Ibarz, A. (2017). Kinetic and thermodynamic study of the photochemical degradation of patulin. *Food Res. Int.* 99: 348–354. https://doi.org/10.1016/j.foodres.2017.05.025.

Jayashree, G.V. and Farhath, K. (2015). Patulin contamination in pure and mixed apple products marketed in Mysore city (India). *Int. J. Curr. Res.* 7 (12): 23508–23511.

Ji, X., Li, R., Yang, H. et al. (2017). Occurrence of patulin in various fruit products and dietary exposure assessment for consumers in China. *Food Control* 78: 100–107. https://doi.org/10.1016/j.foodcont.2017.02.044.

Kabak, B. and Dobson, A.D.W. (2007). Strategies to prevent mycotoxin contamination of food and animal feed: a review. *Crit. Rev. Food Sci. Nutr.* 8398: https://doi.org/10.1080/10408390500436185.

Kadakal, C. and Nas, S. (2003). Effect of heat treatment and evaporation on patulin and some other properties of apple juice. *J. Sci. Food Agric.* 83: 987–990. https://doi.org/10.1002/jsfa.1339.

Kokkinidou, S., Floros, J.D., and Laborde, L.F. (2014). Kinetics of the thermal degradation of patulin in the presence of ascorbic acid. *J. Food Sci.* 79 (1): 108–114. https://doi.org/10.1111/1750-3841.12316.

Lai, T., Wang, Y., Bai, X. et al. (2016). Postharvest biology and technology dissecting inhibitory effect of boric acid on virulence and patulin production of *Penicillium expansum*. *Postharvest Biol. Technol.* 117: 187–196. https://doi.org/10.1016/j.postharvbio.2016.03.003.

Lai, W., Cai, R., Yang, K. et al. (2022). Detoxification of patulin by *Lactobacillus pentosus* DSM 20314 during apple juice fermentation. *Food Control* 131: 108446. https://doi.org/10.1016/j.foodcont.2021.108446.

Lambrese, Y., Sansone, G., Sanz, M.I. et al. (2021). *Kosakonia radicincitans* and *Cryptococcus laurentii* controlled *Penicillium expansum* rot and decreased patulin production at 4 and 25 °C. *Food Microbiol.* 100: 103863. https://doi.org/10.1016/j.fm.2021.103863.

Larsen, T.O., Frisvad, J.C., Ravn, G., and Skaaning, T. (1998). Mycotoxin production by *Penicillium expansum* on blackcurrant and cherry juice. *Food Addit. Contam.* 15: 671–675. 10.1080/02652039809374696.

Leggott, N.L. and Shephard, G.S. (2001). Patulin in south african commercial apple products. *Food Control* 12: 73–76.

Lima, G., Castoria, R., De Curtis, F. et al. (2011). Integrated control of blue mould using new fungicides and biocontrol yeasts lowers levels of fungicide residues and patulin contamination in apples. *Postharvest Biol. Technol.* 60: 164–172. https://doi.org/10.1016/j.postharvbio.2010.12.010.

Liu, B., Peng, X., and Meng, X. (2018). Effective biodegradation of mycotoxin patulin by porcine pancreatic lipase. *Front. Microbiol.* 9: 1–7. https://doi.org/10.3389/fmicb.2018.00615.

Loi, J., Zhou, T., Tsao, R. et al. (2017). Mitigation of patulin in fresh and processed foods and beverages. *Toxins* 9: 157. https://doi.org/10.3390/toxins9050157.

Lopez-Diaz, T.M. and Flannigan, B. (1997). Production of patulin and cytochalasin E by *Aspergillus clavatus* during malting of barley and wheat. *Int. J. Food Microbiol.* 35 (2): 129–136. https://doi.org/10.1016/s0168-1605(96)01211-1.

Lovett, J., Thompson, R.G., and Boutin, B.K. (1975). Patulin production in apples stored in a controlled atmosphere. *J. AOAC* 58: 912–914. https://doi.org/10.1093/jaoac/58.5.912.

Luo, Y., Wang, J., Liu, B. et al. (2015). Effect of yeast cell morphology, cell wall physical structure and chemical composition on patulin adsorption. *PLoS One* 10: 1–16. https://doi.org/10.1371/journal.pone.0136045.

Luo, Y., Li, Z., Yuan, Y., and Yue, T. (2016). Bioadsorption of patulin from kiwi fruit juice onto a superior magnetic chitosan. *J. Alloys Compd.* 667: 101–108. https://doi.org/10.1016/j.jallcom.2016.01.143.

Luo, Y., Zhou, Z., and Yue, T. (2017). Synthesis and characterization of nontoxic chitosan-coated Fe_3O_4 particles for patulin adsorption in a juice-pH simulation aqueous. *Food Chem.* 221: 317–323. https://doi.org/10.1016/j.foodchem.2016.09.008.

Magan, N. (2014). Mycotoxins in food detection and control. *Food Sci. Technol.* https://doi.org/10.1201/9781439823361.

Miller, A. and Silva, C.L.M. (2013). A review on ozone-based treatments for fruit and vegetables preservation. *Food Eng. Rev.* 5: 77–106. 10.1007/s12393-013-9064-5.

Moake, M.M., Padilla-zakour, O.I., and Worobo, R.W. (2005). Review of patulin control methods in foods. *Compr. Rev. Food Sci. Saf.* 4: 8–21.

Moss, M.O., Long, M.T., Moss, M.O., and Long, M.T. (2010). Fate of patulin in the presence of the yeast *Saccharomyces cerevisiae*. *Food Addit. Contam.* 19: 387–399. https://doi.org/10.1080/0265203011009116.

Nagaraja, H., Chennappa, G., Rao, P.C.R.K. et al. (2016). Diversity of toxic and phytopathogenic *Fusarium* species occurring on cereals grown in Karnataka state, India. *3 Biotech* 6: 57.

Opez, E.M., Valle-vargas, G.P., and Palou, E. (2018). *Penicillium expansum* inhibition on bread by Lemongrass essential oil in vapor phase. *J. Food. Protect.* 81 (3): 467–471. https://doi.org/10.4315/0362-028X.JFP-17-315.

Paimard, G., Mohammadi, R., Bahrami, R. et al. (2021). Detoxification of patulin from juice simulator and apple juice via. *LWT* 143: 111146. https://doi.org/10.1016/j.lwt.2021.111146.

Peng, X., Liu, B., Chen, W. et al. (2016). Effective biosorption of patulin from apple juice by cross-linked xanthated chitosan resin. *Food Control* 63: 140–146. https://doi.org/10.1016/j.foodcont.2015.11.039.

Ping, T., Sakai, R., Abdul, N. et al. (2014). High performance liquid chromatography method for the determination of patulin and 5-hydroxymethyl furfural in fruit juices marketed in Malaysia. *Food Control* 38: 142–149. https://doi.org/10.1016/j.foodcont.2013.10.018.

Pittet, D. and Harbarth, S. (1998). What techniques for diagnosis of ventilator-associated pneumonia? *Lancet* 352: 83–84. https://doi.org/10.1016/S0140-6736/(98)85005-8.

Prasad, M.N., Shankara, B.S., and Sreenivasa, M.Y. (2010). Antifungal activity of essential oils against *Phomopsis azadirachtae*- the causative agent of die-back disease of neem. *J. Agric. Technol.* 6 (1): 127–133.

Rao, P.K., Deepti, B.V., Rakesh, S. et al. (2017). Anti-aflatoxigenic potential of cell free supernatant from *Lactobacillus plantarum* MYS44 against *Aspergillus parasiticus*. *Probiot. Antimicrob. Proteins* 11 (1): 55–64.

Reddy, K.R.N., Spadaro, D., and Lore, A. (2010). Potential of patulin production by *Penicillium expansum* strains on various fruits. *Mycotoxin Res.* 26: 257–265. https://doi.org/10.1007/s12550-010-0064-5.

Reid, D.W. and Ware, E.E. (1974). Multidimensionalify of internal versus external control: addition of a third dimension and non-distinction of self versus others. *Can. J. Behav. Sci. Rev. Cancer Sci. Comp.* 6 (2): –131.

Ren, Y., Yao, M., Chang, P. et al. (2021). Isolation and characterization of a *Pseudomonas poae* JSU-Y1 with patulin degradation ability and biocontrol potential against *Penicillium expansum*. *Toxicon* 195: 1–6. https://doi.org/10.1016/j.toxicon.2021.02.014.

Riachy, R.A., Strub, C., Durand, N. et al. (2021). Microbiome status of cider-apples, from orchard to processing, with a special focus on *Penicillium expansum* occurrence and patulin contamination. *J. Fungi* 7 (4): 244. https://doi.org/10.3390/jof7040244.

Ricelli, A., Baruzzi, F., Solfrizzo, M. et al. (2007). Biotransformation of patulin by *Gluconobacter oxydans*. *Appl. Environ. Microbiol.* 73: 785–792. https://doi.org/10.1128/AEM.02032-06.

Ritieni, A. (2003). Patulin in Italian commercial apple products. *J. Agric. Food Chem.* 51: 6086–6090. https://doi.org/10.1021/jf034523c.

Romero-steiner, S., Musher, D.M., Cetron, M.S. et al. (1999). Reduction in functional antibody activity against *Streptococcus pneumoniae* in vaccinated elderly individuals highly correlates with decreased IgG antibody avidity. *Clin. Infect. Dis.* 29: 281–288.

Sadok, I., Szmagara, A., and Staniszewska, M.M. (2017). The validated and sensitive HPLC-DAD method for determination of patulin in strawberries. *Food Chem.* 245: 364–370. https://doi.org/10.1016/j.foodchem.2017.10.093.

Sant'Ana, A.D.S., Rosenthal, A., and Massaguer, P.R.D. (2008). The fate of patulin in apple juice processing: a review. *Food Res. Int.* 41: 441–453. https://doi.org/10.1016/j.foodres.2008.03.001.

Sarubbi, F., Formisano, G., Auriemma, G., and Arrichiello, A. (2016). Patulina patulin in homogenized fruit's and tomato products. *Food Control* 59: 420–423. https://doi.org/10.1016/j.foodcont.2015.06.022.

Saxena, N., Dwivedi, P.D., Ansari, K.M., and Das, M. (2009). Patulin in apple juices: incidence and likely intake in an Indian population. *Food Addit. Contam.* 1: 140–146. https://doi.org/10.1080/02652030802378848.

Scott, P.M. and Somers, E. (1968). Stability of patulin and penicillic acid in fruit juices and flour. *J. Agric. Food Chem.* 16 (3): 483–485.

Sharma, S., Gupta, D., and Sharma, Y.P. (2015). Natural incidence of aflatoxins, ochratoxin a, patulin and their co-occurrence in chilgoza pine nuts marketed in Jammu, India. *Proc. Natl. Acad. Sci. India Sect. B Biol. Sci.* 85 (1): 45–50. https://doi.org/10.1007/s40011-014-0326-7.

Silici, S. and Karaman, K. (2013). Inhibitory effect of propolis on patulin production of *Penicillium expansum* in apple juice. *J. Food Process. Preserv.* 38: 1129–1134. https://doi.org/10.1111/jfpp.12072.

Sommer, N.F., Buchanan, J.R., and Fortlage, R.J. (1974). Production of patulin by *Penicillium expansum*. *J. Appl. Microbiol.* 28 (4): 589–593.

Sreenivasa, M.Y., Dass, R.S., Charith Raj, A.P., and Janardhana, G.R. (2008). PCR-based detection of genus *Fusarium* and Fumonisin-producing isolates from freshly harvested sorghum grains grown in Karnataka, India. *Food Saf.* 28: 236–237.

Sreenivasa, M.Y., Dass, R.S., Charith Raj, A.P., and Janardhana, G.R. (2011a). Mycological evaluation of maize grains produced in Karnataka (India) for the post harvest fungal contamination. *World Appl. Sci. J.* 13 (4): 688–692.

Sreenivasa, M.Y., Dass, R.S., Charith Raj, A.P. et al. (2011b). Assessment of the growth inhibiting effect of some plant essential oils on different *Fusarium* species isolated from sorghum and maize grains. *J. Plant Dis. Protect.* 118 (6): 208–213.

Steiman, R., Sage, L., Krivobok, S. et al. (1989). Production of patulin by micromycetes. *Mycopathologia* 105: 129–133.

Stinson, E.E., Osman, S.F., Huhtanen, C.N., and Bills, D.D. (1978). Disappearance of patulin during alcoholic fermentation of apple juice. *Appl. Env. Microbiol.* 36: 620–622.

Suzuki, T., Takeda, M., and Tanabe, H. (1971). A new mycotoxin produced by *Aspergillus clavatus*. *Chem. Pharm. Bull.* 19 (9): 1786–1788.

Tang, H., Li, X., Zhang, F. et al. (2019). Biodegradation of the mycotoxin patulin in apple juice by Orotate phosphoribosyltransferase from *Rhodotorula mucilaginosa*. *Food Control* 100: 158–164. https://doi.org/10.1016/j.foodcont.2019.01.020.

Tang, X., Zhang, Q., Pividori, M.I. et al. (2022). A sensitive aptasensor using biotin-streptavidin system for patulin detection in apple juice. *Biosensor* 12: 59. https://doi.org/10.3390/bios12020059.

Tangni, E.K., Theys, R., Mignolet, E. et al. (2010). Patulin in domestic and imported apple-based drinks in Belgium: occurrence and exposure assessment. *Food Addit. Contam.* 20: 482–489. https://doi.org/10.1080/0265203031000093204.

Tannous, J., Snini, S.P., El Khoury, R. et al. (2017). Patulin transformation products and last intermediates in its biosynthetic pathway, E - and Z - ascladiol, are not toxic to human cells. *Arch. Toxicol.* 91: 2455–2467. https://doi.org/10.1007/s00204-016-1900-y.

Tolaini, V., Zjalic, S., Reverberi, M. et al. (2010). *Lentinula edodes* enhances the biocontrol activity of *Cryptococcus laurentii* against *Penicillium expansum* contamination and patulin production in apple fruits. *Int. J. Food Microbiol.* 138: 243–249. https://doi.org/10.1016/j.ijfoodmicro.2010.01.044.

Tyllinen, H., Raevuori, M., Karppanen, E., and Garry-Andersson, A.S. (1977). A study on the toxicity of spontaneously molded bread. *Nordisk Vet.* 29 (12): 546–551.

Varga, J., Due, M., Frisvad, J.C., and Samson, R.A. (2007). Taxonomic revision of *Aspergillus* section Clavati based on molecular, morphological and physiological data. *Stud. Mycol.* 59: 89–106. https://doi.org/10.3114/sim.2007.59.11.

Walker, J.L. (1969). The diffusion of innovations among the American states. *Am. Polit. Sci. Rev.* 63: 880–899.

Wallen, L., Lyons, J., and Pridham, G. (1839). Antimicrobial activity of patulin derivatives: a preliminary report. *J. Antibiot.* 33: 767–769.

Wang, L., Yue, T., Yuan, Y. et al. (2015). A new insight into the adsorption mechanism of patulin by the heat-inactive lactic acid bacteria cells. *Food Control* 50: 104–110. https://doi.org/10.1016/j.foodcont.2014.08.041.

Wei, C., Yu, L., Qiao, N. et al. (2020). The characteristics of patulin detoxification by *Lactobacillus plantarum* 13M5. *Food Chem. Toxicol.* 146: 111787. https://doi.org/10.1016/j.fct.2020.111787.

Wheeler, J.L., Harrison, M.A., and Koehler, P.E. (1987). Presence and stability of patulin in pasteurized apple cider. *J. Food Sci.* 52 (2): 479–480.

Wu, S., Duan, N., Zhang, W. et al. (2016). Screening and development of DNA aptamers as capture probes for colorimetric detection of patulin. *Anal. Biochem.* 508: 58–64. https://doi.org/10.1016/j.ab.2016.05.024.

Xing, M., Chen, Y., Li, B., and Tian, S. (2021). Characterization of a short-chain dehydrogenase/reductase and its function in patulin biodegradation in apple juice. *Food Chem.* 348: 129046. https://doi.org/10.1016/j.foodchem.2021.129046.

Yazici, S. and Velioglu, Y.S. (2002). Effect of thiamine hydrochloride, pyridoxine hydrochloride and calcium-d-pantothenate on the patulin content of apple juice concentrate. *Food* 46 (4): 256–257.

Yooussef, M.M., Pham, Q., Achar, P.N., and Sreenivasa, M.Y. (2016). Antifungal activity of essential oils on *Aspergillus parasiticus* isolated from peanuts. *J. Plant Protect. Res.* 56 (2): https://doi.org/10.1515/jppr-2016-0021.

Yuan, Y., Zhuang, H., Zhang, T., and Liu, J. (2010). Patulin content in apple products marketed in Northeast China. *Food Control* 21: 1488–1491. https://doi.org/10.1016/j.foodcont.2010.04.019.

Zbyňovská, K., Petruška, P., Kalafová, A., and Capcarová, M. (2016). Patulin – a contaminant of food and feed: a review. *Acta Fytotechn Zootechn.* 64–67.

Zhang, H., Zheng, X., and Yu, T. (2007). Biological control of postharvest diseases of peach with *Cryptococcus laurentii*. *Food Control* 18: 287–291. https://doi.org/10.1016/j.foodcont.2005.10.007.

Zhang, X., Guo, Y., Ma, Y. et al. (2016). Biodegradation of patulin by a *Byssochlamys nivea* strain. *Food Control* 64: 142–150. https://doi.org/10.1016/j.foodcont.2015.12.016.

Zheng, X., Li, Y., Zhang, H. et al. (2018). Identification and toxicological analysis of products of patulin degradation by *Pichia caribbica*. *Biol. Control* 123: 127–136. https://doi.org/10.1016/j.biocontrol.2018.04.019.

Zheng, X., Wei, W., Rao, S. et al. (2020). Degradation of patulin in fruit juice by a lactic acid bacteria strain *Lactobacillus casei* YZU01. *Food Control* 112: 107147. https://doi.org/10.1016/j.foodcont.2020.107147.

Zhong, L., Carere, J., Lu, Z. et al. (2018). Patulin in apples and apple-based food products: the burdens and the mitigation strategies. *Toxins 10*: 475. https://doi.org/10.3390/toxins10110475.

Zhong, L., Carere, J., Mats, L. et al. (2020). Formation of glutathione patulin conjugates associated with yeast fermentation contributes to patulin reduction. *Food Control* https://doi.org/10.1016/j.foodcont.2020.107334.

Zhou, T., Wang, X., Ye, B. et al. (2018). Postharvest biology and technology effects of essential oil decanal on growth and transcriptome of the postharvest fungal pathogen *Penicillium expansum*. *Postharvest Biol. Technol.* 145: 203–212. https://doi.org/10.1016/j.postharvbio.2018.07.015.

Zhu, R., Feussner, K., Wu, T. et al. (2015). Detoxification of mycotoxin patulin by the yeast *Rhodosporidium paludigenum*. *Food Chem.* 179: 1–5. https://doi.org/10.1016/j.foodchem.2015.01.066.

5

Trichothecenes: Toxigenic Effects and Detoxification Strategies

Monica C. Paul and Regina S. Dass

Fungal Genetics and Mycotoxicology Laboratory, Department of Microbiology, School of Life Sciences, Pondicherry University, Pondicherry, India

CONTENTS

Abstract

Trichothecene is a toxic secondary metabolite produced by the fungi belonging to the order of Hypocreales – *Fusarium*, *Myrothecium*, *Stachybotrys*, and *Trichoderma* species. It is made and secreted during the interaction with the host plants. The food products, namely wheat, corn, meat, and milk of livestock, are majorly contaminated by this mycotoxin. Trichothecene is a

Anti-Mycotoxin Strategies for Food and Feed, First Edition. Edited by Deepa Nagaraju, Sreenivasa Marikunte Yanjarappa, Premila N. Achar, and Angel Medina Vaya.

tetracyclic sesquiterpenoid compound with a core structure with a three-ring molecule known as 12,13-epoxytrichothec-9-ene (EPT). It is classified into four groups, i.e. types A, B, C, and D, depending on the substitution pattern of EPT. The major mycotoxins in the trichothecene group are deoxynivalenol (DON), nivalenol (NIV), and T-2 mycotoxin. Highly sensitive quantification methods, for example, gas or liquid chromatography-tandem mass spectrometry (GC-MS, LC-MS), high-resolution MS (HRMS), radioimmunoassay, enzymatic immunoassay, fluorescent immunoassay, etc., are used for the detection of the toxin in samples. The toxin is easily absorbed into the gastrointestinal membrane and distributed to other body organs such as the skin, kidney, liver, and immune and hematopoietic progenitor cellular systems, causing emesis, anorexia, neuroendocrine changes, immunotoxicity, to name a few. Various detoxification strategies involving physical, chemical, and biological methods can be implemented to decontaminate this toxin from food and feed. Microbial biotransformation is also an effective method that replaces physical and chemical processes. The following chapter discusses the structure and biosynthetic pathway and the physical, chemical, and biological methods of detoxification strategies.

Keywords *Trichothecenes, detoxification strategies, DON, T-2 toxin,* Fusarium

Graphical Representation

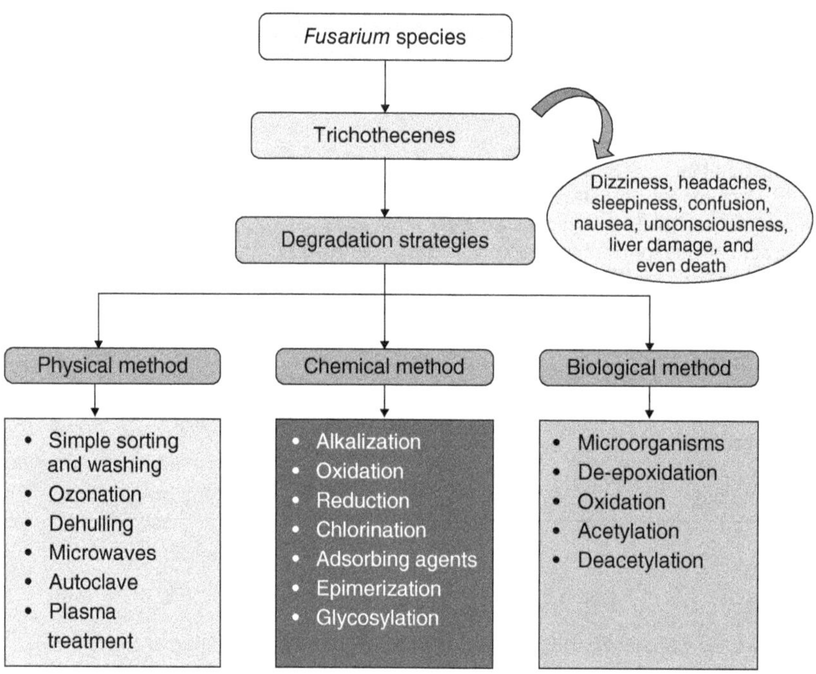

5.1 Introduction

Trichothecenes are sesquiterpenoid mycotoxins that share the 12,13-epoxytrichothecene skeleton as a common structural feature. The term trichothecene is derived from trichothecene, the first member of the family to be identified. Trichothecenes are classified into four subgroups, A, B, C, and D, based on different numbers and positions of hydroxyl moieties present at the primary trichothecene nucleus; types A and B are significant in food commodities. These are commonly found in cereal products (Figure 5.1). Type A-trichothecenes are T-2 toxin, T-2 triol, T-2 tetraol, HT-2 toxin, and neosolaniol (NEO), diacetoxyscirpenol (DAS), harzianum A, and trichodermin. Type B constitutes DON, trichothecin, 3-acetyl-DON (3-ADON), 15-acetyl DON (15-ADON), NIV, and fusarenon X (FUS-X). Type C comprises crotocin, and Type D comprises satratoxin G&H, roridin A, and verrucarin A (Deepa et al. 2016; Deepa and Sreenivasa 2017; Mahato et al. 2022). Type A and Type B are economically essential and have been studied extensively. The various fungal genera that produce this toxin are *Cryptomela*, *Fusarium*, *Myrothecium*, *Stachybotrys*, *Trichoderma/Hypocrea*, *Trichothecium*, and *Verticimonosporium* (Niessen 2007; Polak-Śliwińska and Paszczyk 2021) Aspergillus, Penicillium (Liu et al. 2022). However, *Fusarium* spp. like *Fusarium graminearum*, *Fusarium asiaticum*, *Fusarium culmorum*, *Fusarium cerealis*, *Fusarium pseudograminearum*, *Fusarium sporotrichioides*, *Fusarium sibiricum*, *Fusarium langsethiae*, *Fusarium acuminatum*, and *Fusarium poae* (Gottschalk et al. 2007; Li et al. 2011) produce the widest variety of trichothecene compounds. Despite this, *Fusarium* species causing Fusarium Head Blight (FHB) is the primary trichothecene producer (Foroud et al. 2019).

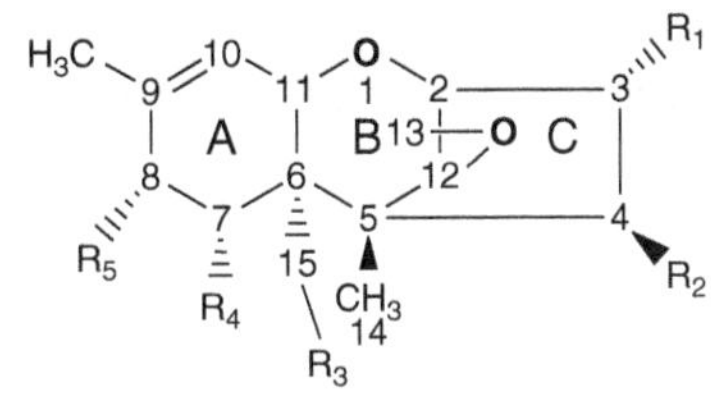

Figure 5.1 Chemical structure of trichothecenes.

The detailed studies of the structural analysis of trichothecenes help understand their toxicity as the toxin's structure is responsible for the toxicity. The methods used to study trichothecene structure are crystallography, nuclear magnetic resonance (NMR), solid-state NMR, and NMR crystallography (Shank et al. 2011). Trichothecenes are a large group of sesquiterpenoid fungal metabolites that contain a common core known as 12,13-epoxytrichothec-9-ene (EPT) (Gutiérrez et al. 2021) consisting of a rigid tetracyclic ring system comprising cyclohexene, A-ring with a double C—C bond between C-9 and C-10, a tetrahydropyranyl B-ring, a cyclopentyl C-ring and an epoxide at C-12/13 (Shank et al. 2011). All the isolated compounds of trichothecenes fall into two main classes, i.e. simple and macrocyclic. The simple trichothecenes are further divided into three types – A, B, and C. Type A is the simplest group because it is neither non-substituted, hydroxylated, nor esterified. Type B has a ketone present at C-8. Type C has a second epoxide ring at C-7/8. A fourth-class type D has a cyclic diester or triester linkage of C-4–C-15. The macrocyclic class has a macrolide ring (Shank et al. 2011; Gutiérrez et al. 2021).

The double bond between C-9–C-10 and the 12,13-epoxy ring system is responsible for the toxicity of trichothecenes. Therefore, its absence makes it non-toxic, and substituting other groups increases or decreases the toxicity. For example, a hydroxyl group at C-3 enhances toxicity, but the activity reduces when substituted with hydrogen or an acetoxy group. Similarly, the hydroxyl group at C-4 decreases toxicity compared to the acetoxy group at the same position. For type B trichothecenes, there is reduced harmful activity when acetoxy is substituted with hydroxyl or hydrogen at the C4 position. Also, it exhibits similar activity when substituting groups with hydroxyl and hydrogen than the acetoxy group at the C-15 position. However, toxicity increases when a macrocyclic ring is between

C-4 and C-15 positions. At C-8, a change from isovaleroyloxy to hydrogen or hydroxyl group decreases toxicity. The presence of a second epoxy at C-7–C-8 also decreases toxicity, whereas epoxidation at C-9–C-10 of some macrocyclic trichothecenes increases harmful activity. In animals, conjugated trichothecenes release toxic precursors after hydrolysis, posing an additional threat.

5.2 Structure and Biosynthesis of Trichothecenes

Studying the genetics and biochemistry of trichothecene biosynthesis in *Fusarium* is vital due to its impact on agriculture and the health hazards posed to humans and animals. The initial steps in trichothecene biosynthesis are similar in *Fusarium*, *Myrothecium*, and *Trichoderma* species. A temperature ranging from −2 to 35 °C with a preferred water activity (a_W) above 0.88 makes it favorable for growing, and the biosynthesis of T-2 toxin occurs between 20 and 30 °C with a water activity (a_W) between 0.980 and 0.995 (Wu et al. 2013; Proctor et al. 2018). Trichothecene biosynthesis and regulatory genes (*TRI* genes) are found in clusters in the genome of *Fusarium* species and other trichothecene-producing genera. Though most *TRI* genes are present in the core cluster, four are located at three different loci, i.e. the TRI1-TRI16 two-gene cluster and two independent loci for *TRI101* and *TRI15*. An enzyme sesquiterpene cyclase initiates trichothecene biosynthesis by producing trichodiene with the help of a substrate farnesyl pyrophosphate. The next four steps in the pathways, viz. C-2 hydroxylation, C-12 and C-13 epoxidation, and C-11 and C-3 hydroxylation are catalyzed by an enzyme P450 monooxygenase, which *TRI4* encodes. Isotrichotriol is the product formed at the end of it. It undergoes two non-enzymatic isomerization steps to create the central ring of isotrichodermol consisting of the basic trichothecene skeleton structure with a C-3 hydroxyl group. *TRI1–TRI16* clusters arrange the functional group at C-8 to differentiate Type A from Type B trichothecenes (Figure 5.2). *TRI1* is required for oxygenation at C-8; this happens by catalyzing the addition of a hydroxyl group. In *Fusarium graminearum*, this group is esterified by TRI16 to an isovalerate group, as in T-2 and HT-2 toxin, whereas *TRI16* is non-functional in *F. graminearum* (Foroud et al. 2019).

The allelic variations in *TRI1* differentiate NX (Northland toxin) and DON chemotypes in *F. graminearum*. *Tri13* and *Tri7* genes are essential for oxygenation and acetylation at the C-4 position. It produces NIV in *F. graminearum* and T2 toxin in *F. sporotrichioides*. Also, *Tri13* and *Tri7* genes are non-functional in DON chemotypes toxin; hence C-4 hydroxyl toxin is absent. The chemotypes of DON produce acetylated derivatives like 3-ADON or 15-ADON from C-3 or C-15 de-acetylation of 3,15-ADON from its acetylated state, which was acetylated by *TRI101* and *TRI3* genes. The allelic variation of *FgTRI8* is responsible for the stereospecificity of the esterase; hence it determines if the DON chemotype in the *F. graminearum* strain produces 3-ADON or 15-ADON. However, in *F. sporotrichioides*, the *FsTR18* gene is a C-3 esterase carrying a hydroxyl group essential for the biosynthesis of the T-2 toxin (Foroud et al. 2019).

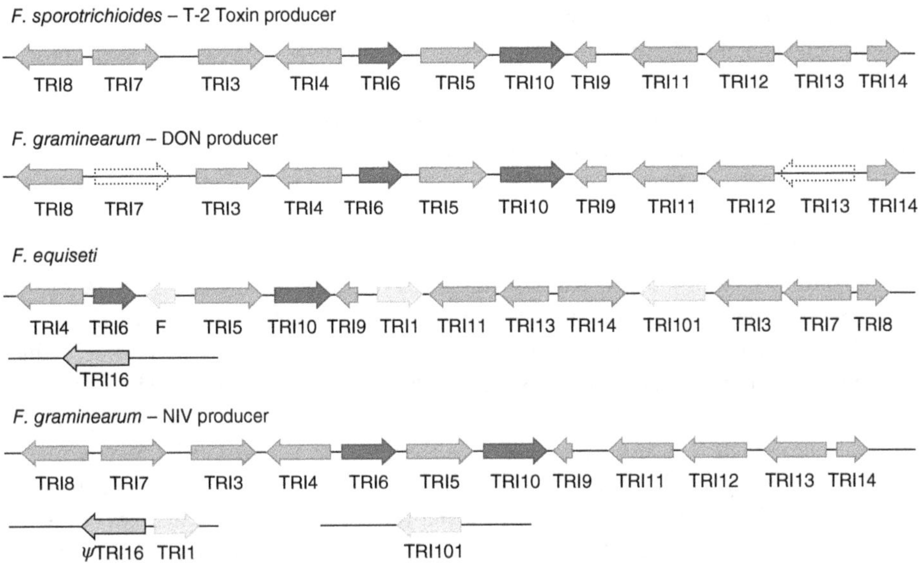

Figure 5.2 Gene cluster of trichothecene producing *Fusarium* species. (*Source:* Villafana et al. (2019)/MDPI/CC BY 4.0).

5.3 Occurrence and Distribution

Climatic conditions, agricultural practices, and cultivar susceptibility influence the distribution of *Fusarium* species and their dominance over other fungi in wheat. Other species like *Alternaria* spp., *Cladosporium* spp., *Epicoccum* spp., and *Rhizopus* spp. infect wheat grain, causing quality loss due to undesirable color and odor (Alkadri et al. 2013). *Stachybotrys atra* produces verrucarin B, verrucarin J, roridin E, and satratoxins F, G, and H, trichoverrins A and B. Among these, trichovarrin A and B are the biosynthetic precursor to the macrocyclic trichothecene in *Myrothecium* sp. The building material of high cellulose and low nitrogen content that are moist and subject to temperature fluctuations makes an ideal environment for *Stachybotrys atra* to grow and produce toxins. This macrocyclic trichothecene is a potent antibiotic agent with phytotoxic, cytotoxic action due to the inhibition of protein synthesis (Croft et al. 1986).

5.4 Toxic Effects of Trichothecenes

Trichothecene toxins pose a risk to animals, plants, poultry, and human beings (Niessen 2007). The toxins affect the eukaryotic cells by inhibiting protein synthesis, causing cytotoxicity and apoptosis (Karlovsky 2011). Poultry is more sensitive than ruminants; 9 mg DON/kg feed is sufficient to cause an adverse effect in chickens. Whereas 1 mg/NIV causes minor pathological changes in chicken, indicating that NIV is more toxic than DON. Swine among farm animals are the most sensitive to trichothecenes, i.e. DON, NIV, and T-2 (Eriksen and Pettersson 2004; Dass et al. 2007; Janardhana et al. 2009; Sreenivasa et al. 2011). Swine are more susceptible to toxins because of their differences in DON metabolism, and males are more sensitive than females (Rotter 1996). T-2 occurs in moldy grains, corn, oats, barley, maize, and animal feed (Li et al. 2022), especially in cold regions and wet storage conditions, causing T-2 toxicosis when ingested by animals. It is broadly reported in swine, cattle, dogs, ducks, chickens, monkeys, etc. (Sun et al. 2014). These toxins are amphipathic molecules that pass across the cell membrane, causing damage to mammals' digestive and immune systems, leading to feed refusal, immunological problems, haemorrhagic lesions, reproductive disorders, and producing harmful levels of free radicals (Karlovsky 2011; Proctor et al. 2020), cytotoxicity, hepatotoxicity, genotoxicity, metabolism modulation, immunotoxicity, gastrointestinal toxicity, etc. (Li et al. 2022) and weight loss, decrease in blood cell and leukocyte count, reduction in plasma glucose, and pathological changes in the liver and stomach (Li et al. 2011). Toxicokinetic studies in broiler chicken revealed that the T-2 triol and HT-2, the primary metabolites of the T-2 toxin, are rapidly absorbed, have high plasma concentrations, and have long elimination half-lives (Sun et al. 2014) and trigger metabolic transformations (Nathanail et al. 2015). DON, 3-DON, 15-ADON, and FUS-X toxins are produced by *F. graminearum* and *Fusarium culmorum*. DON is the most abundant contaminant in animal feed. When ingested by animals, it causes acute and chronic toxic effects, leading to feed refusal, weight loss, and vomiting. 3-ADON and 15-ADON are the acetylation products of DON, and fungi could directly produce this, and these co-occur with DON. It forms a more potent toxin than the parent DON in combination with mammalian digestion. FUS-X is frequently observed with DON, which induces adverse health effects, especially apoptosis in mice (Fan et al. 2016).

In humans, T-2 is associated with increased infection rate, alimentary toxic aleukia (ATA), DNA damage, and induction of apoptosis, causing emesis, diarrhea, lethargy, weight loss, hemorrhage, inhibition of immunity, necrosis, damage of cartilaginous tissues, apoptosis, and death, making it the most acutely toxic member of the trichothecene family. It is also considered the cause of ATA and Kashin-Beck disease (KBD) (Li et al. 2011). It changes the permeability of the cell membrane of myoblasts at concentrations as low as 4 pg/mL (Eriksen and Pettersson 2004). However, the severity of the disease caused by trichothecenes depends on the toxin's type, purity, dose, and duration of exposure. Dermal exposure may lead to burning pain, redness, and blisters. Oral exposure results in vomiting and diarrhea due to damage caused in the digestive and immune systems. Inhalation leads to nasal irritation and cough, and ocular exposure results in blurred vision. Systemic symptoms include weakness, ataxia, hypotension, coagulopathy, and death (CDC 2019). NIV and FUS-X are more hazardous to humans and domestic animals than DON; esophageal and gastric carcinomas have been reported due to consuming food contaminated with this toxin (Gab-Allah et al. 2023). T-2 triol and HT-2 are the primary metabolites of the T-2 toxin found in animals. The metabolic pathway it follows is hydrolysis, hydroxylation, de-epoxidation, and conjugation. Humans are exposed to this toxin by consuming animal products, and toxicokinetic studies help evaluate and control human exposure to T-2 (Sun et al. 2014), triggering metabolic transformations (Nathanail et al. 2015).

In plants, trichothecenes cause chlorosis and growth inhibition. It is the leading cause of wheat head blight and Gibberella ear rot (GER) in maize, a worldwide economic disease

Table 5.1 Evolution of trichothecenes.

Year	Occurrence
430–426 BC	Plague of Athens
1730	New Hampshire disease
1932, 1935	The outbreak in Russian territory
1994	Increased mortality

(Woloshuk and Shim 2013; Proctor et al. 2020), and also prevents protein translation and host responses to infection by exhibiting symptomless conditions (Brown et al. 2015). Toxin accumulated in infested crop debris contaminates agricultural run-off, feeding into aquatic environments (Mahato et al. 2022). T-2 is the trichothecene toxin that typically occurs in farm crops like wheat, oats, barley, maize, and animal feeds, and it can reach up to hundreds μg/kg (Li et al. 2022). HT-2 toxin is the deacetylated form of T-2 toxin. It inhibits plant protein synthesis and cell proliferation (Nathanail et al. 2015). In aquatic systems, fish are affected by aquaculture, and it affects growth, reproduction, and other physiological function and health, which lead to weight gain, body composition, biochemical processes, and the health of the fish in general. The factors like fish species, type of toxin, dose in feeds, and duration of exposure influence the toxic effect on fish. Fish that are majorly affected are rainbow trout (*O. mykiss*) and common carp (*V. carpio* L.), where a feed diet containing 1.8–5.8 mg T-2 toxin/kg induces oxidative stress in the liver impairing its functions, immunotoxicity, and decreased hemoglobin level when consumed for nearly one month (Pietsch and Burkhardt-Holm 2015; Matejova et al. 2016; Modra et al. 2020).

The first exposure to trichothecene occurred in the fifth century B.C. during the plague of Athens in 430–426 B.C., and also in the disease reported in New Hampshire in the 1730s. The condition was termed ATA. However, a severe outbreak of ATA occurred in Russian territory between 1932 and 1945, predominantly in Siberia, due to the consumption of grain and straw left in the snow in winter. People suffer from septic angina, leukopenia (aleukia), hemorrhagic rash, necrotic ulcers on the lining of the digestive tract and skin, and bleeding from the nose, throat, and gums, leading to death. Domestic animals also exhibited similar symptoms. The underlying cause was unknown for many years, but the mortality rate increased. The peak was seen in 1994, with cases reaching 173 000, of which 28 000 died. Following this incident, the scientists conducted a detailed study of the mycobiota in the grain samples and concluded that *F. sporotrichioides* were responsible for the outbreak (Table 5.1). Later, it was also identified that ATA has directly associated with type A trichothecenes. Since then, various strains of this toxin have been isolated (Foroud et al. 2019).

5.5 Detoxification Methods of Trichothecenes

Types A and B are of the most concern to humans because of their broad and high toxicity. The naturally occurring trichothecenes in food are HT-2 toxin, T-2 toxin, DON, 3-acetyl DON, 15-acetyl DON, 4,15-DAS, and NIV due to their high toxicity and prevalence. DON is the most commonly occurring trichothecene in nature. Still, the T-2 toxin, though not as prevalent as DON, has a higher toxicity than DON (Li et al. 2020); hence the detoxification strategies focus more on these toxins. It is important to practice prevention strategies to reduce trichothecene contamination. These are usually carried out at the initial level of food production, i.e. plant growth, harvest, storage, and distribution. The prevention strategy should be employed before fungal infestation or during mold invasion. The Codex Alimentarius has developed several codes of practice for preventing and reducing mycotoxins in cereals and raw materials. These are good manufacturing practices (GMP) and hazard analysis and critical control points (HACCP) (Vila-Donat et al. 2018; Deepa et al. 2021). These systems are used in manufacturing, packaging, and labeling, which includes cleanliness and sanitation, equipment function and use, recordkeeping, personnel, operations and processes, product testing, and addressing errors and complaints (Chin and Lee 2008). A system where food safety is addressed through analysis and control of biological, chemical, and physical hazards from raw material production, procurement, and handling to manufacturing, distribution, and consumption of the finished product (FDA). The decontamination procedures like physical, chemical, and biological methods are employed when prevention methods fail.

5.6 Physical Methods for Detoxification of Trichothecene Toxins

Toxins also remain on the outer surface of the grains. Physical detoxification removes the toxin without the involvement of chemical or biological detoxification processes (Deepa and Sreenivasa 2019a, b). It is done to preserve the quality of cereal foods for long-term use and is carried out as a post-harvest detoxification method (Table 5.2).

The various methods involved in physical detoxification are:

5.6.1 Simple Sorting and Washing

Simple sorting and washing cereal grains are regular practices in the food industry before food processing begins. Sorting separates the poor-quality grains from the healthy and high-quality ones based on their differences in shape, color, density, and size. The types of sorting machines used are flotation and color sorting. Flotation is a segregation method based on the thickness of kernel difference of cereal grains, which reduces DON toxin in corn and wheat by removing the floating kernels. Water-soluble toxins on the surface of the grains can be removed by washing, thus reducing half of the initial concentration (Shanakhat et al. 2018). Washing barley and maize thrice with distilled water reduces DON level by 65–69%. It is an essential method before wet milling or ethanol fermentation (Kabak et al. 2006).

5.6.2 Ozonation

It reduces 78% of DON at 180 minutes with an increased moisture content of 25% in wheat flour. This is done before using the wheat flour as dough to minimize microbial contamination due to its moisture content. Ozonation also decreases DON concentration in wheat grains. However, it becomes more effective only when applied directly to ground or crushed products due to the larger surface area. Moreover, it significantly reduced wet milling

Table 5.2 Strategies against trichothecene in food and feed.

S. No.	Trichothecenes		Methodology	Percent of reduction (%)	References
1.	Physical	Post-harvest strategies	GAPs, GMPs, HACCP	80	Agriopoulou (2020)
		Simple sorting and washing	Cleaning, removal of poor-quality grains, washing with distilled water	65	Shanakhat et al. (2018) and Kabak et al. (2006)
		Dehulling	Removal of the outer layer of the grain	78	Shanakhat et al. (2018)
		Storage	In controlled conditions	60	Agriopoulou (2020)
		Heating	Mild alkaline condition	60	Kumar et al. (2022)
		Irradiation	Gamma rays, UV light, and microwave rays	40	Karlovsky et al. (2016) and Shanakhat et al. (2018)
2.	Chemical	Inhibitors	Sodium azide, 2-deoxy glucose, 2-4 dinitrophenol and ouabain	40	Adhikari et al. (2017)
		Alkalization	Ammonia, sodium hydroxide	˃80	He et al. (2010) and Feizollahi and Roopesh (2021)
		Oxidation	Sodium hypochlorite, sulfur agents	˂70	He et al. (2010)
		Reduction	Sodium bisulfite, sodium metasulfite	˂60	He et al. (2010)
		Chlorination	Chlorine dioxide	˃50	Feizollahi and Roopesh (2021) and Wilson et al. (2005)
		Adsorbing agents	Montmorillonite	66	Li et al. (2022)
			Bentonite feed	50	
		Ozone treatment	*Ozone gas*	29–57	Agriopoulou et al. (2020)

(*Continued*)

Table 5.2 (Continued)

S. No.	Trichothecenes		Methodology	Percent of reduction (%)	References
3.	Biological	Microorganisms	*Geotrichum candidum, Fusarium langsethiae*	93	Wu et al. (2013)
			Saccharomyces pastorianus	31–34	Liu et al. (2022)
			Lactobacillus fermentum	84	Agriopoulou et al. (2020)
			Eubacterium BBSH 797, *Butyrivibrio fibrisolvens, Pelagiabacterium halotolerans, Aspergillus oryzae, Rhizopus oryzae,* Lactic acid bacteria	90	Vanhoutte et al. (2016) and Eriksen and Pettersson (2004)
		Transgenic plant	*Arabidopsis*	89–98	Hao et al. (2021)
4.	Advanced strategy	Cold plasma	Treatment for 5 s	100	Wu et al. (2013) and Hojnik et al. (2017)
		Nanoparticles	Activated carbon, bentonite, aluminum oxide; selenium chondroitin sulfate nanoparticles	87 80	Agriopoulou (2020) and Adhikari et al. (2017)

effluent, proving that moist ozone is more effective than dry. Ozone attacks the C9–C10 double bond in the DON molecule (Alexandre et al. 2017; Afsah-Hejri et al. 2020). Limitations on using ozone, it is used on an industrial scale and has low penetration, short life, corrosiveness, temperature dependency, and safety issues. It also must be applied at a constant temperature within a limited range of temperature and humidity. It can be a costly business as changes like packaging houses necessitate a change in design and equipment, process modification, and new training (Afsah-Hejri et al. 2020).

5.6.3 Dehulling

It is the process of removing the outer layer of the grain before grinding. This method helps reduce the fungal load from the bulk, eliminate fungal colonies from the surface of grains, and reduce contamination (Shanakhat et al. 2018).

5.6.4 Other Techniques

These involve microwaving to lower the toxicity of DON at 175 °C, which reduces 40% of the toxin converting it into a less toxic form. The cold plasma, by using the atmospheric pressure argon cold plasma technique, decreased the toxin from 100 µg/mL to a few µg/mL. Plasma treatments of only five seconds can degrade NIV 100% (Hojnik et al. 2017). Methods like irradiation using gamma (ionizing), UV, and microwave (non-ionizing) are still at the research level (Karlovsky et al. 2016; Shanakhat et al. 2018). Autoclave treatment of DON-contaminated maize and wheat with sodium bisulfite reduces DON concentration (Young 1986; Awad et al. 2010). Heating NIV in the presence of mild alkaline conditions degrades NIV into a less toxic compound (Kumar et al. 2022)

The physical detoxification method cannot entirely remove trichothecene from the food and feed. Therefore, more effective chemical and biological methods must be adopted to destroy the trichothecene toxin. In the United States, the advisory level set by FDA is 1 mg/kg of DON intended for human consumption (Wan et al. 2020). These guidelines are selected based on the toxicological data for mycotoxins by considering the possible reduction that occurs during the physical detoxification method, like cleaning, milling, processing, and cooking operations before human consumption (Patey and Gilbert 1989).

5.7 Chemical Method for Trichothecene Detoxification

The chemical method of detoxification involves adopting chemical treatments, which include the use of sodium bisulfite (Na_2SO_3), ammonium carbonate [$(NH_4)_2CO_3$], sodium metabisulfite ($Na_2S_2O_5$), sodium carbonate (Na_2CO_3), alkaline, chlorine, L-ascorbic acid, and L-cysteine (Feizollahi and Roopesh 2021) to detoxify the grains, mainly animal feed (Table 5.2). The various methods used are as follows:

5.7.1 Alkalization

This procedure transforms the DON and NIV into formaldehyde and lactone by opening the 12,13-epoxy group or losing C-15. Alkaline agents like ammonia and sodium hydroxide covert DON and NIV into norDON and norNIV, which are less toxic than the original toxin.

Ammonium carbonate [$(NH_4)_2CO_3$] is used as a leavening agent and a pH controller agent in baking, and the ammonia released during baking degrades DON present in the flour (He et al. 2010; Feizollahi and Roopesh 2021).

5.7.2 Oxidation

Chemical oxidation of trichothecene toxins includes treatment with 0.25% NaOCl-0.025 mol/L NaOH for four hours. This inhibits the biological activity of the T-2 toxin. Biological oxidation is more specific than chemical oxidation. It occurs through hydroxylation in animal bodies where a hydroxyl group is added at the C-3 position of the C-8 substituent in type A trichothecenes (Adhikari et al. 2017) (Figure 5.3). Oxidizing agents like sodium hypochlorite (NaOCl) change the molecular structure, thereby altering their biological activity. Sulfur agents like Na_2SO_3 and $Na_2S_2O_5$ degrade DON better and, in turn, are more effective in degradation when these chemicals are heated at 80 °C. At pH 4–6, DON, 3-ADON, 15-ADON, DAS, MAS, FUS-X, and NEO completely degraded in an ozone-saturated water system (He et al. 2010).

5.7.3 Reduction

This leads to the structural change that influences biological activities; Na_2SO_3 and $Na_2S_2O_5$ transform DON into DON-sulfonate, which is less toxic than DON. This method leads to the de-epoxidation of trichothecene structure by a specific reduction of the C-12,13 epoxy group (He et al. 2010).

5.7.4 Irradiation

When exposed to ionizing radiation, grains destroy microorganisms and other pathogens without making the food radioactive or losing nutrients (da Silva Aquino 2012). Exposure to gamma (γ) and electron-beam radiation changes the molecular structure of DON, A-DON, and T-2. It reduces the concentration of trichothecenes in grains and has been a better approach for large-scale industries (He et al. 2010).

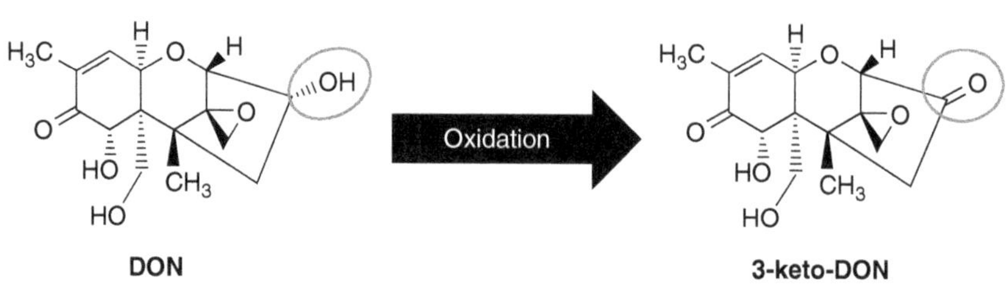

Figure 5.3 Chemical method for detoxification of trichothecene (*Source:* Carere et al. (2017)/John Wiley & Sons).

5.7.5 Chlorination

This method is mainly used for disinfecting the surfaces in food processing facilities, and eliminating the microflora of decayed fruits, vegetables, and poultry (Feizollahi and Roopesh 2021). Chlorine dioxide (ClO_2) in various concentrations is effective against detoxifying verrucarin A and roridin A (trichothecene mycotoxins) (Wilson et al. 2005).

5.7.6 Epimerization

Epimerization of the OH at the C3 OH position of DON changes the R configuration to the S configuration, resulting in a diastereomer interacting strongly with ribosomes. Strains like *Nocardioides*, *Sphingomonas*, and *Devosia* play a role in this method (Xu et al. 2021). About 90% of DON was reduced from wheat when *Nocardioides* sp. was used. The metabolite found was 3-epi-DON (Ikunaga et al. 2010).

5.7.7 Hydroxylation

It occurs in the methyl group at the position of C16 of DON, which was demonstrated in *Sphingomonas* strain KSM1. A fungus named *Blastobotrys capitulate* selectively hydrolyzes at C-8 resulting in the removal of the isovaleryl group to form NEO (Li et al. 2020). Fusarenon-X can be hydrolyzed into NIV via deacetylation in mice and goat, excreted mainly through urine. The liver and kidney convert FX to NIV (Li et al. 2020).

5.7.8 Glycosylation

Glycosylation of OH at the C3 OH position is a phase II detoxification mechanism usually employed in plants, and recent studies showed fungi such as *Trichoderma* sp. and *Clonostachys rosea* adopt a similar method to detoxify DON and its acetylated derivative, 15-acetyl-deoxynivalenol (15-ADON) (Abraham et al. 2022).

5.7.9 Adsorbing Agents

These are also called binding agents, adsorbents, binders, etc. Aluminosilicate-based clays and bacterial/fungal cell walls are the most studied adsorbing agent. Aluminosilicate like zeolites, montmorillonites, and hydrated sodium calcium aluminosilicate (HSCAS) is evaluated for poultry. Zeolites did not prove effective against the toxin's adverse effect. Montmorillonite, however, remains undecided on poultry diet but decontaminates maize *in vitro* up to 66%. The modified HSCAS adsorbent with cetylpyridinium chloride and intercalation of β-glucan prevented T-2-induced damage (Li et al. 2022). Bentonite feed (5–10%) inhibits the toxic effects of T-2 by decreasing intestinal absorption and increasing fecal excretion of the toxin due to its ability to bind to T-2 toxin in farm animals (Adhikari et al. 2017). Sodium montmorillonite clay made by modifying sodium on the surface of the montmorillonite clay is more efficient than montmorillonite in decontaminating T-2 toxin in maize because the clay becomes electrically neutral with the capability to trap T-2 toxin (Olopade et al. 2019).

5.8 Biological Methods for Detoxification of Trichothecenes

Microorganisms like bacteria and fungi isolated from the soil and the digestive tract of ruminants or mycotoxin-contaminated products can degrade many organic compounds and xenobiotics due to their metabolic adaptability and rapid evolution. Hence, these microorganisms and their associated enzymes can transform trichothecenes by modifying their functional group without causing any harm to the environment (Abraham et al. 2022) (Table 5.2).

Biological detoxification methods use bacteria and their secondary metabolites, fungi or yeast, to convert toxins into low-toxic or non-toxic forms by disrupting their basic chemical structure. It is more efficient than chemical and physical detoxification methods, primarily because the enzymes produced by suitable bacteria, fungi, or yeast are used to degrade the toxin and further prevent biosafety issues or animal feed refusal while using live organisms. This method also retains the nutritional value of the food and feed, which is otherwise lost in chemical and physical detoxification methods. It does not produce secondary pollution or nutrient damage, needs mild degradation conditions, and can be done rapidly with low toxicity, high efficiency, and strong specificity. Various biological methods like application of PGPR, essential oils, probiotics, and genetic engineering techniques are in recent trend today for minimizing the trichothecene and growth of *Fusarium* species producing it (Nagendra Prasad et al. 2010; Nagaraja et al. 2016; Achar et al. 2020). Partial fermentation involved in this method improves flavor and nutritional value. The microorganisms are screened to identify the ones that release extracellular enzymes under mild conditions to degrade the toxin. These microbes include *Bacillus* spp., *Devosella*, *Nocardia*, anaerobic bacteria, and fungi that aim to change the epoxy groups at positions C12 and C13 to remove them or open the rings to achieve detoxification (Xu et al. 2021). This occurs through the following mechanisms:

5.8.1 De-epoxidation

It is carried out in the presence of anaerobic bacteria in the digestive tract of ruminants and poultry or from the soil environment. For example, *Eubacterium* BBSH 797, isolated from the ruminal fluid, de-epoxidizes the C12,13 epoxide ring of types A and B trichothecenes (Xu et al. 2021). Also, this bacterial strain BBSH 797 transforms DON into its metabolite DOM-1, a non-toxic de-epoxide of DON (Fuchs et al. 2002). Other strains like *Bacillus* sp. LS100 (isolated from the soil), Eggerthella sp. DII-9, Desulfitobacterium sp. strain PGC-3-9, and *Slackia* sp. D-G6 is also used (Xu et al. 2021). Degradation of T-2 toxin to HT-2 toxin and subsequently to T-2 triol is carried out by *Curtobacterium* sp. Strain 114-2. The reduced form was 23 and 13 times less toxic than the parent toxin. Rat intestinal microflora de-epoxidizes T-2 tetraol and scirpentriol, transforms T-2 toxin into de-epoxy HT-2 toxin, and de-epoxy T-2 triol and DAS into de-epoxymonoacetoxyscirpenol and de-epoxyscirpentriol when mixed cultures were carried for degradation. NIV also can be converted to de-epoxynivalenol with the help of the bacteria *Eubacterium* sp. BBSH 797 (Li et al. 2020) degrades trichothecenes as pure culture isolated from bovine rumen fluid. It has been developed into a commercial product (Biomin® BBSH 797) for detoxifying animal feed. It transforms DON into DOM-1 and de-epoxidizes NIV, T-2 tetraol, scripentriol, and HT-2 toxin (Vanhoutte et al. 2016) (Figure 5.3).

5.8.2 Oxidation

It is carried out by mixed cultures such as *Agrobacterium-Rhizobium* (mixed culture termed D107) and *Pelagibacterium halotolerans* ANSP101. These strains oxidize DON to 3-Keto-DON (Figure 5.3).

5.8.3 Acetylation and De-acetylation

FUS-X and NIV only differ by an acetyl group at the C-4 position. FUS-X gets rapidly acetylated to NIV. The toxic effect of NIV occurred at the same level as that of DON in pigs, but it proved to be more harmful in poultry (Eriksen and Pettersson 2004). T-2 is de-acylated into HT-2 toxin (Vanhoutte et al. 2016). 15-Monoacetoxyscirpenol (15-MAS) and 4,15-Diacetoxyscirpenol (4,15-DAS) can be transformed into 15-MAS 3-glucoside and 14,15-DAS 3-glucoside, which is also called as masked toxins. 4,15-DAS can be hydrolyzed to either 4-MAS or 15 MAS to yield a final product called scirpentriol (SCP) via deacetylation in rats (Li et al. 2020). Acetylation using *F. graminearum* converts DON to 3-acetyl-DON (3-ADON) (Figure 5.4).

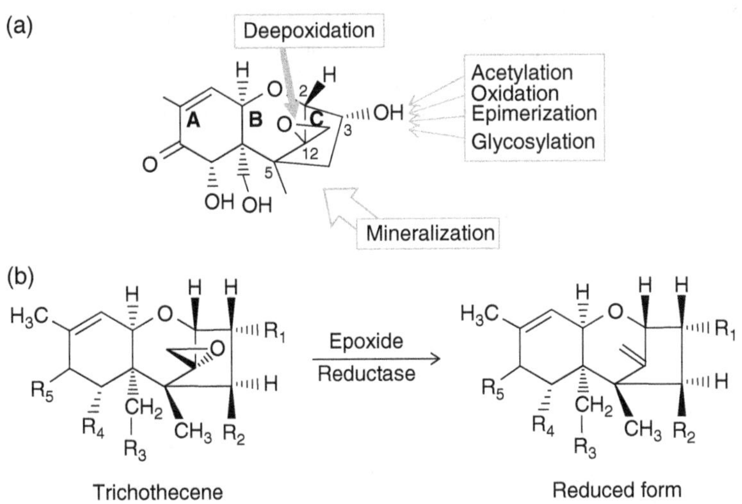

Figure 5.4 Biological methods for detoxification of trichothecenes. (*Source:* Adhikari et al. 2017).

5.9 Advanced Methods for Detoxification of Trichothecenes

They are also used to reduce the biological effect of toxins from the animals' blood, intestines, and other target organs. Microorganisms like fungi and lactic acid bacteria (LAB), yeasts like *Saccharomyces cerevisiae*, *Kluyveromyces marxianus*, and *Geotichum fermentum* show significant adsorption effects on DON; filamentous fungi *Aspergillus oryzae* and *Rhizopus oryzae* absorb DON into the mycelium and degrade it through submerged fermentation with maximum degradation rate after 48 hours. Adsorption occurs through glucomannan on the microbe's cell wall; this material is extracted and used in food and feed industries (Xu et al. 2021). LAB showed the ability to remove DON in a liquid medium, making it more beneficial due to its health benefits and use as a biocontrol agent, and reduced harm associated with mycotoxin ingestion (Franco et al. 2011). Microbial degradation using bacteria is more favorable than fungi because bacteria have a high degradation rate and broad reaction conditions (Abbas 2019). Microorganisms like *Lactobacillus* spp., *Lactococcus lactis*, *Streptococcus thermophilus*, *Pediococcus pentosaceus*, *Propionibacterium freudenreichii*, *S. cerevisiae*, *S. pastorianus*, and *Sporidiobolus pararoseus* can bind to the cell wall components like peptidoglycans, teichoic acid, polysaccharides, and esterified glucomannan are used to protect the poultry from the adverse effect caused by T-2 toxin (Table 5.2).

The indirect detoxifying agents such as Rekicen-RD® (a fructooligosaccharide product) and indoles reduce the toxic effect of T-2 by activating the enzymes like UDP-glucuronosyl transferase for detoxification. A single detoxifying agent might not detoxify T-2 toxin effectively; therefore, the application of multi-component detoxifying agents like a combination of HSCAS and EGM, modified zeolite (clinoptilolite), *Bacillus subtilis*, *B. licheniformis*, *S. cerevisiae* cell wall, and silymarin when added to the diet reduces the toxic effect (Li et al. 2022).

The enzymatic detoxification method combines the features of chemical and biological treatments. It synergizes them, resulting in high efficiency and specificity of action without losing the treated material's aesthetic appearance or food quality. These enzymes are glycosyltransferase, lipase, aldo-keto reductase AKR18A1, and oxidoreductase DepA derived from plants and microorganisms to decontaminate trichothecene toxins (Lyagin and Efremenko 2019). The recent advancement is that *Stachybotrys*, *Podostroma*, and *Myrothecium*, which produce a macrocyclic ring, exhibit other biological activities like antifungal, antimalarial, anticancer, and antitumor properties (Zhu et al. 2020).

5.10 Summary

Trichothecene contamination occurs in food and animal feed through fungi in crops, cereals, nuts, and oilseeds. It enters the animal when the farm animals feed trichothecene-contaminated feed, and from there, it reaches human beings through animal products like milk and eggs. When trichothecenes are ingested, they cause serious human diseases, developmental disorders in animals and poultry, and economic burdens in agriculture due to reduced crop yield and value. Therefore, finding methods to prevent the toxin from entering the food chain is essential. The strategies currently used to detoxify trichothecene toxin involve physical, chemical, and biological detoxification methods. Among these, biological methods involving microorganisms like yeasts, bacteria like *Agrobacterium-Rhizobium*, *Devosia mutans*, *L. plantarum* GT III, and fungi and their enzymes are most favored due to their environmentally friendly mechanisms and retention of nutrients in food and animal feed during detoxification. Heat stability, masked toxin property, and only selected chemicals are helpful toward detoxification, making it challenging to get rid of the toxin post-treatment. Though there are many recent methods like using plant products and nanoparticles to get rid of other mycotoxins, more studies need to be conducted to explore such mediums to detoxify trichothecenes.

5.11 Future Implications

There has to be a detailed study about the genetics of other trichothecenes like T-2, NIV, and HT-2 toxins other than DON, which is widely studied to understand the toxicity better and novel methods for detoxifying trichothecene mycotoxins, as very few methods are available.

5.12 Study Questions

- Trichothecenes and its types
- Degradation of trichothecenes
- Synthesis of trichothecenes
- Recent strategies against trichothecenes

Acknowledgments

The authors gratefully acknowledge the support, guidance, and facilities received at the Fungal Genetics and Mycotoxicology Laboratory, Department of Microbiology, Pondicherry University, India.

Conflict of Interest

The authors declare no conflict of interest

Author Contributions

Monica Paul (MCP) has written the manuscript and Regina Sharmila Dass (RSD) has guided MCP to write the manuscript. RSD has also conceptualized, designed, scrutinized, and corrected the manuscript.

References

Abbas, M. (2019). Co-occurrence of mycotoxins and its detoxification strategies. In: *Mycotoxins - Impact and Management Strategies* (ed. P.B. Njobeh and F. Stepman). Intechopen https://doi.org/10.5772/intechopen.76562.

Abraham, N., Chan, E.T.S., Zhou, T., and Seah, S.Y.K. (2022). Microbial detoxification of mycotoxins in food. *Front. Microbiol.* 13: 957148. https://doi.org/10.3389/fmicb.2022.957148.

Achar, P.N., Quyen, P., Adukwu, E.C. et al. (2020). Investigation of the antifungal and anti-aflatoxigenic potential of plant-based essential oils against *Aspergillus flavus* in peanuts. *J. Fungi* 6 (4): 383. https://doi.org/10.3390/jof6040383.

Adhikari, M., Negi, B., Kaushik, N. et al. (2017). T-2 mycotoxin: toxicological effects and decontamination strategies. *Oncotarget* 8 (20): 15422. https://doi.org/10.18632/oncotarget.

Afsah-Hejri, L., Hajeb, P., and Ehsani, R.J. (2020). Application of ozone for degradation of mycotoxins in food: a review. *Comp. Rev. Food Sci. Food Saf.* 19 (4): 1777–1808. https://doi.org/10.1111/1541-4337.12594.

Agriopoulou, S., Stamatelopoulou, E., and Varzakas, T. (2020). Advances in occurrence, importance, and mycotoxin control strategies: prevention and detoxification in foods. *Foods* 9: 137.

Alexandre, A.P.S., Castanha, N., Calori-Domingues, M.A., and Augusto, P.E.D. (2017). Ozonation of whole wheat flour and wet milling effluent: degradation of deoxynivalenol (DON) and rheological properties. *J. Environ. Sci. Health Part B* 52 (7): 516–524. https://doi.org/10.1080/03601234.2017.1303325.

Alkadri, D., Nipoti, P., Döll, K. et al. (2013). Study of fungal colonization of wheat kernels in Syria with a focus on *Fusarium* species. *Int. J. Mol. Sci.* 14 (3): 5938–5951. https://doi.org/10.3390/ijms14035938.

Awad, W.A., Ghareeb, K., Böhm, J., and Zentek, J. (2010). Decontamination and detoxification strategies for the *Fusarium* mycotoxin deoxynivalenol in animal feed and the effectiveness of microbial biodegradation. *Food Addit. Cont. Part A* 27 (4): 510–520. https://doi.org/10.1080/19440040903571747.

Brown, N.A., Urban, M., and Hammond-Kosack, K.E. (2015). The trans-kingdom identification of negative regulators of pathogen hypervirulence. *FEMS Microbiol. Rev.* 40 (1): 19–40. https://doi.org/10.1093/femsre/fuv042.

Carere, J., Hassan, Y.I., Lepp, D., and Zhou, T. (2017). The enzymatic detoxification of the mycotoxin deoxynivalenol: identification of DepA from the DON epimerization pathway. *Microbiol. Biotechnol.* 11 (6): 1106–1111. https://doi.org/10.1111/1751-7915.12874.

CDC. (2019). CDC | Case definition: trichothecene mycotoxin poisoning. http://emergency.cdc.gov; https://emergency.cdc.gov/agent/trichothecene/casedef.asp.

Chin, R. and Lee, B.Y. (2008). *Principles and Practice of Clinical Trial Medicine*. Elsevier https://doi.org/10.1016/b978-0-12-373695-6.x0001-4.

Croft, W.A., Jarvis, B.B., and Yatawara, C.S. (1986). Airborne outbreak of trichothecene toxicosis. *Atmos. Environ.* 20 (3): 549–552. https://doi.org/10.1016/0004-6981(86)90096-x.

da Silva Aquino, K.A. (2012). Sterilization by gamma irradiation. *Gamma Radiat.* 9: 172–202. https://doi.org/10.5772/34901.

Dass, R.S., Sreenivasa, M.Y., and Janardhana, G.R. (2007). High incidence of *Fusarium verticillioides* in animal and poultry feed mixtures produced in Karnataka, India. *Plant Pathol. J.* 6 (2): 174–178.

Deepa, N. and Sreenivasa, M.Y. (2017). Fumonisins: a review on its global occurrence, epidemiology, toxicity and detection. *J. Vet. Med. Res.* 4 (6): 1093.

Deepa, N., Achar, P.N., and Sreenivasa, M.Y. (2021). Current perspectives of biocontrol agents for management of *Fusarium verticillioides* and its Fumonisin in cereals—a review. *J. Fungi* 7: 776. https://doi.org/10.3390/jof7090776.

Deepa, N. and Sreenivasa, M.Y. (2019a). Biocontrol strategies for effective management of phytopathogenic fungi associated with cereals. In: *New and Future Developments in Microbial Biotechnology and Bioengineering* (ed. J.S. Singh and D.P. Singh), 177–189. Elsevier. ISBN: 9780444641915 10.1016/B978-0-444-64191-5.00013-4.

Deepa, N. and Sreenivasa, M.Y. (2019b). Molecular methods and key genes targeted for the detection of fumonisin producing *Fusarium verticillioides* - an updated review. *Food Biosci.* 32: 100473. https://doi.org/10.1016/j.fbio.2019.100473.

Deepa, N., Charith Raj, A.P., and Sreenivasa, M.Y. (2016). Multiplex PCR method for the early detection of fumonisin producing *Fusarium verticillioides*. *Food Biosci.* 13: 84–88.

Eriksen, G.S. and Pettersson, H. (2004). Toxicological evaluation of trichothecenes in animal feed. *Anim. Feed Sci. Technol.* 114 (1–4): 205–239. https://doi.org/10.1016/j.anifeedsci.2003.08.008.

Fan, Z., Bai, B., Jin, P. et al. (2016). Development and validation of an ultra-high performance liquid chromatography-tandem mass spectrometry method for simultaneous determination of four type B trichothecenes and masked deoxynivalenol in various feed products. *Molecules* 21 (6): 747. https://doi.org/10.3390/molecules21060747.

Feizollahi, E. and Roopesh, M.S. (2021). Mechanisms of deoxynivalenol (DON) degradation during different treatments: a review. *Crit. Rev. Food Sci. Nutr.* 62 (21): 5903–5924. https://doi.org/10.1080/10408398.2021.1895056.

Foroud, N.A., Baines, D., Gagkaeva, T.Y. et al. (2019). Trichothecenes in cereal grains – an update. *Toxins* 11 (11): 634. https://doi.org/10.3390/toxins11110634.

Franco, T.S., Garcia, S., Hirooka, E.Y. et al. (2011). Lactic acid bacteria in the inhibition of *Fusarium graminearum* and deoxynivalenol detoxification. *J. Appl. Microbiol.* 111 (3): 739–748. https://doi.org/10.1111/j.1365-2672.2011.05074.x.

Fuchs, E., Binder, E.M., Heidler, D., and Krska, R. (2002). Structural characterization of metabolites after the microbial degradation of type a trichothecenes by the bacterial strain BBSH 797. *Food Addit. Contam.* 19 (4): 379–386. https://doi.org/10.1080/02652030110091154.

Gab-Allah, M.A., Choi, K., and Kim, B. (2023). Type B trichothecenes in cereal grains and their products: recent advances on occurrence, toxicology, analysis and post-harvest decontamination strategies. *Toxins* 15 (2): 85. https://doi.org/10.3390/toxins15020085.

Gottschalk, C., Barthel, J., Engelhardt, G. et al. (2007). Occurrence of type a trichothecenes in conventionally and organically produced oats and oat products. *Mol. Nutr. Food Res.* 51 (12): 1547–1553. https://doi.org/10.1002/mnfr.200700146.

Gutiérrez, S., McCormick, S.P., Cardoza, R.E. et al. (2021). Distribution, function, and evolution of a gene essential for trichothecene toxin biosynthesis in trichoderma. *Front. Microbiol.* 12: 791641. https://doi.org/10.3389/fmicb.2021.791641.

Hao Z, Zhang Z, Xiang D, Venglat P, Chen J, Gao P, Datla R, Weijers D. Conserved, divergent and heterochronic gene expression during *Brachypodium* and *Arabidopsis* embryo development. *Plant Reprod.* 2021 Sep;34(3):207–224. doi: https://doi.org/10.1007/s00497-021-00413-4.

He, J., Zhou, T., Young, J.C. et al. (2010). Chemical and biological transformations for detoxification of trichothecene mycotoxins in human and animal food chains: a review. *Trends Food Sci. Technol.* 21 (2): 67–76. https://doi.org/10.1016/j.tifs.2009.08.002.

Hojnik, N., Cvelbar, U., Tavčar-Kalcher, G. et al. (2017). Mycotoxin decontamination of food: cold atmospheric pressure plasma versus 'classic' decontamination. *Toxins* 9 (5): 151. https://doi.org/10.3390/toxins9050151.

Ikunaga, Y., Sato, I., Grond, S. et al. (2010). *Nocardioides* sp. strain WSN05-2, isolated from a wheat field, degrades deoxynivalenol, producing the novel intermediate 3-epi-deoxynivalenol. *Appl. Microbiol. Biotechnol.* 89 (2): 419–427. https://doi.org/10.1007/s00253-010-2857-z.

Janardhana, G.R., Dass, R.S., and Sreenivasa, M.Y. (2009). Fumonisins – a new class of fusarial toxins. In: *Frontiers in Fungal Ecology, Diversity and Metabolites* (ed. K.A. Sridhar). New Delhi: I. K. International Publishing House Pvt. Ltd.

Kabak, B., Dobson, A.D.W., and Var, I. (2006). Strategies to prevent mycotoxin contamination of food and animal feed: a review. *Crit. Rev. Food Sci. Nutr.* 46 (8): 593–619. https://doi.org/10.1080/10408390500436185.

Karlovsky, P. (2011). Biological detoxification of the mycotoxin deoxynivalenol and its use in genetically engineered crops and feed additives. *Appl. Microbiol. Biotechnol.* 91 (3): 491–504. https://doi.org/10.1007/s00253-011-3401-5.

Karlovsky, P., Suman, M., Berthiller, F. et al. (2016). Impact of food processing and detoxification treatments on mycotoxin contamination. *Mycotoxin Res.* 32 (4): 179–205. https://doi.org/10.1007/s12550-016-0257-7.

Kumar, P., Mahato, D.K., Gupta, A. et al. (2022). Nivalenol mycotoxin concerns in foods: an overview on occurrence, impact on human and animal health and its detection and management strategies. *Toxins* 14 (8): 527. https://doi.org/10.3390/toxins14080527.

Li, P., Su, R., Yin, R. et al. (2020). Detoxification of mycotoxins through biotransformation. *Toxins* 12 (2): 121. https://doi.org/10.3390/toxins12020121.

Li, S.-J., Zhang, G., Xue, B. et al. (2022). Toxicity and detoxification of T-2 toxin in poultry. *Food Chem. Toxicol.* 169: 113392. https://doi.org/10.1016/j.fct.2022.113392.

Li, Y., Wang, Z., Beier, R.C. et al. (2011). T-2 toxin, a trichothecene mycotoxin: review of toxicity, metabolism, and analytical methods. *J. Agric. Food Chem.* 59 (8): 3441–3453. https://doi.org/10.1021/jf200767q.

Liu, L., Xie, M., and Wei, D. (2022). Biological detoxification of mycotoxins: current status and future advances. *Int. J. Mol. Sci.* 23 (3): 1064. https://doi.org/10.3390/ijms23031064.

Lyagin, I. and Efremenko, E. (2019). Enzymes for detoxification of various mycotoxins: origins and mechanisms of catalytic action. *Molecules* 24 (13): 2362. https://doi.org/10.3390/molecules24132362.

Mahato, D.K., Pandhi, S., Kamle, M. et al. (2022). Trichothecenes in food and feed: occurrence, impact on human health and their detection and management strategies. *Toxicon* 208: 62–77. https://doi.org/10.1016/j.toxicon.2022.01.011.

Matejova, I., Svobodova, Z., Vakula, J. et al. (2016). Impact of mycotoxins on aquaculture fish species: a review. *J. World Aquacul. Soci.* 48 (2): 186–200. https://doi.org/10.1111/jwas.12371.

Modra, H., Palikova, M., Hyrsl, P. et al. (2020). Effects of trichothecene mycotoxin T-2 toxin on haematological and immunological parameters of rainbow trout (*Oncorhynchus mykiss*). *Mycotoxin Res.* 36 (3): 319–326. https://doi.org/10.1007/s12550-020-00396-7.

Nagaraja, H., Chennappa, G., Poorna Chandra Rao, K. et al. (2016). Diversity of toxic and phytopathogenic *Fusarium* species occurring on cereals grown in Karnataka state, India. *3 Biotech* 6: 57.

Nagendra Prasad, M.N., Shankara Bhat, S., and Sreenivasa, M.Y. (2010). Antifungal activity of essential oils against *Phomopsis azadirachtae*- the causative agent of die-back disease of neem. *J. Agric. Technol.* 6 (1): 127–133.

Nathanail, A.V., Varga, E., Meng-Reiterer, J. et al. (2015). Metabolism of the Fusarium mycotoxins T-2 toxin and HT-2 toxin in wheat. *J. Agric. Food Chem.* 63 (35): 7862–7872. https://doi.org/10.1021/acs.jafc.5b02697.

Niessen, L. (2007). PCR-based diagnosis and quantification of mycotoxin producing fungi. *Int. J. Food Microbiol.* 119 (1–2): 38–46. https://doi.org/10.1016/j.ijfoodmicro.2007.07.023.

Olopade, B.K., Oranusi, S.U., Nwinyi, O.C. et al. (2019). Decontamination of T-2 toxin in maize by modified montmorillonite clay. *Toxins* 11 (11): 616. https://doi.org/10.3390/toxins11110616.

Patey, A.L. and Gilbert, J. (1989). Fate of *Fusarium* mycotoxins in cereals during food processing and methods for their detoxification. *Fusarium* 2: 399–420. https://doi.org/10.1016/b978-0-444-87468-9.50028-6.

Pietsch, C. and Burkhardt-Holm, P. (2015). Feed-borne exposure to deoxynivalenol leads to acute and chronic effects on liver enzymes and histology in carp. *World Mycotoxin J.* 8 (5): 619–627. https://doi.org/10.3920/wmj2015.1879.

Polak-Śliwińska, M. and Paszczyk, B. (2021). Trichothecenes in food and feed, relevance to human and animal health and methods of detection: a systematic review. *Molecules* 26 (2): 454. https://doi.org/10.3390/molecules26020454.

Proctor, R.H., McCormick, S.P., and Gutiérrez, S. (2020). Genetic bases for variation in structure and biological activity of trichothecene toxins produced by diverse fungi. *Appl. Microbiol. Biotechnol.* 104 (12): 5185–5199. https://doi.org/10.1007/s00253-020-10612-0.

Proctor, R.H., McCormick, S.P., Kim, H.-S. et al. (2018). Evolution of structural diversity of trichothecenes, a family of toxins produced by plant pathogenic and entomopathogenic fungi. *PLoS Pathog.* 14 (4): 1006946. https://doi.org/10.1371/journal.ppat.1006946.

Rotter, B.A. (1996). Invited review: toxicology of deoxynivalenol (VOMITOXIN). *J. Toxicol. Environ. Health* 48 (1): 1–34. https://doi.org/10.1080/009841096161447.

Shanakhat, H., Sorrentino, A., Raiola, A. et al. (2018). Current methods for mycotoxins analysis and innovative strategies for their reduction in cereals: an overview. *J. Sci. Food Agric.* 98 (11): 4003–4013. https://doi.org/10.1002/jsfa.8933.

Shank, R.A., Foroud, N.A., Hazendonk, P. et al. (2011). Current and future experimental strategies for structural analysis of trichothecene mycotoxins—a prospectus. *Toxins* 3 (12): 1518–1553. https://doi.org/10.3390/toxins3121518.

Sreenivasa, M.Y., Dass, R.S., Raj, A.-P.C. et al. (2011). Assessment of the growth inhibiting effect of some plant essential oils on different *Fusarium* species isolated from sorghum and maize grains. *J. Plant Dis. Protect.* 118 (6): 208–213.

Sun, Y.X., Yao, X., Shi, S.N. et al. (2014). Toxicokinetics of T-2 toxin and its major metabolites in broiler chickens after intravenous and oral administration. *J. Vet. Pharmacol. Ther.* 38 (1): 80–85. https://doi.org/10.1111/jvp.12142.

Vanhoutte, I., Audenaert, K., and De Gelder, L. (2016). Biodegradation of mycotoxins: tales from known and unexplored worlds. *Front. Microbiol.* 7: 561. https://doi.org/10.3389/fmicb.2016.00561.

Vila-Donat, P., Marín, S., Sanchis, V., and Ramos, A.J. (2018). A review of the mycotoxin adsorbing agents, with an emphasis on their multi-binding capacity, for animal feed decontamination. *Food Chem. Toxicol.* 114: 246–259. https://doi.org/10.1016/j.fct.2018.02.044.

Villafana, R., Ramdass, A., and Rampersad, S. (2019). Selection of *Fusarium* trichothecene toxin genes for molecular detection depends on TRI gene cluster organization and gene function. *Toxins* 11 (1): 36. https://doi.org/10.3390/toxins11010036.

Wan, J., Chen, B., and Rao, J. (2020). Occurrence and preventive strategies to control mycotoxins in cereal-based food. *Compr. Rev. Food Sci. Food Saf.* 19 (3): 928–953. https://doi.org/10.1111/1541-4337.12546.

Wilson, S.C., Brasel, T.L., Martin, J.M. et al. (2005). Efficacy of chlorine dioxide as a gas and solution in the inactivation of two trichothecene mycotoxins. *Int. J. Toxicol.* 24 (3): 181–186. https://doi.org/10.1080/10915810590953437.

Woloshuk, C.P. and Shim, W.B. (2013). Aflatoxins, fumonisins, and trichothecenes: a convergence of knowledge. *FEMS Microbiol. Rev.* 37 (1): 94–109. https://doi.org/10.1111/1574-6976.12009.

Wu, Q., Dohnal, V., Kuca, K., and Yuan, Z. (2013). Trichothecenes: structure-toxic activity relationships. *Curr. Drug Met.* 14 (6): 641–660. https://doi.org/10.2174/1389200211314060002.

Xu, H., Wang, L., Sun, J. et al. (2021). Microbial detoxification of mycotoxins in food and feed. *Crit. Rev. Food Sci. Nutr.* 62 (18): 1–19. https://doi.org/10.1080/10408398.2021.1879730.

Young, J.C. (1986). Reduction in levels of deoxynivalenol in contaminated corn by chemical and physical treatment. *J. Agric. Food Chem.* 34 (3): 465–467. https://doi.org/10.1021/jf00069a022.

Zhu, M., Cen, Y., Ye, W. et al. (2020). Recent advances on macrocyclic trichothecenes, their bioactivities and biosynthetic pathway. *Toxins* 12 (6): 417. https://doi.org/10.3390/toxins12060417.

Further Reading

Janik, E., Niemcewicz, M., Podogrocki, M. et al. (2021). T-2 toxin—the most toxic trichothecene mycotoxin: metabolism, toxicity, and decontamination strategies. *Molecules* 26 (22): 6868. https://doi.org/10.3390/molecules26226868.

Kumar, P., Mahato, D.K., Gupta, A. et al. (2022). Nivalenol mycotoxin concerns in foods: an overview on occurrence, impact on human and animal health and its detection and management strategies. *Toxins* 14 (8): 527. https://doi.org/10.3390/toxins14080527.

McCormick, S.P., Price, N.P., and Kurtzman, C.P. (2012). Glucosylation and other biotransformations of T-2 toxin by yeasts of the Trichomonascus clade. *ASM J.* 78 (24): 8694–8702. https://doi.org/10.1128/aem.02391-12.

Muhialdin, B.J., Saari, N., and Meor Hussin, A.S. (2020). Review on the biological detoxification of mycotoxins using lactic acid bacteria to enhance the sustainability of foods supply. *Molecules* 25 (11): 2655. https://doi.org/10.3390/molecules25112655.

Wilson, S.C., Brasel, T.L., Martin, J.M. et al. (2005). Efficacy of chlorine dioxide as a gas and in solution in the inactivation of two trichothecene mycotoxins. *Int. J. Toxicol.* 24 (3): 181–186. https://doi.org/10.1080/10915810590953437.

6

Citrinin: A Potential Mycotoxin in Food and Feed with Possible Management Strategies to Combat Its Contamination

Kadaiah Ajithkumar[1], *Attihalli S. Savitha*[2], *Matapati Renuka*[1], *and Manjunath K. Naik*[2]

[1] *Main Agricultural Research Station, University of Agricultural Sciences, Raichur, Karnataka, India*
[2] *Department of Plant Pathology, College of Agriculture, University of Agricultural Sciences, Raichur, Karnataka, India*

CONTENTS

Abstract

Citrinin, an important mycotoxin, of significant health concern for animals and human beings is synthesized by ubiquitous fungal genera *Penicillium*, *Aspergillus*, and *Monascus*. It is widely distributed across the globe and contaminates agricultural commodities such as stored food grains, beans, fruits, vegetables, black olives, roasted nuts, sunflowers, spices, and spoils dairy products. Tactical management strategies involved in degradation of citrinin including

Anti-Mycotoxin Strategies for Food and Feed, First Edition. Edited by Deepa Nagaraju, Sreenivasa Marikunte Yanjarappa, Premila N. Achar, and Angel Medina Vaya.

physical measures such as filtration, adsorption, heat treatment, light treatment, high hydrostatic pressure, and cold plasma techniques can be utilized. Chemical weapons comprise application of fungicide, ozone treatment, response surface methodology, exogenous ascorbic acid, troxerutin, and genistein. On the contrary, eco-friendly and reliable methods include usage of biocontrol agents such as *Trichoderma hamatum*, *Rhizobium borbori*, *Saccharomyces cerevisiae*, *Rhodotorula mucilaginosa*, and *Klebsiella pneumoniae*. Even some essential oils of *Azadirachta indica* and *Zataria multiflora* significantly suppressed citrinin production. Further, citrinin is detoxified by using probiotics, H_2O_2, and magnetic nanoparticles.

Keywords *Chitosan, citrinin, cold plasmas, hepatotoxic, magnetic nanoparticles, nephrotoxic,* Penicillium citrinum, Saccharomyces cerevisiae

Graphical Representation

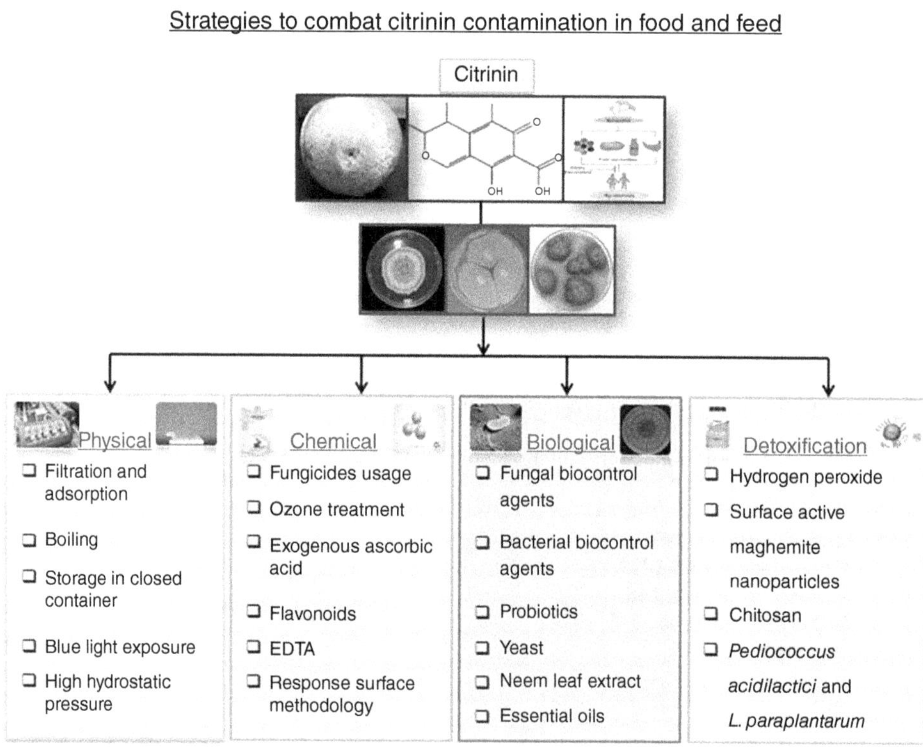

6.1 Introduction

Citrinin (CIT) is a secondary toxic metabolite synthesized by the ubiquitous fungal genera *Penicillium* (*Penicillium citrinum*, *Penicillium expansum*, and *Penicillium verrucosum*), *Aspergillus* (*Aspergillus niveus*, *Aspergillus carneus*, and *Aspergillus terreus*), and *Monascus* (*Monascus purpureus* and *Monascus ruber*). Many agricultural commodities often get contaminated by CIT during pre- and post-harvest stages (Sreenivasa et al. 2008; Zhang et al. 2017). CIT was first discovered by Hetherington and Raistrick (1931) and isolated from *P. citrinum* by Thom (He and Cox 2016). This fungus is a mesophile which requires optimum temperature of 26–30 °C and water activity of 0.8–0.84 a_w (Sweeney and Dobson 1998). It is a polyketide molecule having IUPAC name as (3R, 4S)-4, 6-dihydro-8-hydroxy-3,4,5-trimethyl-6-oxo-3H-2-benzopyran-7-carboxylic acid having molecular formula of $C_{13}H_{14}O_5$ with 250.25 g/mol molecular weight. It exists as acidic lemon-yellow crystals with 172 °C melting point, autofluorescent compound, which easily dissolves in organic solvents, sodium acetate, sodium carbonate, and aqueous sodium hydroxide relatively than water (Poupke et al. 1997). It is having cytotoxic, skin irritant, hepatotoxic, and nephrotoxic effects on humans where it decreases DNA, protein, and glutathione content in the kidney and liver tissues (Blanc et al. 1995). CIT caused cells to produce more reactive oxygen species and less cellular ATP, therefore removing it from food and its products is an incredible undertaking from a health, environmental, and economic standpoint (Stormer and Hoiby 1996). The International Agency for Cancer Research classified CIT as Group 3 of carcinogens because there were limited facts of its carcinogenicity (Flajs and Peraica 2009).

6.2 Occurrence and Distribution of Citrinin

CIT is well known "slow-acting" mycotoxin (Mirocha and Christensen 1974), which naturally occurs in stored food grains (wheat, rice, maize, barley, oats, and rye), beans, fruits, vegetables, black olives, roasted nuts (almonds, peanuts, hazelnuts, pistachio nuts), sunflower seeds, spices (black pepper, cardamom, coriander, cumin, dry ginger, fennel, and turmeric), and herbs, and spoiled dairy products such as cheese often contaminated by CIT producing fungi (Doughari 2015; Deepa et al., 2016a, b) (Figure 6.1). Date back in 1953–1954, a consequence happened in Japan where people suffered from "poisoning by moldy rice" and "yellow rice syndrome," which was indirectly connected with the contamination of food products with CIT toxin (Zhang et al. 2021). Ahamad and Vairamuthu (2000) conducted a survey in Tamil Nadu to know the occurrence of CIT in compounded individual feed ingredients. They came out with the result that out of 63 compounded feed and 43 individual feed samples examined about 44.4–51.0% samples witnessed the CIT contamination. The toxin is often detected in fruits such as oranges, sweet cherries, tomatoes, dried grapes, pears, larger beer, and apples (Wang et al. 2016). The natural occurrence of CIT (49–92 μg/kg) in rice from India, Japan, Vietnam, China, Canada, Malaysia, and Iran was reported by Silva et al. (2021).

The fungus-producing CITs are widely distributed across the world. They readily contaminate the food and feed materials as reported in Denmark, Canada, Tunisia, India, Switzerland, Egypt, Japan, Vietnam, Spain, Iran, China, Taiwan, and Balkan areas such as Albania, Bosnia, Bulgaria, Croatia, Herzegovina, Serbia, Kosovo, North Macedonia, Slovenia, Montenegro, and Romania (Silva et al. 2021). In India, CIT contamination in spices such as black pepper, cumin, fenugreek, and dry ginger was reported for the first time in Bihar state (Jeswal and Kumar 2015). CIT normally possessed antimicrobial properties. However, it is less effective as an antibiotic due to its nephrotoxicity. The toxin primarily affects the kidney in mammals, leading to renal dysfunction. Later, it attacks

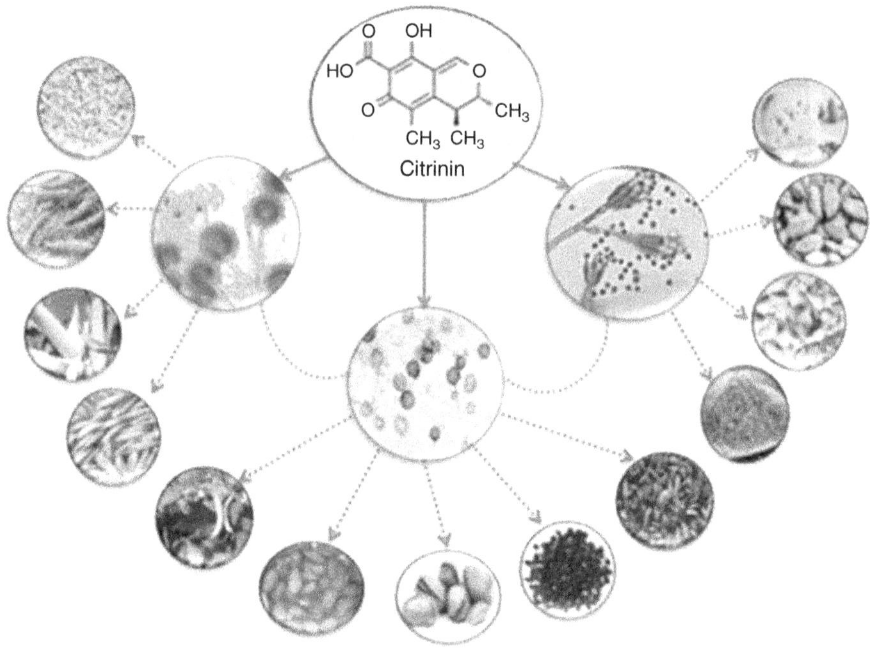

Figure 6.1 Occurrence of CIT in agricultural commodities.

the liver and bone marrow as well (Vella et al. 1995). It was initially named "Monascidin A" as it was obtained from *Monascus* spp. but later based on their structural studies, it was renamed CIT (Pan and Hsu 2014). The lethal dose in oral administration of CIT has been fixed in different animals and birds (35–58 mg/kg), rats (50 mg/kg), rabbits (134 mg/kg), ducks (57 mg/kg), and chicken (95 mg/kg) (Pan and Hsu 2014; Deepa and Sreenivasa 2017a, b).

P. citrinum is a ubiquitous ascomycete fungus belonging to the section *Furcatum* and series *Citrina* (Pitt 1979). It produces a grayish-colored colony with white periphery which exerts granular powdery appearance to the colony, as the pathogen grows rapidly and produces septate, hyaline, and branched mycelium, which further differentiates to form long, septate, biverticillately branched conidiophore bearing metulae and phialides on which chains of globose to sub-globose, finely rough surfaced conidia are arranged in broom shape (Soumya et al. 2022). *Aspergillus* species are the saprophytic fungus which is prevalent across the globe and produces cinnamon-buff to sand brown colonies on potato dextrose agar with yellow to deep dirty brown-colored pigmentation. Morphologically, the pathogen produces septate, branched hyaline mycelia which differentiate to form hyaline, smooth-walled conidiophores on which compact, biseriate, and densely columnar conidial heads are formed, which bear globose to ellipsoidal, smooth-walled light yellow-colored to hyaline conidia (Cornelia 2012). *Monascus* genus vernacularly known as red pigment-producing ascomycete fungi form thin and spreading circular red colonies on PDA media. The mycelium is septate, branched, colored, and has oval-shaped spores (Dogra and Kumar 2017).

6.3 Toxicity and Its Effects of Citrinin in Animals, Birds, and Humans

Once CIT gets entry into host system, it is readily absorbed from the gastrointestinal tract and rapidly distributed across kidney, liver, urinary bladder, blood, lungs, sex organs, and spleen. Kidney has the highest affinity toward binding to chemicals. Hence, it plays a major role in elimination of toxicants from the body. These organs probably act as storage sites for CIT and its degradation products. CIT causes biochemical changes in the host cell that alter enzymes including alkaline phosphatase, glutamate dehydrogenase, and succinic oxidase as well as inhibits active ion transport and respiration activity of kidney slices. The macromolecules such as DNA, RNA, and protein synthesis get diminished by CIT (Pan and Hsu 2014) (Figure 6.2).

Cattle such as cows and calves, when consumed feedstuff consisting of CIT, developed symptoms such as depression, fever, uremia, and diarrhea. Histopathological examination revealed that nephritis and nephrosis, which were characterized by the existence of hyaline casts, birefringent crystals, perirenal edema, pneumonia, and fatty changes in the liver (Lloyd 1980). Griffiths and Done (1991) observed cattle suffering from pruritus, pyrexia, and hemorrhagic syndrome (Figure 6.3). Friis et al. studied the toxic effects of CIT during 1969 in swine that lead to coma because of renal insufficiency and decrease in apatite, which ultimately caused death of pigs. Even Szczech et al. (1974) also recorded renal

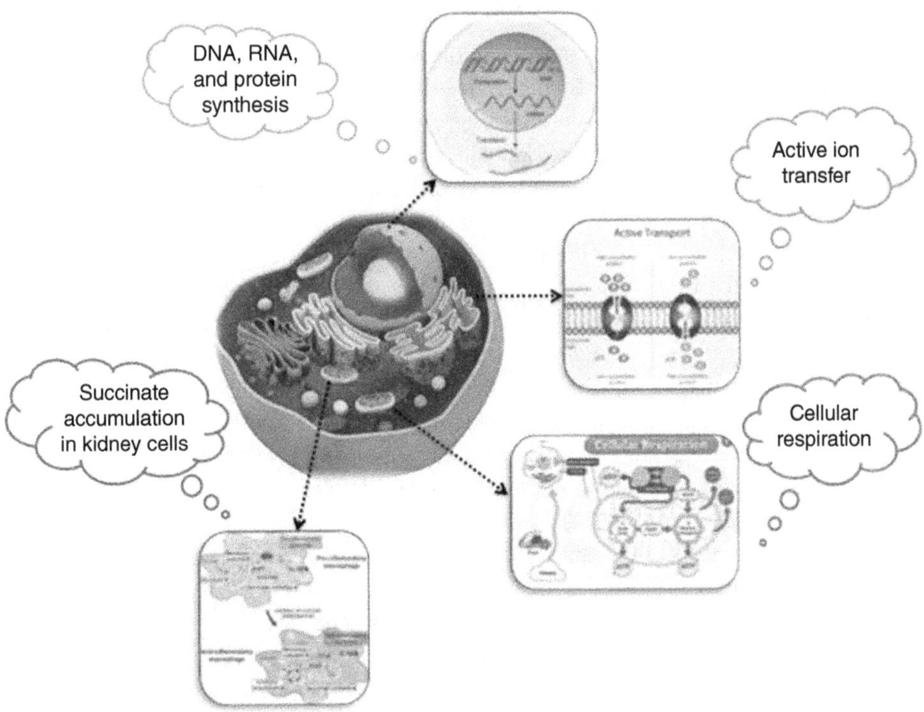

Figure 6.2 Representation of biochemical changes induced by CIT toxicity.

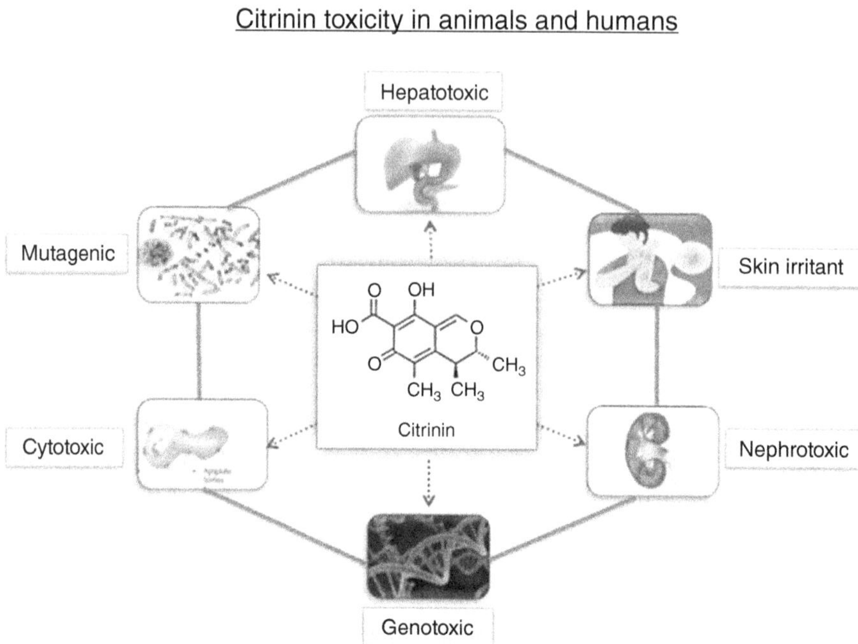

Figure 6.3 Representation of CIT toxicity in animals and humans.

damage. Porcine nephropathy termed as "mold nephrosis" occurred in Denmark due to consumption of CIT-contaminated moldy feed to swine which degenerated the kidney cells (Dunn and Friendman 1994) (Figure 6.3). Guinea pig led to development of gross lesions on kidneys, liver, intestines, skeletal muscles, and radial streaking of the cortex region. Epithelial cells degenerated and necrosis in the proximal tubules, hyperplasia in liver, mucosal inflammation, necrosis, ulceration in intestine, and degeneration and necrosis in skeletal muscles (Thacker et al. 1977) (Figure 6.3). So-Jeo et al. and Kitchen et al. (2007, 1977) reported that consumption of 8.3 μg CIT per kg feed in dogs has resulted in anorexia, emaciation, polydipsia, and vomiting after one month causing renal failure with renal atrophy, congestion of glomerular capillary, diffuse degeneration, necrosis, and calcification of tubular epithelium, which finally led to death in dogs (Figure 6.3).

CIT toxicity in rabbits has developed acute renal failure (azotemia, decreased creatinine clearance) with tubular dysfunction as indicated by glucosuria, cylindruria, anorexia, lethargy, dullness, loose feces, dehydration and polydipsia signs, and isosthenuria (Hanika et al. 1984; Kumar et al. 2007). CIT also has reproductive system toxicity in both male and female mice, as in males, it minimizes the viability and proliferation of Sertoli cells through apoptosis and necrosis. It enhances the production of abnormal sperms and decreases rate of survival of sperms and results in low fertility (Arai and Hibino 1983; Yasemin Aydin et al. 2021), whereas, in females, it causes apoptosis in oocytes through oxidative stress along with decrease in fertilization and *in vitro* embryo development. Even in a mice's bone marrow, it has resulted in chromosomal abnormalities and hypodiploidy (Alexander et al. 2012; Wu et al. 2017) (Figure 6.3).

The CIT toxicity in domestic birds such as chickens, ducks, and turkeys results in watery diarrhea, increased food consumption rate, and decreased weight gain because of degeneration in kidney (Mehdi et al. 1984). Alterations in the morphology of the intestinal villi in broiler chicks were observed and found broilers suffered from depression in growth, polydipsia, diarrhea, dehydration, and hydropic degeneration of renal epithelial cells, renal ultrastructural alterations in proximal tubular epithelial cells, ring-shaped mitochondria, membrane-bound intranuclear inclusions, and cytoplasmic aggregates of smooth endoplasmic reticulum (Witlock et al. 1977; Roberts and Mora 1978; Brown et al. 1986; Abdelhamid and Dorra 1990) (Figure 6.3). Consumption of CIT-contaminated maize and beans by people has resulted in allergies in humans and Balkan endemic nephropathy, which is a chronic tubulointerstitial nephritis disease characterized by high frequency of urothelial atypia. Occasionally, there is formation of tumors in renal pelvis and urethra which ultimately leads to kidney failure, was also considered genotoxic (Berndt et al. 1980; Wichmann et al. 2002; Donmez-Altuntas et al. 2007). Chang et al. (2010) suggested that CIT exposure to human embryonic kidney cells arrests the cell cycle at G2/M due to inhibition of mitotic spindle formation and tubulin polymerization (Figure 6.3).

6.4 Effects of Both Pre- and Post-Harvest Stages on Citrinin Production

Grain or other commodities which enter a godown or storehouse always carry filamentous fungal load whose population dynamics depend on the field climatic conditions and harvesting processes (Magan and Lacey 1986). Fungal infection and contamination of CIT may start from field itself during harvesting, handling, storage, and processing. The critical postharvest factor includes mechanical injury, grain moisture content, time of harvesting and insect infestation, and drying method (Neme and Mohammed 2017). Insect pests are common visitors in storage ecosystem, which produces metabolic heat to generate water via condensation process. This water molecule helps in rapid colonization by fungi which leads to the spoilage of food commodities (Deepa et al. 2021). These storage pests also help in the dissemination of fungal spores and hyphae across the seed lot and result in quick deterioration of grain and easy contamination of mycotoxin (Sinha 1971). There is a report for the production of CIT under indoor environmental conditions as studied by Tuomi et al. (2000) from 79 bulk samples of moldy interior surfaces, which includes wallpaper, cardboard, wood, sand, soil, paint, plasterboard, linoleum, and polyurethane insulation. Out of these, only three samples were contaminated with 20–3500 ng/g of CIT. This data suggests that humans can come across CIT through inhalation or dermal contact.

6.5 Physical Control Measures Against Citrinin

The key factors in avoiding any mycotoxin contamination include four major steps:

i) Preventing contamination
ii) Removing the contaminated material from food

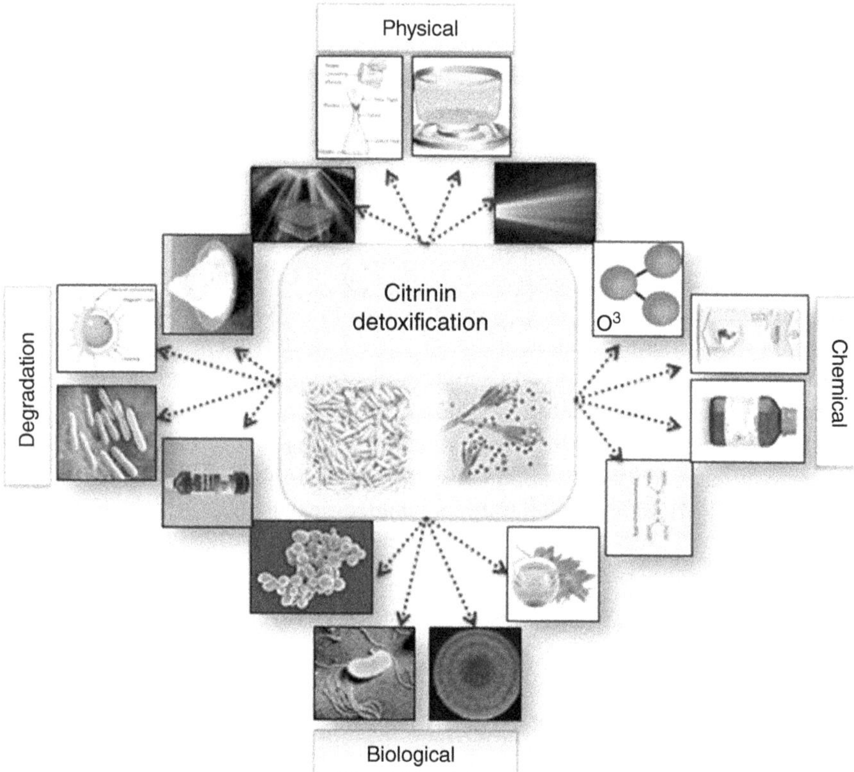

Figure 6.4 CIT detoxification strategies in food and feed.

iii) Mitigating mycotoxin content in the food
iv) Treating the exposed individuals (Karlovasky et al. 2016) (Figure 6.4).

6.5.1 Agronomic Practices

The minimization or prevention of mycotoxin contamination at field level includes employing good agronomic practices such as utilization of resistant varieties, soil tillage, crop rotation, insect pests, and disease management through various biocontrol agents (Choudhari and Kumar 2010). Further, CIT contamination can be prevented by placing the food materials inside a tightly closed container which should be kept in a well-ventilated place (Doughari 2015). Mycotoxin production is highly climate-dependent as the prevailing moisture and temperature during plant growth period as well as in storage conditions regulate the fungal contamination. Therefore, weather forecasts can be used as a reference for early disease prediction and corresponding management strategies for avoiding the disease as well as preventing the toxification of food and feed raw materials, which is more significant than successful treatment (Milani 2013). Cold storage is an often-used physical method for storing fruits and vegetables across the globe as it prolongs shelf life of the commodity along with retention of nutritional and sensory qualities of the produce and suppresses the growth of spoilage fungi *Penicillium* as its growth gets stagnated at a low temperature range of 4–11 °C (Aghdam et al. 2018) (Table 6.1).

Table 6.1 Strategies on detoxification of CIT.

S. No.	Anti-mycotoxin strategy		Methodology	Reduction (%)	References
1.	Physical	Adsorption and filtration	Molecularly imprinted polymer spheres	98–100	Meydan et al. (2021)
		Heat treatment	Citrinin is sensitive to heat	50–100	Pan and Hsu (2014)
		Light treatment	Citrinin is sensitive to light	100	Schmidt-Heydt et al. (2012)
		High hydrostatic pressure	Delayed pathogen growth and reproduction, HPAS	64–100	Tokusoglu et al. (2010) and Awuchi et al. (2023)
		Cold atmospheric pressure plasma	Sulfur hexafluoride gases	100	Durek et al. (2018)
2.	Chemical	Fungicides	Allite, rovral, cantus, ortiva, luna, and mancozeb	100	Schmidt-Heydt (2013)
		Ozone	Oxidizing agent and a potent disinfectant	75	Savi et al. (2015)
		Acids and solvents	Propionic acid, phosphate-ethanol, exogenous ascorbic acid, ethidium dibromide tetra acetic acid	91.6	Gupta et al. (2018), Lee et al. (2007), and Wei et al. (2022)
		Flavonoids	Troxerutin, genistein	87.9	Huang et al. (2019) and He et al. (2020)
		Ammonium salts	Ammonium sulfate, ammonium nitrate	100	Gu et al. (2021)
3.	Biological	Fungal bioagent	*Trichoderma hamatum*	45–100	Ezzat and Abd-Allah (2005)
		Bacterial bioagent	*Rhizobium borbori* PS45, *Pseudomonas fluorescens*, *Bacillus subtilis*, *Glucanobacter oxydans*	32–65	Kanpiengjai et al. (2015), Wallace et al. (2017), Mohammadi et al. (2017), and Markov et al. (2019)
		Yeast	*Saccharomyces cerevisiae*, *Rhodotorula mucilaginosa*, *Wickerhamomyces anomalus*, *Yarrowia lipolytica*	90–100	Moghdam et al. (2019), Ahima et al. (2019), Zhang et al. (2019), and Wang et al. (2019)
		Natural essential oils	Neem leaf extract, *Zataria multiflora*, Mint aqueous solution	73–89.6	Mossini and Kemmelmeier (2008), Mohajeri et al. (2018), and Panda et al. (2018)

(*Continued*)

Table 6.1 (Continued)

S. No.	Anti-mycotoxin strategy		Methodology	Reduction (%)	References
4.	Detoxification	Hydrogen peroxide	Strong oxidizing agent affects fungal respiratory mechanism	100	Fouler et al. (1994)
		Probiotics	*Pediococcus acidilactici* and *Lactobacillus paraplantarum*	100	Okeke et al. (2015)
		Magnetic nanoparticles	Chelating properties of citrinin toward iron (III) atoms on the surface of SAMNs	70	Magro et al. (2016)
		Chitosan	Antifungal and antimicrobial activity	50–70	Abd-Allah and Hashem (2006) and Coutinho et al. (2020)
		Enzymes	Manganese peroxidase	100	Wang et al. (2022)

6.5.2 Adsorption and Filtration

Traditionally, mycotoxin contamination can be managed by following physical measures such as adsorption and filtration. Adsorption is a surface phenomenon characterized by adhesion of adsorbate molecules onto the surface of a solid absorbent material. Whereas, filtration is a process in which solid particles in a liquid fluid are removed by means of a filter medium that only permits the fluids to pass through but retains the solid particles. Meydan et al. (2021) found that molecularly imprinted polymer spheres specifically bind to the CIT through adsorption process and have maximum adsorption capacity of 38.6 mg/g with 98–100% removal of CIT.

6.5.3 Heat Treatment

CIT is highly sensitive to heat which becomes unstable upon heat treatment as it gets converted into CIT H1 and CIT H2, which are less cytotoxic compared to CIT. This decomposition generally takes place at 175 °C under dry conditions and > 100 °C with moisture (Clark et al. 2006). Even a simple hot water treatment for 20 minutes has reduced CIT by half in *Monascus*-fermented products (Pan and Hsu 2014).

6.5.4 Light Treatment

CIT is also highly sensitive to light as blue and white lights of 455 and 470 nm wavelengths, respectively, can completely degrade the CIT content (Schmidt-Heydt et al. 2012).

6.5.5 High Hydrostatic Pressure (HHP)

It is a non-thermal preservation technology which can completely eradicate the *P. citrinum* load at 4 °C and CIT content degraded 64–100% at 35 ± 2 °C as HHP enables the food processing at ambient or lower temperature which results in death of pathogen, and the moderate pressure of 200–300 Mpa utilized here resulted in delayed pathogen growth and reproduction (Tokusoglu et al. 2010). High-pressure acidified steaming (HPAS) is a novel method composed of three techniques – high pressure, steaming, and acidification. In HPAS, aqueous citric acid (pH 5) is added to water and subjected to steaming at 15 lbs pressure, when maize samples are treated with HPAS significantly reducing CIT to the extent of 30–51% (Awuchi et al. 2023).

6.5.6 Cold Atmospheric Pressure Plasma (CAP)

It is a newly emerging potential technique for detoxification of CIT from feed samples as reported by Vaseghi et al. (2017). They observed that application of sulfur hexafluoride gases at 20 Kv voltage, 100 W power for two minutes resulted in complete destruction of *Penicillium* and CIT. Cold plasmas are generated under low pressure and low power conditions and have lower temperatures. It can be used as an effective tool for inactivation of *Aspergillus niger* and *Penicillium verrucosum* inoculated onto barley (Durek et al. 2018).

6.6 Chemical Control Measures Against Citrinin

6.6.1 Fungicides

Chemical ways of control include the application of fungicides such as aliette, rovral, cantus, ortiva, luna, and mancozeb, which completely prevent the growth of the fungus and avoid CIT accumulation in food products (Schmidt-Heydt 2013).

6.6.2 Ozone (O_3) Treatment

Ozone is an oxidizing agent and a potent disinfectant used to maintain food surface hygiene. It acts on unsaturated lipids present in the cell membrane of the fungus causing leakage of their cellular component and finally lead to death. Even it causes oxidation of cellular proteins which results in reduction in fungal growth and causes death. Savi et al. (2015) found that application of ozone at 60 μmol/mol for 180 minutes resulted in complete inhibition of *P. citrinum* and corresponding reduction in the CIT production of 42.90 μg/kg compared to control 173.51 μg/kg.

6.6.3 Acids and Solvents

Propionic acid is added as a preservative to the barley in order to prevent fungal contamination and further CIT production by those fungi (Gupta et al. 2018). Response surface methodology is an extraction technique of CIT where phosphate (1.5%) – ethanol (45%) extractant solvent was utilized for removing 91.6% CIT from red mold rice within 70 minutes (Lee et al. 2007). Exogenous ascorbic acid (EAA) is water-soluble antioxidant, scavenges the damaging oxidants and manages oxidative stress as CIT biosynthesis from *M. ruber* was highly induced by the oxidative stress condition. Therefore, addition of 16 mg/L of EAA to culture media has reduced the CIT yield by 67% (Wei et al. 2022). Even addition of ethidium dibromide tetra acetic acid (EDTA) completely inhibited CIT production by *Aspergillus oryzae* and *A. niger* due to its chelating nature as EDTA binds to the metal ions such as Zn^{+2}, Fe^{+2}, and Mn^{+2} required for the growth of these fungi.

6.6.4 Flavonoids

Huang et al. (2019) found that addition of 15 g/L of troxerutin flavonoid to liquid fermentation media with low-starch peptone reduced CIT yield by 87.9% 14 days post fermentation of *Monascus aurantiacus* Li AS3.4384 (MALA) culture. Genistein is also another major soy isoflavonoid that has antioxidant and anticancer properties. Addition of this compound during fermentation has affected glutamic acid pathway, pyruvate synthesis pathway, aspartic acid, tricarboxylic acid (TCA) cycle, and lysine degradation pathway which in turn contributed to reduction of CIT from *Monascus* because of change in the precursor needed for CIT biosynthesis (He et al. 2020).

6.6.5 Ammonium Salts

Ammonium sulfate and ammonium nitrate completely destroyed CIT as both ammonium salts decrease the pH of the media dropped to 4.3 and 4.8, respectively, which automatically reduced the toxin synthesis as both are positively correlated (Gu et al. 2021).

6.7 Biological Control Measures Against Citrinin

Microorganisms as detoxification activity:

6.7.1 Fungal Bioagents

Biological control measures are environmentally friendly and reliable methods which make use of several microorganisms such as *T. hamatum* decreasing CIT content (45–100%) in the rice grain through the drop in the viability of *Penicillium viridicatum* and lysis by cell wall lytic enzymes (Ezzat and Abd-Allah 2005; Prasad et al. 2010).

6.7.2 Bacterial Bioagents

R. borbori PS45 reduced the CIT concentration up to 60–65% (Kanpiengjai et al. 2015). Wallace et al. (2017) explained the antifungal activity of *Pseudomonas fluorescens* against *P. expansum* causing blue mold decay on the apple fruits as it minimized the decay incidence through mechanism of nutrients and space competition, release of growth inhibitory metabolites which mainly targets the conidial germination and mycelia inhibition. Another investigation was carried out by Mohammadi et al. (2017) to evaluate the antifungal activity of *Bacillus subtilis* and *Agrobacterium radiobacter* against *Penicillium digitatum* on lemon fruits. They found that the disease severity was diminished due to inhibition of mycelial growth and conidial germination resulting from the cell wall lytic enzymes such as chitinase and glucanase. *Gluconobacter oxydans* has a positive role in suppressing CIT content as both viable and heat-treated *G. oxydans* cells can bind to CIT from a liquid medium and eliminates 32.6% and 26.4% toxins, respectively (Markov et al. 2019). Plant growth-promoting bacteria plays a major role in degradation of mycotoxins like patulin, aflatoxins, fumonisin, and trichothecene associated with food and feed (Sreenivasa et al. 2011a; Chennappa et al. 2014, 2016; Nagaraja et al. 2016).

6.7.3 Yeast

Saccharomyces cerevisiae has the ability to decrease the level of CIT from 1.1–35.5 ppb to 0.8–30 ppb in flour within 48 hours (Azizi et al. 2014). Heat-treated *S. cerevisiae* (10^5 cells/mL) at 121 °C has reduced 98% CIT content from *Monascus purpurea* as the common yeast is having binding ability to several toxins through adsorption process where the cell wall components such as glucans and proteins involved in provision of numerous easily accessible binding sites to CIT (Moghdam et al. 2019).

Rhodotorula mucilaginosa orange pigmented yeast was also efficient in degrading 91.61% CIT *in vitro* as it hindered the growth of *P. digitatum* (Ahima et al. 2019) due to their fast proliferation ability, rapid colonization, and production of huge extracellular matrix, which helps in survival for longer duration, and quick host nutrient utilization capacity makes them compete with pathogens. Hence, all these parameters contribute for yeast to be a good biocontrol agent (Richard and Prusky 2002). Zhang et al. (2019) recorded antagonistic yeast *Wickerhamomyces anomalus* against blue mold *Penicillium* decay of pears as it reduced spore germination and germ tube length, hence minimizing disease incidence to 5.56% in pears treated with 1×10^8 cells/mL, as compared with 100% disease occurrence in the control. Another novel antagonist yeast *Yarrowia lipolytica* exhibited bioprotection ability against grapes decay incited by *Penicillium rubens*. They found that this yeast has a positive role in reducing disease incidence through restraining spore germination, and germ tube elongation and also activated pathogen defense-related gene expression in fruits (Wang et al. 2019). The combined action of activated charcoal (0.4%) and lyophilized yeast culture (0.2%) were effective in ameliorating the impact of CIT on blood parameters (Priyadarshini and Narasareddy 2010).

6.7.4 Natural Essential Oils

Neem leaf extract (3.12 mg/mL) was efficient in reduction of CIT production by up to 80% as it retarded the *P. citrinum* growth (Mossini and Kemmelmeier 2008; Yooussef et al. 2016). The essential oil (150 ppm) obtained from *Z. multiflora* Boiss significantly concealed the mycelial growth (88.6%) and CIT production (89.6%) of *P. citrinum* (Mohajeri et al. 2018). The mint aqueous solution has inhibited up to 73% CIT production by *P. citrinum* (Sreenivasa et al. 2011b; Panda et al. 2018; Deepa and Sreenivasa 2019a, b; Achar et al. 2020).

6.8 Detoxification/Degradation/Binding Methods of Citrinin

6.8.1 Hydrogen Peroxide (H_2O_2)

CIT was completely detoxified by prior incubation with 0.05% hydrogen peroxide (H_2O_2) at room temperature for 30 minutes and upon heating CIT at 100 °C, it will form some toxic molecules which can be further detoxified upon reheating with it with H_2O_2 (Fouler et al. 1994) as it is a strong oxidizing agent resulting in generation of ROS and OH^{-1} radicals, which affects fungal respiratory mechanism leading to death.

6.8.2 Probiotics

CIT content in white maize was degraded completely during fermenting for 72 hours as the toxin was bound on the peptidoglycan surface of *Pediococcus acidilactici* and *Lactobacillus paraplantarum* along with the acidic condition created by these bacteria which also has harsh effect on fungal growth (Okeke et al. 2015).

6.8.3 Magnetic Nanoparticles

They are well known as "surface active maghemite nanoparticles" (SAMNs) and are an efficient and reliable means for CIT removal (70%) from Monascus-treated foods because the chelating properties of CIT toward iron (III) atoms on the SAMNs were exploited for the recognition and magnetic removal of CIT (Magro et al. 2016).

6.8.4 Chitosan

It is a bioactive, non-toxic polymer made up of 3-1, 4 glucosamine obtained from the chitin in crustacean shell wastes. It could be utilized as an alternative application for managing seed-borne *Penicillium* in lentils as it has antifungal activities and activates plant defense responses. This compound even interferes with negatively charged macromolecule residues present on the fungal cell surface resulting in alteration of permeability of plasma membranes. It completely destroyed CIT on lentil seeds stored for six months (Abd-Allah and Hashem 2006). Further, Coutinho et al. (2020) employed chitosan antifungal edible coating for postharvest preservation of oranges obtained from deacetylation of chitin which is produced from crustacean-processing waste as a promising tool for managing 50–70% of *P. citrinum* growth in orange fruits due to its antimicrobial nature, enhancing the shelf-life of the commodity through reduced respiration rate and water loss.

6.8.5 Enzymes

Manganese peroxidase (MnP) obtained from *Moniliophthora roreri* is a special heme-containing peroxidase which oxidizes phenolic lignin molecules via direct interaction or indirectly with the help of Mn^{+3} elements. Chemically, CIT consists of phenolic hydroxyl group which acts as a substrate for MnP. Therefore, upon action of this enzyme, CIT is converted into less toxic compound, i.e. dihydrocitrinone. The treatment of MnP to red yeast rice degraded CIT completely within 72 hours (Wang et al. 2022).

6.9 Summary

CIT is a potent and powerful mycotoxin synthesized by the ubiquitous fungal genera *Penicillium*, *Aspergillus*, and *Monascus*, which readily contaminate many agricultural food and feed commodities across the world. CIT mainly targets kidney, liver, and cytosol as well as acts as a skin irritant even though it is also having carcinogenic properties. In order to eliminate CIT contamination from food and feed, various management measures including physical, chemical, biological, and detoxification methods were employed. Each method has its own specialty as physical measures include thermal, light, and pressure application; on the contrary, chemical measures utilize various fungicides, flavinoids, ascorbic acid, and ozone to combat CIT contamination. However, the biological tactics are environmentally friendly and highly reliable, which make use of some fungal and bacterial biocontrol agents along with plant extracts that are being exploited for reducing and degrading the toxin. Recent advanced strategies including cold plasmas, ozone treatment, magnetic nanoparticles, flavinoids, EAA, EDTA, MnP, HPAS treatment, and chitosan application are explained in this chapter.

6.10 Future Implications

- Future studies should concentrate on development of advanced CIT detoxification methods with higher efficacy.
- Essential for the development of detailed degradation mechanisms for citrinin.
- More emphasis should be given to the advanced biological degradation approaches.

6.11 Study Questions

1) Write the physicochemical properties of CIT.
2) What are the harmful effects of CIT on humans?
3) Write the mode of action of baker's yeast on CIT degradation.
4) What are SAMNs and how do they control CIT?
5) How do cold plasmas detoxify CIT?

Acknowledgments

The authors thank for the support given by one and all on successful completion of the chapter.

Conflict of Interest

The authors confirm that they have no conflict of interest.

Author Contributions

Conceptualization and editing: A. K. and S. A. S.; Writing and review: R. M. and A. K.; Supervision: N. M. K.

References

Abd-Allah, E.E. and Hashem, A. (2006). Seed mycoflora of *Lens esculenta* and their biocontrol by chitosan. *Phytoparasitica* 34 (2): 213–218.

Abdelhamid, A.M. and Dorra, T.M. (1990). Study on the effects of feeding hens on mycotoxins (aflatoxin, patulin or citrinin)-contaminated diets on the egg quality and tissue constituents. *Arch. Anim. Nutr.* 40: 305–316.

Achar, P.N., Quyen, P., Adukwu, E.C. et al. (2020). Investigation of the antifungal and anti-aflatoxigenic potential of plant-based essential oils against *Aspergillus flavus* in peanuts. *J. Fungi* 6 (4): 383.

Aghdam, M.S., Jannatizadeh, A., Luo, Z., and Paliyath, G. (2018). Ensuring sufficient intracellular ATP supplying and friendly extracellular ATP signaling attenuates stresses, delays senescence and maintains quality in horticultural crops during postharvest life. *Trends Food Sci. Technol.* 76: 67–81.

Ahamad, D.B. and Vairamuthu, S. (2000). Occurrence of citrinin mycotoxin in compounded feeds and various feed ingredients of poultry ration in Nammakal area (Tamil Nadu). *Indian J. Environ. Toxicol.* 10 (2): 84–86.

Ahima, J., Zhang, H., Apaliya, M.T. et al. (2019). The effect of Rhodotorula mucilaginosa on degradation of citrinin production by *Penicillium digitatum* and its toxin *in vitro*. *J. Food Measure. Character.* 13: 2998–3004.

Alexander, J., Benford, D., Boobis, A. et al. (2012). Scientific opinion on the risks for public and animal health related to the presence of citrinin in food and feed. *EFSA J.* 10 (3): 1–82.

Arai, M. and Hibino, T. (1983). Tumorigenicity of citrinin in male F344 rats. *Cancer Lett.* 17: 281–287.

Awuchi, C.G., Nwozo, O.S., Aja, P.M., and Odongo, G.A. (2023). High pressure acidified steaming with varied citric acid dosing can successfully detoxify mycotoxins. *Food Sci. Nutr.* 11: 1–9.

Azizi, I.G., Gorgi, M., Rouhi, S. et al. (2014). Effect of *Saccharomyces cerevisiae* yeast in reducing of amount of citrinin fungal toxin in wheat flour. *Iran Public Health* 43 (2): 241–247.

Berndt, W.O., Hayes, A.W., and Phillips, R.D. (1980). Effects of mycotoxins on renal function: mycotoxic nephropathy. *Kidney Int.* 18: 656–664.

Blanc, P.J., Laussac, J.P., Le, B.J. et al. (1995). Characterization of monascidin a from *Monascus* as citrinin. *Int. J. Food Microbiol.* 27: 201–213.

Brown, T.P., Manning, R.O., Fletcher, O.J., and Wyatt, R.D. (1986). The individual and combined effects of citrinin and ochratoxin a on renal ultrastructure in layer chicks. *Avian Dis.* 30: 191–198.

Chang, C.H., Yu, F.Y., Wu, T.S. et al. (2010). Mycotoxin citrinin induced cell cycle G2/M arrest and numerical chromosomal abberrations associated with distruption of microtubule formation in human cells. *Toxicol. Sci.* 119 (1): 84–92.

Chennappa, G., Adkar-Purushothama, C.R., Suraj, U. et al. (2014). Impact of pesticides on PGPR activity of *Azotobacter* sp. isolated from pesticide flooded paddy soils. *Greener J. Agric. Sci.* 4 (4): 117–129.

Chennappa, G., Naik, M.K., Adkar-Purushothama, C.R. et al. (2016). PGP, abiotic stress tolerant and antifungal activity of *Azotobacter* sp. isolated from paddy soils. *Indian J. Exp. Biol.* 54 (5): 322–331.

Choudhari, A.K. and Kumar, P. (2010). Management of mycotoxin contamination in preharvest and postharvest crops: present status and future perspective. *J. Phytol.* 2: 37–52.

Clark, B.R., Capon, R.J., Lacey, E. et al. (2006). Citrinin revisited: from monomers to dimers and beyond. *Org. Biomol. Chem.* 4: 1520–1528.

Cornelia, L.F. (2012). *Aspergillus terreus*: how inoculum size and host characteristics affects its virulence. *J. Infect. Dis.* 205 (8): 1192–1194.

Coutinho, T.C., Ferreira, M.C., Rose, L.H. et al. (2020). *Penicillium citrinum* and *P. mallochii*: new phytopathogens of orange fruits and their control using chitosan. *Carbohydr. Polym.* 15: 234–244.

Deepa, N. and Sreenivasa, M.Y. (2017a). *Fusarium verticillioides*, a globally important pathogen of agriculture and livestock: a review. *J Vet. Med. Res.* 4 (4): 1084.

Deepa, N. and Sreenivasa, M.Y. (2017b). Fumonisins: a review on its global occurrence, epidemiology, toxicity and detection. *J. Vet. Med. Res.* 4 (6): 1093.

Deepa, N. and Sreenivasa, M.Y. (2019a). Biocontrol strategies for effective management of phytopathogenic fungi associated with cereals. In: *New and Future Developments in Microbial Biotechnology and Bioengineering* (ed. J.S. Singh and D.P. Singh), 177–189. Elsevier. ISBN: 9780444641915 10.1016/B978-0-444-64191-5.00013-4.

Deepa, N. and Sreenivasa, M.Y. (2019b). Molecular methods and key genes targeted for the detection of fumonisin producing *Fusarium verticillioides* - an updated review. *Food Biosci.* 32: 100473. https://doi.org/10.1016/j.fbio.2019.100473.

Deepa, N., Nagaraja, H., and Sreenivasa, M.Y. (2016a). Prevalence of fumonisin producing *Fusarium verticillioides* associated with cereals grown in Karnataka (India). *Food Sci. Human Well.* 5: 156–162. https://doi.org/10.1016/j.fshw.2016.07.001.

Deepa, N., Charith Raj, A.P., and Sreenivasa, M.Y. (2016b). Multiplex PCR method for the early detection of fumonisin producing *Fusarium verticillioides*. *Food Biosci.* 13: 84–88.

Deepa, N., Achar, P.N., and Sreenivasa, M.Y. (2021). Current perspectives of biocontrol agents for management of *Fusarium verticillioides* and its Fumonisin in cereals—a review. *J. Fungi* 7: 776. https://doi.org/10.3390/jof7090776.

Dogra, P. and Kumar, D. (2017). Characterization of *Monascus purpureus* isolated from red yeast rice and its evaluation for the production of cholesterol lowering lovastatin. *Biol. Forum Int. J.* 9 (1): 70–76.

Donmez-Altuntas, H., Dumlupinar, G., Imamoglu, N. et al. (2007). Effects of the mycotoxin citrinin on micronucleus formation in a cytokinesis-block genotoxicity assay in cultured human lymphocytes. *J. Appl. Toxicol.* 27: 337–341.

Doughari, S.H. (2015). The occurrence, properties and significance of citrinin mycotoxin. *J. Plant Pathol. Microbiol.* 6 (11): 1–6.

Dunn, B.B. and Friendman, L. (1994). Distribution and metabolism of citrinin: a review. *Biodegr. Res.* 4: 27–40.

Durek, J., Schluter, O., Roscher, A. et al. (2018). Inhibition or stimulation of ochratoxin a synthesis on inoculated barley triggered by diffuse coplanar surface barrier discharge plasma. *Front. Microbiol.* 9: 1–9.

Ezzat, S.M. and Abd-Allah, E.F. (2005). Natural occurrence of citrinin in rice grains and biocontrol of its producing fungus by *Trichoderma hamatum*. *Phtoparasitica* 33: 73–84.

Flajs, D. and Peraica, M. (2009). Toxicological properties of citrinin. *Arh. High Rada Toksikol.* 60: 457–464.

Fouler, S.G., Trivedi, A.B., and Kitabatake, N. (1994). Detoxification of citrinin and ochratoxin a by hydrogen peroxide. *J. AOAC Int.* 77 (3): 631–637.

Friis, P., Hasslager, E., and Krogh, P. (1969). Isolation of citrinin and oxallic acid from *Penicillium veridicatum* westling and their nephrotoxicity in rats and pigs. *Acta Pathol. Microbiol. Scand.* 77 (3): 559–560.

Griffiths, I.B. and Done, S.H. (1991). Citrinin as a possible cause of the pruritis, pyrexia, haemorrhagic syndrome in cattle. *Vet. Rec.* 129 (6): 113–117.

Gu, S., Chen, Z., Wang, F., and Wang, X. (2021). Characterization and inhibition of four fungi producing citrini in various culture media. *Biotechnol. Lett.* 43: 701–710.

Gupta, R.C., Srivastava, A., and Lall, R. (2018). Ochratoxins and citrinin. *Vet. Toxicol.* 72: 1019–1027.

Hanika, C., Carlton, W.W., Boon, G.D., and Tuite, J. (1984). Citrinin mycotoxicosis in the rabbit: clinicopathologic alterations. *Food Chern. Toxicol.* 22: 999–1008.

He, Y. and Cox, R.J. (2016). The molecular steps of citrinin biosynthesis in fungi. *Chem. Sci.* 7 (3): 2119–2127.

He, S., Liu, X., Wang, Y. et al. (2020). Metabolomics analysis based on UHPLC-Q-TOF-MS/MS reveals effects of genistein on reducing mycotoxin citrinin production by *Monascus aurantiacus* Li AS3.4384. *Food Sci. Technol.* 130: 1–8.

Hetherington, A.C. and Raistrick, H. (1931). Biochemistry of micro-organisms. XIV. Production and chemical constitution of a new yellow coloring matter, citrinin, produced from dextrose by *Penicillium citrinum* Thon. *Philos. Trans. R. Soc. Lond., Series B* 220: 269.

Huang, Z., Zhang, L., Wang, Y. et al. (2019). Effects of rutin and its derivatives on citrinin production by *Monascus aurantiacus* Li AS3.4384 in liquid fermentation using different types of media. *Food Chem.* 284: 205–212.

Jeswal, P. and Kumar, D. (2015). Mycobiota and natural incidence of aflatoxins, ochratoxin a and citrinin in Indian spices confirmed by LC-MS/MS. *Int. J. Microbiol.* 3: 1–8.

Kanpiengjai, A., Mahawan, R., and Khanongnuch, C. (2015). A soil bacterium *Rhizobium borbori* and its potential for citrinin degrading application. *Ann. Microbiol.* 66: 807–816.

Karlovasky, P., Suman, M., Berthiller, F. et al. (2016). Impact of food processing and detoxification treatments on mycotoxin contamination. *Mycotoxin Res.* 32: 179–205.

Kitchen, D.O., Carlton, W.W., and Hinsman, E.J. (1977). Ochratoxin a and citrinin induced nephrosis in beagle dogs, terminal renal ultrastructure alterations. *Vet. Pathol.* 14 (4): 392–406.

Kumar, M., Dwivedi, P., Sharma, A.K. et al. (2007). Ochratoxin a and citrinin nephrotoxicity in New Zealand white rabbits: an ultrastructural assesment. *Mycopathologia* 163: 21–30.

Lee, C.L., Chen, W.P., Wang, J.J., and Pan, T.M. (2007). A simple and rapid method for removing citrininwhile retaining monocolin K in red mold rice. *J. Agric. Food Chem.* 55: 11101–11108.

Lloyd, W.E. (1980). Citrinin and ochratoxin toxicosis in cattle in United States. *Proc. 2nd Symp. Vet. Lab. Diagnost.* 25: 435–439.

Magan, N. and Lacey, J. (1986). The phylloplane microbial populations of wheat and effect of late fungicide applications. *Ann. Appl. Biol.* 109: 117–128.

Magro, M., Moritz, D.E., Bonaiuto, E. et al. (2016). Citrinin mycotoxin recognition and removal by naked magnetic nanoparticles. *Food Chem.* 203: 503–512.

Markov, K., Frece, J., Pleadin, J. et al. (2019). *Gluconobacter oxydans* - potential biological agent for binding or biotransformation of mycotoxins. *World Mycotoxin J.* 12 (2): 153–161.

Mehdi, N.A.Q., Carlton, W.W., Boon, G.D., and Tuite, J. (1984). Studies on the sequential development and pathogenesis of citrinin mycotoxicosis in turkeys and ducklings. *Vet. Pathol.* 21: 216–223.

Meyden, I., Bilici, M., Turan, E., and Zengin, A. (2021). Selective extraction and determination of citrinin in rey samples by a molecularly imprinted polymers (MIP) using reversible addition fragmentation chain transfer precipitation polymerization (RAFTTP) with high performance liquid chromatography (HPLC) detection. *Anal. Lett.* 54: 1697–1708.

Milani, J.M. (2013). Ecological conditions affecting mycotoxin production in cereals: a review. *Vet. Med.* 58 (8): 405–411.

Mirocha, C.J. and Christensen, C.M. (1974). Fungus metabolites toxic to animals. *Ann. Rev. Phytopathol.* 12: 303–330.

Moghadam, D.H., Shahid, F., Yazdi, T.F. et al. (2019). Biological detoxification of *Monascus purpureus* pigments by heat treated *Saccharomyces cerevisiae*. *J. Food Sci. Agric.* 99 (9): 4439–4444.

Mohajeri, F.A., Misaghi, A., Gheisari, H. et al. (2018). The effect of *Zataria multiflora* Boiss essential oil on the growth and citrinin production by *Penicillium citrinum* in culture media and mozerella cheese. *Food Chem. Toxicol.* 118: 691–694.

Mohammadi, P., Tozlu, E., Kotan, R., and Kotan Senol, M. (2017). Potential of some bacteria for biological control of postharvest citrus green mould caused by *Penicillium digitatum*. *Plant Protect. Sci.* 53: 1–10.

Mossini, S.A.G. and Kemmelmeier, C. (2008). Inhibition of citrinin production in *Penicillium citrinum* cultures by neem [*Azadiractin indica* A. Juss (Meliaceae)]. *Int. J. Mol. Sci.* 9 (9): 1676–1684.

Nagaraja, H., Chennappa, G., Poorna Chandra Rao, K. et al. (2016). Diversity of toxic and phytopathogenic *Fusarium* species occurring on cereals grown in Karnataka state, India. *3 Biotech* 6: 57.

Neme, K. and Mohammed, A. (2017). Mycotoxin occurrence in grains and the role of post harvest management as a mitigation stratergies. A review. *Food Control* 78: 412–425.

Okeke, E.C.N., Nwangburuka, C.C., Sulyok, M. et al. (2015). Bacterial diversity and mycotoxin reduction during maize fermentation (steeping) for ogi production. *Front. Microbiol.* 6: 1–12.

Pan, T.M. and Hsu, W.H. (2014). Monascus-fermented products. *Encyclo. Food Microbiol.* 2: 815–825.

Panda, P., Aika, V., and Mehta, A. (2018). Effect of aqueous extracts of *Mentha arvensis* (mint) and *Piper betle* (betel) on the growth and citrinin production from toxigenic *Penicillium citrinum*. *J. Food Sci. Technol.* 52: 3466–3474.

Pitt, J.I. (1979). *The Genus Penicillium and its Telomorphic States Eupenicillium and Talaromyces*, 1–634. London: Academic.

Poupke, R., Luz, Z., and Destro, R. (1997). Carbon-13 NMR of citrinin in the solid state and solutions. *J. Phys. Chem.* 101 (28): 5097–5102.

Prasad, M.N.N., Shankara Bhat, S., and Sreenivasa, M.Y. (2010). Antifungal activity of essential oils against *Phomopsis azadirachtae*- the causative agent of die-back disease of neem. *J. Agric. Technol.* 6 (1): 127–133.

Priyadarshini, C.H. and Narasareddy, G.V. (2010). Amelioration of toxic effects of aflatoxin and citrinin by adsorbents in broilers. *Indian Vet. J.* 87 (1): 23–25.

Richard, W.J. and Prusky, D. (2002). Expression of an antifungal peptide in *Saccharomyces*, a new approach for biological control of the postharvest disease caused by *Colletotrichum coccodes*. *Phytopathology* 92: 33–37.

Roberts, W.T. and Mora, E.C. (1978). Toxicity of *Penicillium citrinum* AUA-532 contaminated corn and citrinin in broiler chicks. *Poult. Sci.* 57: 1221–1226.

Savi, G.D., Piacentini, K.C., and Scussel, V.M. (2015). Ozone treatment efficiency in *Aspergillus* and *Penicillium* growth inhibition and mycotoxin degradation of stored wheat grains (*Triticum aestivum* L.). *J. Food Process Preserv.* 39 (6): 940–948.

Schmidt-Heydt, M., Cramer, B., Graf, I. et al. (2012). Wavelength-dependant degradation of ochratoxin and citrinin by light in vitro and in vivo and its implications on *Penicillium*. *Toxins* 4: 1535–1551.

Schmidt-Heydt, M., Stoll, D., and Geisen, R. (2013). Fungicides effectively used for growth inhibition of several fungi could induce mycotoxin biosynthesis in toxigenic species. *Int. J. Food Microbiol.* 166: 407–412.

Silva, L.J.G., Pereira, A.M.P.T., Pena, A., and Lino, C.M. (2021). Citrinin in foods and suppliments: a review of occurrence and analytical methodologies. *Foods* 10 (1): 1–33.

Sinha, R.N. (1971). Fungus as food for some stored product insect. *J. Econ. Entom.* 64: 3–6.

So-Jeo, A., Seok-Young, J., Man-Su, L. et al. (2007). Canine renal failure caused by ochratoxin a and citrinin in the commercial dog food. *J. Vet. Clin.* 24 (2): 82–87.

Soumya, R.S., Warke, V.G., Mahajan, G.B. et al. (2022). Isolation and identification of *Penicillium citrinum* strains from the leaves of *Fragaria xananassa* cultivated by nutrient film technique. *Acta Sci. Microbiol.* 5 (6): 28–33.

Sreenivasa, M.Y., Dass, R.S., Charith Raj, A.P., and Janardhana, G.R. (2008). PCR-based detection of genus *Fusarium* and Fumonisin-producing isolates from freshly harvested sorghum grains grown in Karnataka, India. *J. Food Saf.* 28: 236–237.

Sreenivasa, M.Y., Dass, R.S., Charith Raj, A.P., and Janardhana, G.R. (2011a). Mycological evaluation of maize grains produced in Karnataka (India) for the post-harvest fungal contamination. *World Appl. Sci. J.* 13 (4): 688–692.

Sreenivasa, M.Y., Dass, R.S., Charith Raj, A.P. et al. (2011b). Assessment of the growth inhibiting effect of some plant essential oils on different *Fusarium* species isolated from sorghum and maize grains. *J. Plant Dis. Protect.* 118 (6): 208–213.

Stormer, F.C. and Hoiby, E.A. (1996). Citrinin, ochratoxin a and iron. Possible implications for their biological function and induction of nephropathy. *Mycopathologia* 134: 103–107.

Sweeney, M.J. and Dobson, A.D.W. (1998). Mycotoxin production by *Aspergillus*, *Fusarium* and *Penicillium* species. *Int. J. Food Microbiol.* 43: 141–158.

Szczech, G.M., Carlton, W.W., and Lund, J.E. (1974). Determination of enzyme concentration in urine for diagnosis of renal damage. *J. Am. Anim. Hosp. Assoc.* 10: 171–174.

Thacker, H.L., Carlton, W.W., and Sansing, G.A. (1977). Citrinin mycotoxicosis in the Guinea pig. *Food Cosmet. Toxicol.* 15: 553–561.

Tokusoglu, O., Alpas, H., and Bozoglu, F. (2010). High hydrostatic pressure effects on mold flora, citrinin mycotoxin, hydroxytyrosol, oleuropein, phenolics and antioxident activity of black table olives. *Innov. Food Sci. Emerg. Technol.* 11: 250–258.

Tuomi, T., Reijula, K., Johnson, T. et al. (2000). Mycotoxins in crude building materials from water damaged buildings. *Appl. Environ. Microbiol.* 66: 1899–1904.

Vaseghi, N., Bayat, M., Nosrati, A.C. et al. (2017). Plasma jet impacts on citrinin production in isolates belonging to *Penicillium* spp. *Int. J. Mol. Clin. Microbiol.* 7 (2): 875–889.

Vella, F., Kpodo, K., Sorensen, A.K., and Jokebson, M. (1995). The occurrence of mycotoxins in fermented maize products. *Food Chem.* 56: 147–153.

Wallace, R.L., Hirkala, D.L., and Nelson, L.M. (2017). Postharvest biological control of blue mold of apple by *Pseudomonas fluorescens* during commercial storage and potential modes of action. *Postharvest Biol. Tec.* 133: 1–11.

Wang, M., Jiang, N., Xian, H. et al. (2016). A single-step solid phase extraction for the simultaneous detection of eight mycotoxins in fruits by ultra-high performance liquid chromatography-tandem mass spectrometry. *J. Chromatogr. A* 1429: 22–29.

Wang, M., Zhao, L., Zhang, X. et al. (2019). Study on biocontrol of postharvest decay of table grapes caused by *Penicillium rubens* and the possible resistance mechanisms by *Yarrowia lipolytica*. *Biol. Control* 130: 110–117.

Wang, S., Wang, X., Huang, H. et al. (2022). Detoxification of the mycotoxin citrinin by a manganese peroxidase from *Moniliophthora roreri*. *Toxins* 14: 1–11.

Wei, S., He, Y., Yang, J. et al. (2022). Effects of exogenous ascorbic acid on the yields of citrinin and pigments, antioxidant capacities and fatty acid composition of *Monascus ruber*. *Food Sci. Technol.* 154: 1–7.

Wichmann, G., Herbarth, O., and Lehmann, I. (2002). The mycotoxins citrinin, gliotoxin and patulin affect interferon-γ rather than interleukin-4 production in human blood cells. *Environ. Toxicol.* 17: 211–218.

Witlock, D.R., Wyatt, R.D., and Ruff, M.D. (1977). Morphological changes in the avian intestine induced by citrinin and lack of effect of aflatoxin and T-2 toxin as seen with scanning electron microscopy. *Toxicon* 15: 41–44.

Wu, Y., Zhang, N., Li, Y.H. et al. (2017). Citrinin exposure affects oocyte maturation and embryo development by inducing oxidative stress-mediated apoptosis. *Oncotarget* 8: 34525–34533.

Yasemin Aydin, Y., Yilmaz, B.O., Yildizbayrak, N. et al. (2021). Evaluation of citrinin-induced toxic effects on mouse Sertoli cells. *Drug Chem. Toxicol.* 44 (6): 559–565.

Yooussef, M.M., Pham, Q., Achar, P.N., and Sreenivasa, M.Y. (2016). Antifungal activity of essential oils on *Aspergillus parasiticus* isolated from peanuts. *J. Plant Protect. Res.* 56 (2): 139–142. https://doi.org/10.1515/jppr-2016-0021.

Zhang, X., Lin, Z., Apaliya, M.T. et al. (2017). The possible mechanisms involved in citrinin elimination by *Cryptococcus podzolicus* Y3 and the effects of extrinsic factors on the degradation of citrinin. *J. Microbiol. Biotechnol.* 27 (12): 2119–2128.

Zhang, Q., Zhao, L., Li, Z. et al. (2019). Screening and identification of an antagonistic yeast controlling postharvest blue mold decay of pears and the possible mechanisms involved. *Biol. Control* 133: 26–33.

Zhang, H., Ahima, J., Yang, Q. et al. (2021). A review on citrinin: its occurrence, risk implications, analytical techniques, biosynthesis, physiochemical properties and control. *Food Res. Int.* 141: 1–16.

Further Reading

Dunn, B.B. and Friendman, L. (1994). Distribution and metabolism of citrinin: a review. *Biodegr. Res.* 4: 27–40.

Mehdi, N.A.Q., Carlton, W.W., Boon, G.D., and Tuite, J. (1984). Studies on the sequential development and pathogenesis of citrinin mycotoxicosis in turkeys and ducklings. *Vet. Pathol.* 21: 216–223.

Neme, K. and Mohammed, A. (2017). Mycotoxin occurrence in grains and the role of post-harvest management as mitigation strategies. A review. *Food Control* 78: 412–425.

7

Detoxification and Control Strategies of Zearalenone in Food and Feed

Rouaa Daou[1], André El Khoury[1], and Ali Atoui[2]

[1] *Centre d'Analyses et de Recherche (CAR), Unité de Recherche Technologies et Valorisation Agro-Alimentaire (UR-TVA), Faculty of Sciences, Saint-Joseph University of Beirut, Campus of Sciences and Technologies, Mar Roukos, Lebanon*
[2] *Laboratory of Microbiology, Department of Life and Earth Sciences, Faculty of Sciences, Hadath Campus, Lebanese University, Beirut, Lebanon*

CONTENTS

Abstract

Zearalenone is a mycotoxin produced by *Fusarium* species that contaminates cereal products used for food and feed such as maize, wheat, oats, and barley. Zearalenone is an estrogenic mycotoxin that can lead to several health problems including decreased reproduction in livestock causing economic losses. Zearalenone is a resistant and heat-stable molecule and its complete removal from food and feed is unachievable. Hence, control measures should be applied throughout the whole food chain. Nonetheless, decontamination processes that are

Anti-Mycotoxin Strategies for Food and Feed, First Edition. Edited by Deepa Nagaraju, Sreenivasa Marikunte Yanjarappa, Premila N. Achar, and Angel Medina Vaya.

discussed in this chapter have been established including physical, chemical, and biological ones. Physical decontamination includes removal of Zearalenone through physical degradation methods, while chemical methods involve the usage of strong oxidants or chemicals to inactivate the mycotoxin's structure. However, both physical and chemical methods can negatively affect food quality. Therefore, biological methods can be adopted by using microorganisms and enzymes to degrade Zearalenone.

Keywords *Zearalenone, physical, chemical, biological, decontamination*

Graphical Representation

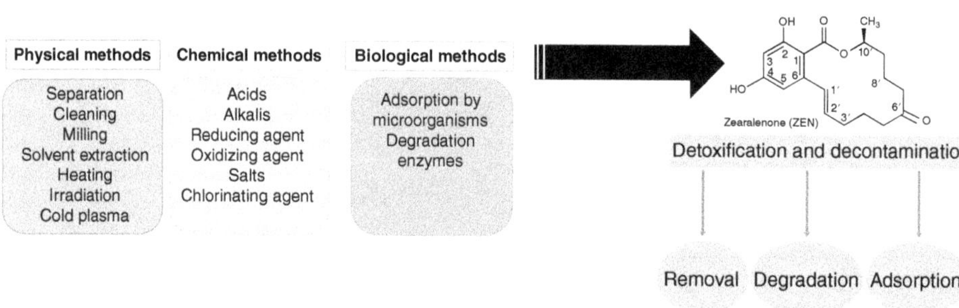

7.1 Introduction

Zearalenone (ZEN) is a non-steroidal estrogenic mycotoxin produced by *Fusarium* species including *Fusarium graminearum* spp. *complex*, *Fusarium culmorum*, *Fusarium cerealis*, *Fusarium equiseti*, *Fusarium crookwellense*, *Fusarium semitectum*, *Fusarium sporotrichioides*, *Fusarium oxysporum*, and *Fusarium acuminatum* (Zinedine et al. 2007; Deepa and Sreenivasa 2017a; Ropejko and Twarużek 2021). *Fusarium* that are known as soil fungi are affected by environmental conditions and are typically frequent in temperate and warm climates as their invasion and development are promoted by temperatures ranging from 20 to 30 °C and by a high relative humidity of 90% (Stanciu et al. 2019). *Fusarium* fungi are also promoted by weather conditions, mainly rainfall, during and after flowering. So, ZEN mostly occurs in high-moisture crops during late autumn and winter (Bianchini and Bullerman 2014; Stanciu et al. 2019). ZEN is mostly produced in crops on field. However, it might occur post-harvest specifically if the crops were not dried properly before storage (Zinedine et al. 2007). Mainly, it contaminates maize and can be found in other crops such as oats, barley, wheat, sorghum, rice, and rye (Zinedine et al. 2007; Gil-Serna et al. 2014). ZEN has also been detected in some food products such as flour, chocolate, bread, oil, milk, and others (Deepa and Sreenivasa 2017b; Rogowska et al. 2019).

ZEN is a resorcyclic acid lactone with a chemical formula of $C_{18}H_{22}O_5$ that resembles and is similar to natural estrogen structure such as 17β-estradiol (Rogowska et al. 2019; Kailasa et al. 2020; Wu et al. 2021). In other words, ZEN belongs to the family of xenoestrogens that can act in a manner that imitates estrogen *in vivo* and initiate chemical reactions the way those hormones do, or block hormonal receptors which disrupt the function of natural estrogen. Hence, ZEN can act as endocrine-disrupting compound in a way according to Rogowska et al. (2019) that "disrupts secretion, synthesis, metabolism, transport, or the action of endogenous hormones responsible for homeostasis, growth, and reproduction" (Rogowska et al. 2019). This disruption in the hormonal balance caused *in vivo* can lead to infertility and different diseases of the reproductive system (Rogowska et al. 2019; Wu et al. 2021). Different studies have also reported the ability of ZEN to bind to mammary gland receptors causing breast cancer (Minervini et al. 2005; Yu et al. 2005; Wu et al. 2021). Exposure to ZEN can also cause other health effects since it was reported to be immunotoxic, genotoxic, teratogenic, carcinogenic, hematotoxic, and hepatotoxic (Bai et al. 2017) (Figure 7.1).

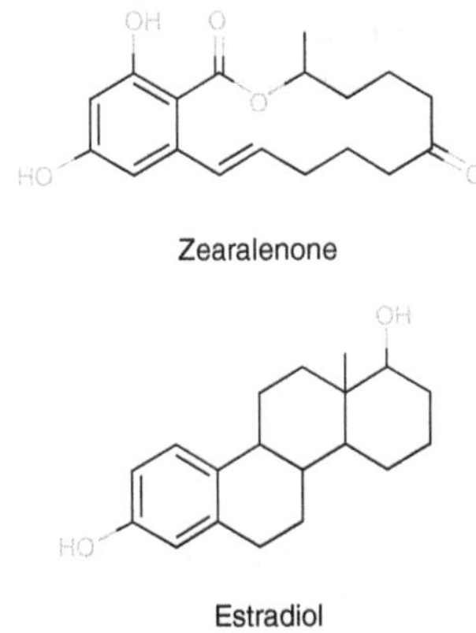

Figure 7.1 Chemical structure of zearalenone and estradiol.

Due to its different health effects, the European Union has determined a maximum ZEN tolerable level of 50 μg/kg in cereals and maize-based foods including bread, 200 μg/kg in unprocessed maize, and 20 μg/kg in infant's and children's foods (European Commission 2006).

ZEN presence in the food system is mostly inevitable as it also exhibits high stability during different food chain levels including storage. ZEN is also heat resistant, which prevents its degradation when exposed to high temperatures including those achieved during pasteurization (Sreenivasa et al. 2008; Rogowska et al. 2019). Applying good measures throughout the whole food chain such as good agricultural practices, good drying practices, and good storage practices remains the most effective strategy in controlling contamination of ZEN and other mycotoxins in the final food product (Daou et al. 2021). However, this approach might not be certainly effective against the produced mycotoxins. Therefore, different detoxification and decontamination strategies have been evolved to decrease ZEN contamination in agricultural products including physical, chemical, and biological methods that will be explored in this chapter. Decontamination is more comprehensive and includes detoxification methods. So, while the first involves the removal of contaminated parts' and mycotoxins' removal and/or inactivation, the latter refers to post-harvest treatments that aim to reduce the ultimate toxic effects of mycotoxins (Jemmali 1980).

7.2 Occurrence and Distribution

ZEN is present in the food chain and has been extensively studied. Due to its toxicity and resistant nature, the European Commission has set a maximum tolerance limit for ZEN in food products. This level differs from one product to another as it was set at 100, 350, and

75 μg/kg in unprocessed cereals, unprocessed maize, and cereals intended for direct human consumption, respectively (European Commission 2006). Other levels are also set for different types of food products (European Commission 2006). ZEN has been found in different foods including cereals, mainly maize, wheat, rye, barley, and sorghum (Ropejko and Twarużek 2021). It has also been found in rice, flour, soybeans, and other food by-products such as pasta, bread, breakfast cereal, beer, and maize oil (Deepa et al. 2016a, b; Ropejko and Twarużek 2021). ZEN can contaminate milk as well if found in cows' feed (Prelusky et al. 1990).

Occurrence studies have reported the contamination of ZEN in several food products in different countries. ZEN was found in maize in Croatia, Argentina, and Bulgaria in 80%, 100%, and 21.1% of samples, respectively (Domijan et al. 2005; Manova and Mladenova 2009; Scudamore and Patel 2009). In Germany and Morocco, 85% and 15% of maize samples were contaminated with ZEN at a mean level of 48 and 14 μg/kg, respectively (Schollenberger et al. 2006; Zinedine et al. 2006). As for wheat samples, ZEN was detected in 1.9% of samples in Bulgaria and 63% of samples in Germany at a mean level of 10 and 15 μg/kg, respectively (Schollenberger et al. 2006; Manova and Mladenova 2009). Contamination with ZEN in rice has been explored in several studies; 6%, 80%, 7%, and 47% positive samples were reported in Malaysia, Bahrain, Uruguay, and Nigeria, respectively (Abbas et al. 2000; Abdullah et al. 1998; Makun et al. 2007; Musaiger et al. 2008). As for other cereals, ZEN was found in 24% of oat samples in Germany, 11.1% of barley samples in Bulgaria, 100% of beans, and 77% of grain samples in South Korea (Chang et al. 2017; Schollenberger et al. 2006; Manova and Mladenova 2009). In byproducts, ZEN was found in 43% of maize bread samples in Pakistan at a mean of 9.45 μg/kg, and in 43.6%, 14.3%, and 11.3% of sliced bread, pasta, and beer samples from Spain (Cano-Sancho et al. 2010; Iqbal et al. 2014).

In animal-based products, ZEN was detected in 41.42% and 68.57% of buffalo meat and liver in Iran at ranges of 0.1–2.5 ng/mL, and 0.1–4.34 ng/mL, respectively (Mahmoudi 2014). ZEN was found as well in 52% of chicken meat samples and 45% of egg samples from Pakistan (Iqbal et al. 2014). It was also detected in 44% of egg samples in China at a mean of 2.23 μg/kg (Wang et al. 2018). In Italy, ZEN was found in cow's milk infant formula in 9% of samples (Meucci et al. 2011).

7.3 Physical Detoxification and Decontamination Methods

Mycotoxin physical control methods involve mainly the removal of contaminated and harmed crops using methods like sorting, sieve cleaning, density segregation, and steeping. They also include further thermal processing such as heating, microwave heating, extrusion, etc., and non-thermal processes such as irradiation and cold plasma treatment. Physical strategies applied to remove ZEN have two different action mechanisms as they either aim at physical removal of the toxin or physical-induced degradation (Wu et al. 2021). Methods involved in physical removal are usually applied in cereal processing and those include steps like separation, solvent extraction, and adsorption that are based on removing the outer contamination on the coat of the kernel (Daou et al. 2021; Wu et al. 2021). On the other hand, physical-induced degradation strategies depend on destroying the chemical formation of ZEN leading to the production of non-toxic or less toxic compounds (Wu et al. 2021). Such strategies comprise heating, irradiation, and low-pressure cold plasma (Wu et al. 2021).

7.3.1 Separation, Cleaning, and Milling

Physical control techniques include the separation of damaged or contaminated crops from healthy ones or the removal of the outer contaminated crop cover through methods like sorting, sieve cleaning, density segregation, washing, dehulling, and steeping (Pleadin et al. 2019; Daou et al. 2021). Grain separation is considered an efficient strategy that is widely used without altering grain quality or inducing further damage (Pascale et al. 2022). Through this process, and by using water or water-based solutions, mycotoxins, specifically water-soluble ones, can be partially removed from the grain's outer surface. Solubility should be considered before applying those methods and in the case of ZEN, its hydrophobic nature renders water-washing processes less effective. However, ZEN is soluble in basic pH solutions such as alcohols, acetonitrile, acetone, or benzene (Ropejko and Twarużek 2021). Different studies have reported varying results on the application of physical washing methods. Trenholm et al. (1992) reported a decrease of ZEN upon washing with distilled water and sodium bicarbonate by 2–61% and 80–87%, respectively (Trenholm et al. 1992). Washing maize with water reduced ZEN by 44–50% while soaking it. Washing it in sodium carbonate further removed 35% with an additional decrease of 4% upon the removal of floating kernels (Rotter et al. 1995).

As for other cleaning and milling procedures, it is important to consider that ZEN is heterogeneously distributed in crops with most of the contamination found in the epidermis and germ fractions of the grains. Since in the production of refined wheat products, those two layers are removed, ZEN concentration can be therefore decreased after mechanical peeling and degerming (Wu et al. 2021). This was shown in different studies; milling procedure along with cleaning and sieving was reported to reduce ZEN by 50% in wheat flour and by more than 50% in artificially contaminated Japanese wheat patent flour (Palpacelli et al. 2007; Zheng et al. 2014). While in a third study, significant difference was found in the distribution of ZEN among different milling fractions of wheat with ZEN being higher in bran than flour (Schwake-Anduschus et al. 2015). Similar results were reported by Zhang et al. (2018) in which ZEN was found to be concentrated in fiber-rich parts of the grain after milling (Karlovsky et al. 2016; Zhang et al. 2018).

7.3.2 Solvent Extraction

ZEN is insoluble in water but can dissolve in alkaline solutions such as ether, benzene, methanol, and ethanol (Mróz et al. 2022). Hence, ZEN can be extracted using an organic solvent mixture with water including 90% acetone, 80% isopropanol, pure acetonitrile, and pure methanol as reported in some studies (Wu et al. 2021). Nonetheless, the extraction procedure has its drawbacks, most importantly, the decrease in the nutritional quality of cereals and others including pollution, high cost, and the need for large-scale processing equipment (Wu et al. 2021). A study by Pallaroni et al. (2002) reported that by using microwave-assisted extraction at different temperatures, ZEN was significantly extracted at 80 °C. The extraction varied while using different solutions; for example, ZEN in maize was removed by 90% regardless of the solution used, whereas in wheat, it was mostly extracted by methanol-acetonitrile mixture, followed by methanol, and acetonitrile at removal rates of 89%, 77%, and 72%, respectively (Pallaroni et al. 2002). Therefore, more studies are still needed in this domain to test the efficacy of several solvents in extraction.

7.3.3 Adsorption

The addition of sorbent material in animal feed is the dominant approach in the industry. It is used to achieve selective removal of mycotoxins at the level of the GI tract (Jard et al. 2011). Feed additives acting as adsorbents were defined by the European Commission in regulation (EC) No. 386/2009 as "substances that suppress or reduce the absorption, promote the excretion of mycotoxins, or modify their mode of action and thereby mitigate possible adverse effects of mycotoxins on animal health" (European Commission 2009). As reported in the literature, the adsorbents that have a high affinity toward mycotoxins and are mostly studied are activated carbons, hydrated sodium calcium aluminosilicates, zeolites, bentonites, and certain clays (Kabak et al. 2006). These adsorbents differ in their mode of action as they either reduce the bioavailability of mycotoxins or degrade them by transforming them into less toxic compounds (Jard et al. 2011). Similarly, ZEN can be removed from the feed using adsorption methods that have been explored and reported in several studies. Avantaggiato et al. (2003) reported a reduction in pig GI model of 43–85% and 19–52% upon the addition of activated carbon or cholestyramine, respectively (Avantaggiato et al. 2003). Similarly, several studies reported the efficacy of activated diatomaceous clay, organo-montmorillonites, graphene oxide, and polymers in adsorbing ZEN (Wu et al. 2021). Diatomaceous clay was found to decrease ZEN contamination by 79.8% when added to feed (Denli et al. 2015). In different studies, organo-montmorillonites had the ability to adsorb more than 70% of ZEN, graphene oxide removed 95% contamination in maize oil, while imprinted polymers adsorbed 74.95–88.41% in maize (Bai et al. 2017; Huang et al. 2020; Sun et al. 2020). Hence, adsorbents proven as safe can be used in animal feed to reduce ZEN in the food system.

7.3.4 Heating

ZEN is a heat-stable compound that can tolerate temperatures up to 160 °C causing it to resist conventional heat treatment methods such as pasteurization and sterilization (Zhang et al. 2018; Wu et al. 2021). According to Wu et al. (2021), decontaminating ZEN through heating depends on several factors including temperature, time, moisture content, and food matrix (Wu et al. 2021). Thermal processes include steam heating, infrared, microwave, radiofrequency, extrusion heating, etc. (Daou et al. 2021). Extrusion studies have shown significant reductions in ZEN. Ryu et al. (1999) reported a decrease in ZEN concentration in maize grits ranging from 66% to 83% at different temperatures of 120, 140, and 160 °C and mixing or non-mixing options (Ryu et al. 1999). Another study reported a concentration decrease ranging between 67% and 81% at different temperatures of 150, 175, and 200 °C at different mixing speeds (Cetin and Bullerman 2005). Heating effects on ZEN were explored in buffer solution at different pH levels (4, 7, and 10) and different temperatures (100, 125, 150, 175, 200, and 225 °C). Most reduction was achieved at 200 and 225 °C in which complete destruction was observed while the solution was heated for 60 minutes regardless of the pH (Ryu et al. 2003). No significant decreases were found in heating ground maize of different moisture content at different temperatures ranging from 20 to 110 °C for 2 to 12 days, where only 13% reduction was achieved at 110 °C after 12 days (Lauren and Smith 2001). In a third study that used crust-like model imitating maize bread, reductions of 0%, 27%, 7%, 30%, 32%, and 28% were achieved at the temperature/time combination of 100 °C/6 hours, 150 °C/180 minutes, 200 °C/10 minutes, 200 °C/20 minutes, 200 °C/30 minutes, and 250 °C/15 minutes, respectively (Numanoglu et al. 2013). Additionally, a heating numerical model reported by Gbashi et al. (2019) found that the optimal decontamination conditions of ZEN were 216.57 °C/63.28 minutes and 210.85 °C/54.71 minutes for pure standards and spiked maize, respectively (Gbashi et al. 2019). On the other hand, microwave heating was applied to spiked maize oil samples that were cooked for 2.5, 5, and 10 minutes, respectively, and reduction was reported to be ranging from 9% to 38% (Sadeghi et al. 2020). Therefore, different heating methods can be used to control ZEN in foods where heating does not affect the nutritional quality.

7.3.5 Irradiation

Irradiation involves non-thermal treatment which might be practical on the industrial scale. ZEN can be destroyed by irradiation by breaking the chemical bonds in the mycotoxin structure and degrading it into smaller non-toxic molecules. Several studies have been reported on the effect of gamma and UV irradiation that proved to be effective in decreasing ZEN. Additionally, Calado et al. (2020) reported that a reduction in concentration after irradiation was followed by a general decrease in ZEN toxicity (Calado et al. 2020). Despite health concerns, the European Commission approved a maximum allowable dose of 10 kGy as a safe level to be applied to food without posing danger to human health (Pleadin et al. 2019). Additionally, the World Health Organization (WHO) and the Food and Agriculture Organization (FAO) of the United Nations have approved using the dose of 25 kGy in some food products (Kalagatur et al. 2018). A reduction in ZEN was reported to be 6%, 8%, 25%, and 31% upon exposing maize to gamma-irradiation at doses of 5, 7.5, 10, and 20 kGy, respectively (Hooshmand and Klopfenstein 1995). Similarly, ZEN was found to be reduced by 49%, 54.6%, 63.7%, and 97% in wheat samples at radiation doses of 5, 10, 15, and 20 kGy, respectively (Sebaei et al. 2022). In yellow maize samples, the reduction was 28.9%, 24.8%, 34.4%, and 51.1%, respectively, while in white maize samples, ZEN was decreased by 26.6%, 50.1%, 20.3%, and 59.9%, respectively, at the mentioned doses of 5, 10, 15, and 20 Kgy, respectively (Sebaei et al. 2022). As for UV irradiation, it has reduced 58–78% of ZEN in maize at 4 and 6 kGy, respectively, as reported by Aziz et al. (2004) and 71.1% reduction was achieved in a second study at UV dose of 50 kGy for maize samples (Aziz et al. 2004; Luo et al. 2017). Additionally, reductions of 75.4%, 52%, and 48% were reported on filter paper, maize, and wheat kernels, respectively, after being exposed to varying UV doses (Popović et al. 2018). Hence, irradiation can be used in safe limits recommended below 20 kGy at an industrial scale.

7.3.6 Cold Plasma

Cold plasma comprises a non-thermal technique that involves the usage of an ionized gas containing partially ionized atoms and molecules of approximately zero net charge that have the ability to partially or completely destroy mycotoxins (Misra et al. 2019). Cold plasma treatments have been applied to ZEN in some studies with promising results. Three studies explored the effect of cold plasma treatment on ZEN standards; complete degradation was achieved at 60 seconds, 8 minutes, and 20 minutes in the first, second, and third studies, respectively (Ten Bosch et al. 2017; Hojnik et al. 2019; Wielogorska et al. 2019). Cold plasma treatments allow for fast decontamination at ambient temperature and pressure combination. It also does not alter food quality. However, cold plasma treatments may not be practical on an industrial scale (Daou et al. 2021).

7.4 Chemical Detoxification and Decontamination Methods

Chemical decontamination and detoxification treatments involve using organic or synthetic chemicals, mainly acids, alkalis, reducing and oxidizing agents, salts, and chlorinating agents (Colovic et al. 2019; Daou et al. 2021). Those chemicals can be introduced to food or feed through processes of mixing, packing, fumigation, or immersion and they can destroy the chemical bonds of mycotoxins or work on neutralizing their active groups (Karlovsky et al. 2016; Wu et al. 2021). Examples of such chemicals include ozone, hydrogen peroxide, calcium hypochlorite, chlorine, and sodium hypochlorite (Liu et al. 2022). Several studies have shown chemical methods to be effective at ZEN removal. However, the concern that chemicals might alter food quality remains prevalent. An additional concern is their tendency to remain in food, hence affecting the health of humans and animals (Liu et al. 2022). Chemical methods can also release mycotoxins from their masked forms, making them more bioavailable (Karlovsky et al. 2016).

Some chemicals studied for ZEN detoxification include ones like ozone (O_3), methylamine, sodium sulfite, cyclodextrin, and other natural plant extracts.

Ozone treatment was suggested to attack the double bond found in ZEN chemical structure. Afterward, degradation products are expected that are similar in structure to ZEN. Nevertheless, those byproducts were found to possess less toxic effects than their parent molecule (Xu et al. 2019). Ozone treatment was found effective in several studies (Table 7.1). Added to that, it is a highly degradable molecule that can decompose to oxygen automatically ensuring safe application (Yang et al. 2020). However, several drawbacks exist such as prolonged treatment times that lead to fat oxidation and deterioration of food quality. Some research suggest the opposite. Nonetheless, more studies are needed in this aspect especially since ozone treatment results can be affected and reduced by different parameters including sample's physical characteristics, initial ZEN concentration, exposure duration, ozone flow rate, and commodity's moisture content (Santos Alexandre et al. 2018).

On the other hand, other chemicals such as methylamine, sodium sulfite, and cyclodextrin can be used for detoxification of feed and have shown promising results in some studies. However, methylamine, specifically in combination with calcium hydroxide, can alter the nutritional value and palatability leading to less feed consumption by animals, in addition to reduced digestibility and gastrointestinal availability (Rempe et al. 2013). Sodium sulfite, on the other hand, has been used widely as a food additive but some studies suggest that thiamine concentration was affected in the blood and urine by increasing sodium sulfite rates in food or feed (Bahrenthien et al. 2020). Additionally, other natural food product alternatives have been tested such as grape pomace that can act by adsorbing ZEN at a lower cost and in safer ways (Greco et al. 2019) (Table 7.1).

Table 7.1 Examples of studies reporting chemical means for ZEN removal.

Method	Commodity	Treatment conditions	Result	References
Ozone	Wheat grains	O_3 generated at maximum flow until maximum concentration of 20 mg/L was reached and study was conducted for 80 and 130 min at room temperature	58.6% average reduction	Reinholds et al. (2016)
	Maize	O_3 generated at 100 mg/L for 180 min	86% reduction at 180 min	Qi et al. (2016)
	Wheat bran	O_3 was at concentration of 62 mg/L at 25 °C	52% concentration decrease at 15 min	Santos Alexandre et al. (2018)
	Maize flour	Contaminated maize flour was exposed to 60 mg/L of O_3 for 90 min at 20 °C	95.1% degradation at 90 min	Xu et al. (2019)
	Maize flour	Naturally contaminated whole maize flour was exposed to 51.5 mg/L O_3 for 5, 10, and 60 min, respectively, at 25 °C	Reduction: At 5 min: 37.9% At 10 min: 55.7% At 60 min: 62.3%	Alexandre et al. (2019)
	Ground maize	Naturally contaminated maize were ground and exposed to varying O_3 levels of 40, 85, and 99 mg/L, respectively, at different durations ranging from 20 to 180 min	Highest percentage reduction was observed at 40 mg/L of 68.1% and 70.3% at 120 and 180 min, respectively	Krstović et al. (2021)
Treatment with sodium metabisulfite and methylamine	Maize	Contaminated maize were treated using six different scenarios consisting of three doses of methylamine (2.5, 5, and 10 g/kg, respectively, of maize) at a fixed dose of 5 g sodium metabisulfite/kg, in the presence or absence of 20 g calcium hydroxide ($Ca(OH)_2$)/kg	ZEN concentrations were reduced by 72%, 85%, and 95% within the first 5 min of the treatment at methylamine dosages of 2.5, 5, and 10 g/kg maize, respectively	Rempe et al. (2013)
Adsorption using B-cyclodextrin bead polymers	Standard aqueous solution of ZEN (10 μM)	Sodium acetate, sodium borate, and phosphate buffered saline with ZEN standards were incubated with B-cyclodextrin bead polymers in a thermo-mixer at different temperatures for different time durations	ZEN can be significantly reduced by incubating with B-cyclodextrin bead polymers: 85–90% reduction after 60 min 70–80% reduction after 5 min	Poór et al. (2018)

(*Continued*)

Table 7.1 (Continued)

Method	Commodity	Treatment conditions	Result	References
Treatment with sodium sulfite	Maize	Contaminated maize were fortified with 5 g sodium sulfite/kg and preserved for 79 days and then included in the diet of male piglets	ZEN was not affected by sodium sulfite treatment	Tran et al. (2018)
Adsorption with grape pomace	Standard aqueous solutions of ZEN (1 μg/mL)	A suspension of ZEN standards, grape pomace, and buffer at different pH was mixed and shaken for 90 min at constant temperature of 37 °C and constant speed of 250 rpm	Maximum adsorption was 70% ZEN adsorption was not affected by pH	Avantaggiato et al. (2014)
Adsorption by agricultural byproducts	*In vivo* study	Piglets were administered feed contaminated with ZEN and containing agricultural byproducts Urine samples were collected and analyzed for ZEN biomarkers during 24 h	Malvasia grape pomace reduced ZEN biomarkers by 69%	Gambacorta et al. (2016)
Adsorption by grape and olive pomace	Standard aqueous solutions of ZEN (0.05, 0.5, 1, 2, 4, 6, and 10 μg/mL)	Adsorbents and mycotoxin standard mixture were incubated at 37 °C for 1 h with rotary agitation at 40 rpm	Micronized dry grape stems: 99% Dry olive pomace: 93%	Fernandes et al. (2019)
Adsorption using plant food material	Standard aqueous solutions of ZEN (1 μg/mL)	ZEN standards and multiple mycotoxin standards were prepared. Food plant materials were suspended in the solution and shaken for 90 min at constant temperature of 37 °C and constant speed of 250 rpm and different pH (4 and 7)	ZEN's best adsorbents were grape pomaces, artichoke waste, and almond hulls with % adsorption of 84%, 89%, and 76%, respectively The adsorption by those agents did not change with pH and absorbed ZEN was not released after pH change from acidic to neutral	Greco et al. (2019)

7.5 Biological Detoxification and Decontamination Methods

Biological means of decontamination involve the usage of microorganisms like bacteria, molds, yeasts, and algae. Biological methods have gained interest as the most favorable application particularly since physical and chemical methods were shown to have several drawbacks such as being impractical, expensive, time-consuming, and limited to large-scale production. In addition, possible health side effects could result from chemical methods as well as lower nutritional quality in food and possible environmental effects (Deepa and Sreenivasa 2019a, b; Daou et al. 2021; Deepa et al. 2021). Biological methods do not pose any serious threat to the environment. However, their effectiveness in several studies was limited to laboratory settings. Their usage is also impractical in the removal of several mycotoxins in a single treatment (Sreenivasa et al. 2011a, b; Daou et al. 2021).

For ZEN removal, mostly three biological methods are studied. The first one involves adsorption through cell walls of different microorganisms, the second one involves degradation by microorganisms, while the third one relies on enzymes for ZEN degradation (Dass et al. 2007; Wu et al. 2021).

7.5.1 Adsorption

Several microorganisms have been tested for adsorption based on their ability to bind mycotoxins through their wall structures by different chemical bonds such as non-covalent, ionic, and hydrogen bonds, as well as hydrophobic interactions (Chennappa et al. 2014; Wu et al. 2021; Nahle et al. 2022). This process binds the mycotoxin and reduces its bioavailability. However, this bond might be weak leading to release of the mycotoxin back into food. Therefore, further studies are needed to establish its strength (Nagaraja et al. 2016; Yooussef et al. 2016; Achar et al. 2020; Nahle et al. 2022).

Generally, lactic acid bacteria strains that are recognized as safe by the Scientific Committee on Animal Nutrition of the European Union and that are a natural part of the GI microflora showed promising results on ZEN adsorption (Sangsila et al. 2016). However, its effectiveness is still not well established at high mycotoxin concentrations in food.

In addition, other yeast strains such as *Saccharomyces* have proved effective and a correlation was found between the amount of cell wall and ZEN binding capacity (Król et al. 2018) (Table 7.2).

7.5.2 Degradation

The degradation of ZEN is facilitated by several microorganisms (Table 7.3) and enzymes that have diverse characteristics and degradation abilities (Ju et al. 2019). Degradation is mainly achieved by transforming ZEN into less toxic metabolites that have lower oestrogenic activity through different processes of glycosylation, sulfation, and hydrolyzation (Wu et al. 2021). Additionally, it has been reported that ZEN loses its estrogenic activity by the lactone ring cleavage which could be an effective degradation method specifically by enzymatic actions of lactone hydrolase and laccase (Figure 7.2) (Table 7.3).

7.6 Summary

ZEN can cause several toxic health effects posing a significant threat to public health. Additionally, economic losses and food waste could increase as a result of contamination. Control methods developed that include physical, chemical, and biological methods have been explored and showed different results. Physical and chemical methods were reported to be effective. However, the preferred method of decontamination and ZEN removal is

Table 7.2 Studies on adsorption of ZEN by microorganisms.

Microorganism	Commodity	Treatment conditions	Result	References
Saccharomyces cerevisiae	Buffer solution	Incubation for 60 min at 25 °C	Binding of ZEN at pH 3 and 6.5 was 75.1% and 77.5%, respectively	Campagnollo et al. (2015)
Lactobacillus pentosus	MRS broth	Eight strains of *Lactobacillus pentosus* were incubated in MRS broth at 37 °C for 24 h in a 5% CO_2 incubator	Highest adsorption was found for three strains at 83.17%, 82.78%, and 81.69%, respectively Adsorption differed between strains and increased as ZEN initial concentration increased	Sangsila et al. (2016)
LAB isolates and yeast from Kefir	UHT cows' milk, MRS, and YPD broths	Incubation at 25 °C for 24 h LAB strains were incubated in MRS and yeasts were incubated in YPD	ZEN adsorption: 100% in milk 100% in MRS 0–44% in YPD	Taheur et al. (2017)
Lactococcus lactis *Bifidobacterium* sp.	Tryptone soya agar	Incubation at 37 °C with shaking for different time durations ranging from 0 to 1200 min	90% at 20 min 88% at 720 min	Król et al. (2018)
Lactococcus sakei *Pediococcus acidilactici* Two strains of *Pediococcus peotosaceus*	Wheat	Each culture was incubated at its optimal temperature for 48 h	12% adsorption ability 38% adsorption ability Between 25% and 37% adsorption ability	Juodeikiene et al. (2018)
Saccharomyces strains (*S. cerevisiae* and *S. pastorianus*)	Wort	Fermentation was performed for 96 h at 20 °C	The yeast adsorbed 31% of ZEN	Wall-Martínez et al. (2019)
Lactococcus paracasei	MRS broth	Incubated at 37 °C for 24 h with or without stress conditions	Maximum adsorption In non-stress conditions: 53.3% In stress conditions: 55.3%	Rogowska et al. (2019)
Lactococcus lactis	Tryptic soy broth		Maximum adsorption In non-stress conditions: 41.0% In stress conditions: 47.4%	
Saccharomyces cerevisiae	Yeast extract-peptone-dextrose broth		Maximum adsorption In non-stress conditions: 36.5% In stress conditions: 57.0%	

Table 7.3 Different studies on degradation of ZEN by microorganisms.

Microorganism	Commodity	Treatment conditions	Degradation %	References
Saccharomyces cerevisiae	Yeast extract-peptone-dextrose medium	Incubation at 30 °C for 72 h with shaking at 150 rpm	More than 90% of ZEN was degraded	Keller et al. (2015)
Bacillus pumilus	Culture medium	Incubation at 37 °C for 24 h with shaking at 180 rpm	Degradation up to 95.7%	Wang et al. (2017)
Bacillus cereus	LB medium	Incubation at 37 °C for 24 h	Degradation by 100%	Wang et al. (2018)
	Simulated gastric fluid		Degradation by 89.31%	
Bacillus subtilis and other *Bacillus* strains	Maize	Incubation at 37 °C for 24 h	Maximum degradation of 56% of ZEN achieved by a *B. subtilis* strain	Chen et al. (2019)
Bacillus subtilis *Candida utilis* *Aspergillus oryzae*	YPD broth	Bacillus strains were mixed together and incubated at 37 °C for 48 h while placed in a rotary shaker at 180 rpm	Degradation of 92.27% was achieved by the *Bacillus* strain mixture With the addition of *A. orayzae*, 95.15% of ZEN were degraded	Liu et al. (2019)
Bacillus subtilis	Culture of soy beans, wheat, and maize. Liquid food of maize oil, soybean oil, beer, and milk	For liquid food: incubation at 30 °C for 24 h For solid culture: incubation at 37 °C for 48 h	Maize oil: 56% Soybean oil: 49% Beer: 65% Milk: 57% Soybean: 61% Wheat: 51% Maize: 75%	Ju et al. (2019)

(*Continued*)

Table 7.3 (Continued)

Microorganism	Commodity	Treatment conditions	Degradation %	References
Bacillus natto		For liquid food: incubation at 30 °C for 24 h For solid culture: incubation at 37 °C for 48 h	Maize oil: 51% Soybean oil: 53% Beer: 73% Milk: 69% Soybean: 70% Wheat: 39% Maize: 59%	
Bacillus strains	ZEN standard solution	Incubation at 30 °C for 24, 48, and 72 h, respectively	Degradation of 58–96.9% by all strains at 72 h The most effective strain in this study was *B. mycoides* with 89.53% degradation achieved	González Pereyra et al. (2020)

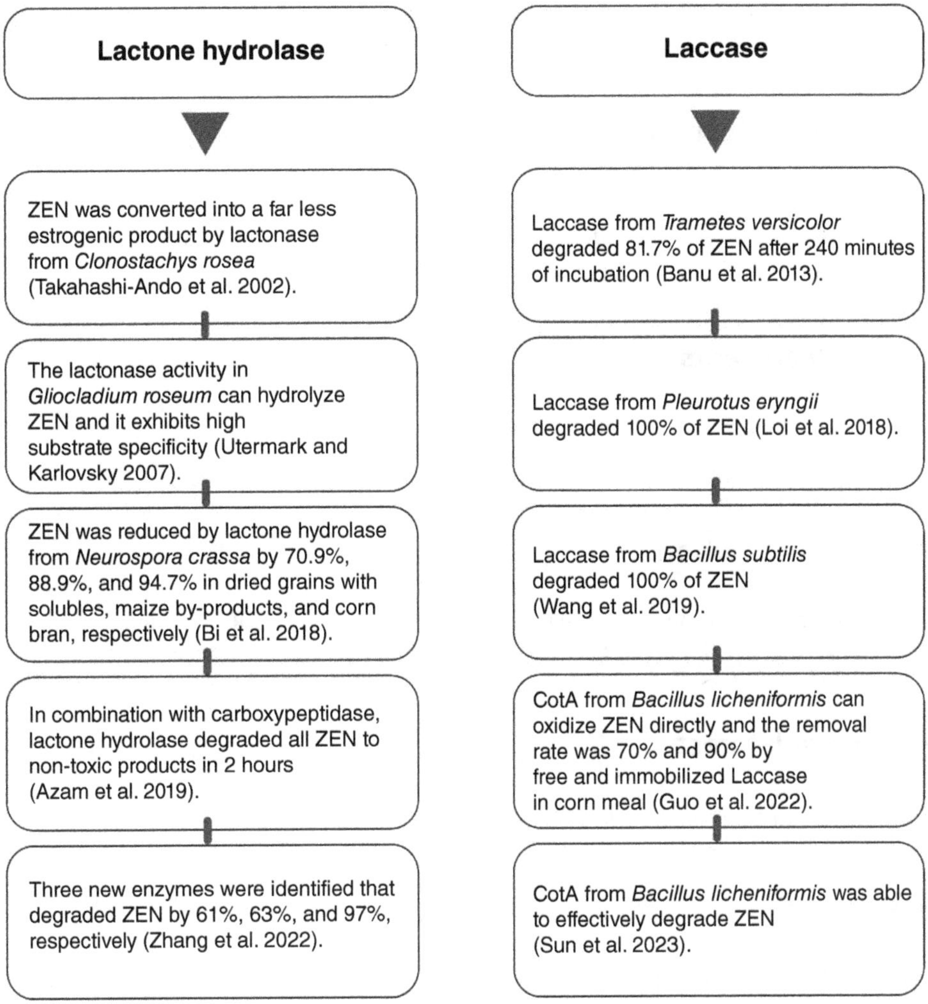

Figure 7.2 Studies that summarize enzymatic actions of lactone hydrolase and laccase on ZEN and their degradation results.

through the activity of natural microorganisms and enzymes used in biological decontamination due to their high specificity and safety. However, those methods still need more studies and development specifically to explore their byproducts' toxicity and find ways to increase their efficiency and applicability in the food industry.

7.7 Future Implications

Among all detoxification methods, biological methods present many advantages. More studies are needed to test the potential of direct use of microorganisms for ZEN detoxification in food products without affecting their nutritional and organoleptic characteristics.

Besides, it is of utmost importance to better characterize the microbial enzymes showing high efficiency in ZEN detoxification in terms of their mechanism of action.

7.8 Study Questions

1) Do ZEN detoxification and decontamination methods apply in food systems?
2) What is the best detoxification method for ZEN detoxification in foods in terms of toxin removal and quality attribute preservation?

Acknowledgments

The authors thank one and all for their kind support in successfully publishing the chapter.

Author Contributions

Original draft preparation, conceptualization, writing, and editing R.D., review and editing A.A. and A.K., coordinating A.A.

Conflict of Interest

The authors confirm that they have no conflicts of interest.

References

Abbas, H.K., Cartwright, R.D., Windham, G.L. et al. (2000). The presence of mycotoxins and fungi in rice and corn in the southern united states. *Bull. Inst. Compr. Agric. Sci.* 8: 21–34.

Abdullah N, Nawawi A, Othman I. (1998). Survey of fungal counts and natural occurrence of aflatoxins in Malaysian starch-based foods. *Mycopathologia* 143 (1): 53–58.

Achar, P.N., Quyen, P., Adukwu, E.C. et al. (2020). Investigation of the antifungal and anti-aflatoxigenic potential of plant-based essential oils against *Aspergillus flavus* in peanuts. *J. Fungi* 6 (4): 383. https://doi.org/10.3390/jof6040383.

Alexandre, A.P.S., Castanha, N., Costa, N.S. et al. (2019). Ozone technology to reduce zearalenone contamination in whole maize flour: degradation kinetics and impact on quality. *J. Sci. Food Agric.* 99: 6814–6821.

Avantaggiato, G., Havenaar, R., and Visconti, A. (2003). Assessing the zearalenone-binding activity of adsorbent materials during passage through a dynamic in vitro gastrointestinal model. *Food Chem. Toxicol.* 41: 1283–1290.

Avantaggiato, G., Greco, D., Damascelli, A. et al. (2014). Assessment of multi-mycotoxin adsorption efficacy of grape pomace. *J. Agric. Food Chem.* 62: 497–507.

Aziz, N.H., Moussa, L.A.A., and Far, F.M.E. (2004). Reduction of fungi and mycotoxins formation in seeds by gamma-radiation. *J. Food Saf.* 24 (2): 109–127.

Bahrenthien, L., Kluess, J., Berk, A. et al. (2020). Detoxifying deoxynivalenol (DON)-contaminated feedstuff: consequences of sodium sulphite (SoS) treatment on performance and blood parameters in fattening pigs. *Mycotoxin Res.* 36 (2): 213–223.

Bai, X., Sun, C., Xu, J. et al. (2017). Detoxification of zearalenone from corn oil by adsorption of functionalized go systems. *Appl. Surf. Sci.* 430: 198–207.

Bianchini, A. and Bullerman, L.B. (2014). MYCOTOXINS | Classifications. In: *Encyclopedia of Food Microbiology*, 2e (ed. C.A. Batt and M.L.B.T. Tortorello), 854–861. Oxford: Academic Press.

Calado, T., Abrunhosa, L., Cabo Verde, S. et al. (2020). Effect of gamma-radiation on zearalenone-degradation, cytotoxicity and estrogenicity. *Foods* 9 (11): 1658–1674.

Campagnollo, F.B., Franco, L.T., Rottinghaus, G.E. et al. (2015). In vitro evaluation of the ability of beer fermentation residue containing *Saccharomyces cerevisiae* to bind mycotoxins. *Food Res. Int.* 77 (3): 643–648.

Cano-Sancho, G., Marin, S., Ramos, A.J., et al. (2010). Occurrence of aflatoxin m1 and exposure assessment in catalonia (spain). *Revista Iberoamericana de Micologia* 27 (3): 130–135.

Cetin, Y. and Bullerman, L.B. (2005). Evaluation of reduced toxicity of zearalenone by extrusion processing as measured by the MTT cell proliferation assay. *J. Agric. Food Chem.* 53 (16): 6558–6563.

Chang, H., Kim, W., Park, J.H., et al. (2017). The occurrence of zearalenone in south korean feedstuffs between 2009 and 2016. *Toxins* 9 (7): 223–238.

Chen, S.-W., Wang, H.-T., Shih, W.-Y. et al. (2019). Application of Zearalenone (ZEN)-detoxifying bacillus in animal feed decontamination through fermentation. *Toxins* 11 (6): 330–341.

Chennappa, G., Adkar-Purushothama, C.R., Suraj, U. et al. (2014). Impact of pesticides on PGPR activity of *Azotobacter* sp. isolated from pesticide flooded paddy soils. *Greener J. Agric. Sci.* 4 (4): 117–129.

Colovic, R., Puvača, N., Cheli, F. et al. (2019). Decontamination of mycotoxin-contaminated feedstuffs and compound feed. *Toxins* 11 (11): 617–635.

Daou, R., Joubrane, K., Maroun, R.G. et al. (2021). Mycotoxins: factors influencing production and control strategies. *AIMS Agric. Food.* 6 (1): 416–447.

Dass, R.S., Sreenivasa, M.Y., and Janardhana, G.R. (2007). High incidence of *Fusarium verticillioides* in animal and poultry feed mixtures produced in Karnataka, India. *Plant Pathol J.* 6 (2): 174–178.

Deepa, N. and Sreenivasa, M.Y. (2017a). *Fusarium verticillioides*, a globally important pathogen of agriculture and livestock: a review. *J. Vet. Med. Res.* 4 (4): 1084.

Deepa, N. and Sreenivasa, M.Y. (2017b). Fumonisins: a review on its global occurrence, epidemiology, toxicity and detection. *J. Vet. Med. Res.* 4 (6): 1093.

Deepa, N. and Sreenivasa, M.Y. (2019a). Biocontrol strategies for effective management of phytopathogenic fungi associated with cereals. In: *New and Future Developments in Microbial Biotechnology and Bioengineering* (ed. J.S. Singh and D.P. Singh), 177–189. Elsevier. ISBN: 9780444641915 10.1016/B978-0-444-64191-5.00013-4.

Deepa, N. and Sreenivasa, M.Y. (2019b). Molecular methods and key genes targeted for the detection of fumonisin producing *Fusarium verticillioides* - an updated review. *Food Biosci.* 32: 100473. https://doi.org/10.1016/j.fbio.2019.100473.

Deepa, N., Nagaraja, H., and Sreenivasa, M.Y. (2016a). Prevalence of fumonisin producing *Fusarium verticillioides* associated with cereals grown in Karnataka (India). *Food Sci. Human Well.* 5: 156–162. https://doi.org/10.1016/j.fshw.2016.07.001.

Deepa, N., Charith Raj, A.P., and Sreenivasa, M.Y. (2016b). Multiplex PCR method for the early detection of fumonisin producing *Fusarium verticillioides*. *Food Biosci.* 13: 84–88.

Deepa, N., Achar, P.N., and Sreenivasa, M.Y. (2021). Current perspectives of biocontrol agents for management of *Fusarium verticillioides* and its Fumonisin in cereals—a review. *J. Fungi* 7: 776. https://doi.org/10.3390/jof7090776.

Denli, M., Blandon, J.C., Guynot, M.E. et al. (2015). Efficacy of activated diatomaceous clay in reducing the toxicity of zearalenone in rats and piglets. *J. Anim. Sci.* 93 (2): 637–645.

Domijan, A.M., Peraica, M., Cvjetković, B. et al. (2005). Mould contamination and co-occurrence of mycotoxins in maize grain in Croatia. *Acta Pharm.* 55 (4): 349–356.

European Commission (2006). Regulation (EC) no 1881/2006 of 19 December 2006 setting maximum levels for certain contaminants in foodstuffs. *Off. J. Eur. Union* L364: 5.

European Commission. (2009). Commission Regulation (EC) No 384/2009 of 12 May 2009 amending Regulation (EC) No 1831/2003 of the European Parliament and of the Council as regards the establishment of a new functional group of feed additives 2009.

Fernandes, J.-M., Calado, T., Guimarães, A. et al. (2019). In vitro adsorption of aflatoxin B(1), ochratoxin A, and zearalenone by micronized grape stems and olive pomace in buffer solutions. *Mycotoxin Res.* 35 (3): 243–252.

Gambacorta, L., Pinton, P., Avantaggiato, G. et al. (2016). Grape pomace, an agricultural byproduct reducing mycotoxin absorption: in vivo assessment in pig using urinary biomarkers. *J. Agric. Food Chem.* 64: 6762–6771.

Gbashi, S., Madala, N.E., De Saeger, S. et al. (2019). Numerical optimization of temperature-time degradation of multiple mycotoxins. *Food Chem. Toxicol. Int. J. Publ. Br. Ind. Biol. Res. Assoc.* 125: 289–304.

Gil-Serna, J., Vázquez, C., González-Jaén, M.T., Patiño, B., 2014. MYCOTOXINS | Toxicology. In: Batt, C.A., Encyclopedia of Food Microbiology (2) Tortorello, M.L.B.T.-E. of F.M. (Second E. (Eds.)). Academic Press, Oxford, pp. 887–892.

González Pereyra, M.L., Di Giacomo, A.L., Lara, A.L. et al. (2020). Aflatoxin-degrading *Bacillus* sp. strains degrade zearalenone and produce proteases, amylases and cellulases of agro-industrial interest. *Toxicon* 180: 43–48.

Greco, D., D'Ascanio, V., Santovito, E. et al. (2019). Comparative efficacy of agricultural by-products in sequestering mycotoxins. *J. Sci. Food Agric.* 99 (4): 1623–1634.

Hojnik, N., Modic, M., Tavčar-Kalcher, G. et al. (2019). Mycotoxin decontamination efficacy of atmospheric pressure air plasma. *Toxins* 11 (4): 219–231.

Hooshmand, H. and Klopfenstein, C.F. (1995). Effects of gamma irradiation on mycotoxin disappearance and amino acid contents of corn, wheat, and soybeans with different moisture contents. *Plant Foods Hum. Nutr.* 47 (3): 227–238.

Huang, Z., He, J., Li, H. et al. (2020). Synthesis and application of magnetic-surfaced pseudo molecularly imprinted polymers for zearalenone pretreatment in cereal samples. *Food Chem.* 308: 125696.

Iqbal, S.Z., Nizar, S., Asi, M.R., Jinap, S. (2014). Natural incidence of aflatoxins, ochratoxin a, and zearalenone in chicken meat and eggs. *Food Control* 43 (-): 98–103

Jard, G., Liboz, T., Mathieu, F. et al. (2011). Review of mycotoxin reduction in food and feed: from prevention in the field to detoxification by adsorption or transformation. *Food Addit. Contam. Part A Chem. Anal. Control. Expo. Risk Assess.* 28 (11): 1590–1609.

Jemmali, M. (1980). Decontamination and detoxification of mycotoxins. *Pure Appl. Chem.* 52: 175–181.

Ju, J., Tinyiro, S.E., Yao, W. et al. (2019). The ability of *Bacillus subtilis* and *Bacillus natto* to degrade zearalenone and its application in food. *J. Food Process. Preserv.* 43 (10): 1–9.

Juodeikiene, G., Bartkiene, E., Cernauskas, D. et al. (2018). Antifungal activity of lactic acid bacteria and their application for *Fusarium* mycotoxin reduction in malting wheat grains. *LWT* 89: 307–314.

Kabak, B., Dobson, A.D.W., and Var, I. (2006). Strategies to prevent mycotoxin contamination of food and animal feed: a review. *Crit. Rev. Food Sci. Nutr.* 46 (8): 593–619.

Kailasa, S.K., Park, T.J., Singhal, R.K., and Basu, H. (2020). Nanoparticle-integrated electrochemical devices for identification of mycotoxins. In: *Handbook of Nanomaterials in Analytical Chemistry* (ed. C.B.T.-H. Mustansar Hussain) of N. in A.C. (Ed.), 275–296. Elsevier.

Kalagatur, N.K., Kamasani, J.R., and Mudili, V. (2018). Assessment of detoxification efficacy of irradiation on zearalenone mycotoxin in various fruit juices by response surface methodology and elucidation of its in-vitro toxicity. *Front. Microbiol.* 9: 1–13.

Karlovsky, P., Suman, M., Berthiller, F. et al. (2016). Impact of food processing and detoxification treatments on mycotoxin contamination. *Mycotoxin Res.* 32: 179–205.

Keller, L., Abrunhosa, L., Keller, K. et al. (2015). Zearalenone and its derivatives α-Zearalenol and β-Zearalenol decontamination by *Saccharomyces cerevisiae* strains isolated from bovine forage. *Toxins* 7 (8): 3297–3308.

Król, A., Pomastowski, P., Rafińska, K. et al. (2018). Microbiology neutralization of zearalenone using *Lactococcus lactis* and *Bifidobacterium* sp. *Anal. Bioanal. Chem.* 410 (3): 943–952.

Krstović, S., Krulj, J., Jakšić, S. et al. (2021). Ozone as decontaminating agent for ground corn containing deoxynivalenol, zearalenone, and ochratoxin A. *Cereal Chem.* 98 (1): 135–143.

Lauren, D.R. and Smith, W.A. (2001). Stability of the fusarium mycotoxins nivalenol, deoxynivalenol and zearalenone in ground maize under typical cooking environments. *Food Addit. Contam.* 18 (11): 1011–1016.

Liu, C., Chang, J., Wang, P. et al. (2019). Zearalenone biodegradation by the combination of probiotics with cell-free extracts of *Aspergillus oryzae* and its mycotoxin-alleviating effect on pig production performance. *Toxins* 11 (10): 552–567.

Liu, M., Zhao, L., Gong, G. et al. (2022). Invited review: remediation strategies for mycotoxin control in feed. *J. Anim. Sci. Biotechnol.* 13: 19–35.

Luo, X., Qi, L., Liu, Y. et al. (2017). Effects of electron beam irradiation on zearalenone and ochratoxin A in naturally contaminated corn and corn quality parameters. *Toxins* 9 (3): 84–95.

Mahmoudi, R. (2014). Occurrence of Zearalenone in raw animal origin food produced in North-West of Iran. *J. Food Qual. Hazards Control* 1 (1): 25–28.

Makun, H., Timothy, A.G., Akanya, H. et al. (2007). Fungi and some mycotoxins contaminating rice (Oryza Sativa) in Niger State, Nigeria. *Afr. J. Biotechnol.* 6 (2): 99–108.

Manova, R. and Mladenova, R. (2009). Incidence of zearalenone and fumonisins in Bulgarian cereal production. *Food Control* 20 (4): 362–365.

Meucci, V., Soldani, G., Razzuoli, E., et al. (2011). Mycoestrogen pollution of Italian infant food. *J. Pediatr.* 159 (2): 278–283. https://doi.org/10.1016/j.jpeds.2011.01.028.

Minervini, F., Giannoccaro, A., Cavallini, A., and Visconti, A. (2005). Investigations on cellular proliferation induced by zearalenone and its derivatives in relation to the estrogenic parameters. *Toxicol. Lett.* 159 (3): 272–283.

Misra, N.N., Yadav, B., Roopesh, M.S., and Jo, C. (2019). Cold plasma for effective fungal and mycotoxin control in foods: mechanisms, inactivation effects, and applications. *Compr. Rev. Food Sci. Food Saf.* 18 (1): 106–120.

Mróz, M., Gajęcka, M., Brzuzan, P. et al. (2022). Carry-over of zearalenone and its metabolites to intestinal tissues and the expression of CYP1A1 and GSTπ1 in the colon of gilts before puberty. *Toxins* 14 (5): 354–375.

Musaiger, A.O., Al-Jedah, J.H., and D'souza, R. (2008). Occurrence of contaminants in foods commonly consumed in Bahrain. *Food Control* 19 (9): 854–861.

Nagaraja, H., Chennappa, G., Poorna Chandra Rao, K. et al. (2016). Diversity of toxic and phytopathogenic *Fusarium* species occurring on cereals grown in Karnataka state, India. *3 Biotech* 6: 57.

Nahle, S., El Khoury, A., Savvaidis, I. et al. (2022). Detoxification approaches of mycotoxins: by microorganisms, biofilms and enzymes. *Int. J. Food Contam.* 9: 3–17.

Numanoglu, E., Yener, S., Gökmen, V. et al. (2013). Modelling thermal degradation of zearalenone in maize bread during baking. *Food Addit. Contam. Part A Chem. Anal. Control. Expo. Risk Assess.* 30 (3): 528–533.

Pallaroni, L., Björklund, E., and von Holst, C. (2002). Alternative extraction methods for zearalenone: microwave assisted extraction and accelerated solvent extraction. *Mycotoxin Res.* 1: 74–77.

Palpacelli, V., Beco, L., and Ciani, M. (2007). Vomitoxin and zearalenone content of soft wheat flour milled by different methods. *J. Food Protect.* 70 (2): 509–513.

Pascale, M., Logrieco, A.F., Lippolis, V. et al. (2022). Industrial-scale cleaning solutions for the reduction of *Fusarium* toxins in maize. *Toxins* 14 (11): 728–744.

Pleadin, J., Frece, J., and Markov, K. (2019). Mycotoxins in food and feed. *Adv. Food Nutr. Res.* 89: 297–345.

Poór, M., Faisal, Z., Zand, A. et al. (2018). Removal of zearalenone and zearalenols from aqueous solutions using insoluble beta-cyclodextrin bead polymer. *Toxins* 10 (6): 216–228.

Popović, V., Fairbanks, N., Pierscianowski, J. et al. (2018). Feasibility of 3D UV-C treatment to reduce fungal growth and mycotoxin loads on maize and wheat kernels. *Mycotoxin Res.* 34 (3): 211–221.

Prelusky, D.B., Scott, P.M., Trenholm, H.L., and Lawrence, G.A. (1990). Minimal transmission of zearalenone to milk of dairy cows. *J. Environ. Sci. Health B.* 25 (1): 87–103. https://doi.org/10.1080/03601239009372678.

Qi, L., Li, Y., Luo, X. et al. (2016). Detoxification of zearalenone and ochratoxin A by ozone and quality evaluation of ozonised corn. *Food Addit. Contam. Part A Chem. Anal. Control. Expo. Risk Assess.* 33 (11): 1700–1710.

Reinholds, I., Gražina, J., Bartkiene, E. et al. (2016). Evaluation of ozonation as a method for mycotoxins degradation in malting wheat grains. *World Mycotoxin J.* 9 (3): 1–10.

Rempe, I., Kersten, S., Valenta, H., and Dänicke, S. (2013). Hydrothermal treatment of naturally contaminated maize in the presence of sodium metabisulfite, methylamine and calcium hydroxide; effects on the concentration of zearalenone and deoxynivalenol. *Mycotoxin Res.* 29 (3): 169–175.

Rogowska, A., Pomastowski, P., Sagandykova, G., and Buszewski, B. (2019). Zearalenone and its metabolites: effect on human health, metabolism and neutralisation methods. *Toxicon* 162: 46–56.

Ropejko, K. and Twarużek, M. (2021). Zearalenone and its metabolites-general overview, occurrence, and toxicity. *Toxins* 13 (1): 1–12.

Rotter, R.G., Rotter, B.A., Thompson, B.K. et al. (1995). Effectiveness of density segregation and sodium carbonate treatment on the detoxification of Fusarium-contaminated corn fed to growing pigs. *J. Sci. Food Agric.* 68: 331–336.

Ryu, D., Hanna, M.A., and Bullerman, L.B. (1999). Stability of zearalenone during extrusion of corn grits. *J. Food Protect.* 62 (12): 1482–1484.

Ryu, D., Hanna, M.A., Eskridge, K.M., and Bullerman, L.B. (2003). Heat stability of zearalenone in an aqueous buffered model system. *J. Agric. Food Chem.* 51 (6): 1746–1748.

Sadeghi, E., Oskoei, L., Nejatian, M., and Mehr, S. (2020). Effect of microwave, deep frying and oven cooking on destruction of zearalenone in spiked maize oil. *World Mycotoxin J.* 13 (4): 515–522.

Sangsila, A., Faucet-Marquis, V., Pfohl-Leszkowicz, A., and Itsaranuwat, P. (2016). Detoxification of zearalenone by *Lactobacillus pentosus* strains. *Food Control* 62: 187–192.

Santos Alexandre, A.P., Vela-Paredes, R.S., Santos, A.S. et al. (2018). Ozone treatment to reduce deoxynivalenol (DON) and zearalenone (ZEN) contamination in wheat bran and its impact on nutritional quality. *Food Addit. Contam. Part A Chem. Anal. Control. Expo. Risk Assess.* 35 (6): 1189–1199.

Schollenberger, M., Müller, H.M., Rüfle, M., et al. (2006). Natural occurrence of 16 fusarium toxins in grains and feedstuffs of plant origin from Germany. *Mycopathologia* 161 (1): 43–52. https://doi.org/10.1007/s11046-005-0199-7.

Schwake-Anduschus, C., Proske, M., Muenzing, K. et al. (2015). Distribution of deoxynivalenol, zearalenone, and their respective modified analogues in milling fractions of naturally contaminated wheat grains. *World Mycotoxin J.* 8 (4): 433–443.

Scudamore, K.A. and Patel, S. (2009). Occurrence of Fusarium mycotoxins in maize imported into the UK, 2004–2007. *Food Addit. Contam. A.* 26 (3): 363–371. https://doi.org/10.1080/02652030802406219.

Sebaei, A.S., Sobhy, H.M., Fouzy, A.S.M., and Hussain, O.A. (2022). Occurrence of zearalenone in grains and its reduction by gamma radiation. *Int. J. Environ. Anal. Chem.* 102 (11): 2503–2511.

Sreenivasa, M.Y., Dass, R.S., Charith Raj, A.P., and Janardhana, G.R. (2008). PCR-based detection of genus *Fusarium* and Fumonisin-producing isolates from freshly harvested sorghum grains grown in Karnataka, India. *J. Food Saf.* 28: 236–237.

Sreenivasa, M.Y., Dass, R.S., Charith Raj, A.P., and Janardhana, G.R. (2011a). Mycological evaluation of maize grains produced in Karnataka (India) for the post-harvest fungal contamination. *World Appl. Sci. J.* 13 (4): 688–692.

Sreenivasa, M.Y., Dass, R.S., Charith Raj, A.P. et al. (2011b). Assessment of the growth inhibiting effect of some plant essential oils on different *Fusarium* species isolated from sorghum and maize grains. *J. Plant Dis. Protect.* 118 (6): 208–213.

Stanciu, O., Juan, C., Berrada, H. et al. (2019). Study on trichothecene and zearalenone presence in Romanian wheat relative to weather conditions. *Toxins* 11 (3): 163–180.

Sun, Z., Lian, C., Li, C., and Zheng, S. (2020). Investigations on organo-montmorillonites modified by binary nonionic/zwitterionic surfactant mixtures for simultaneous adsorption of aflatoxin B1 and zearalenone. *J. Colloid Interface Sci.* 565: 11–22.

Taheur, F.B., Fedhila, K., Chaieb, K. et al. (2017). Adsorption of aflatoxin B1, zearalenone and ochratoxin A by microorganisms isolated from kefir grains. *Int. J. Food Microbiol.* 251: 1–7.

Ten Bosch, L., Pfohl, K., Avramidis, G. et al. (2017). Plasma-based degradation of mycotoxins produced by *Fusarium*, *Aspergillus* and *Alternaria* Species. *Toxins* 9 (3): 97–109.

Tran, A.T., Kluess, J., Berk, A. et al. (2018). Detoxification of Fusarium-contaminated maize with sodium sulphite - in vivo efficacy with special emphasis on mycotoxin residues and piglet health. *Arch. Anim. Nutr.* 72: 58–75.

Trenholm, H.L., Charmley, L.L., Prelusky, D.B., and Warner, R.M. (1992). Washing procedures using water or sodium carbonate solutions for the decontamination of three cereals contaminated with deoxynivalenol and zearalenone. *J. Agric. Food Chem.* 40: 2147–2151.

Wall-Martínez, H.A., Pascari, X., Bigordà, A. et al. (2019). The fate of Fusarium mycotoxins (deoxynivalenol and zearalenone) through wort fermenting by *Saccharomyces* yeasts (*S. cerevisiae* and *S. pastorianus*). *Food Res. Int.* 126: 1–8.

Wang, G., Yu, M., Dong, F. et al. (2017). Esterase activity inspired selection and characterization of zearalenone degrading bacteria Bacillus pumilus ES-21. *Food Control* 77: 57–64.

Wang, Y., Zhang, J., Wang, Y. et al. (2018). Occurrence and quantitative risk assessment of twelve mycotoxins in eggs and chicken tissues in China. *Toxins* 10 (11): 2–18.

Wielogorska, E., Ahmed, Y., Meneely, J. et al. (2019). A holistic study to understand the detoxification of mycotoxins in maize and impact on its molecular integrity using cold atmospheric plasma treatment. *Food Chem.* 301: 1–8.

Wu, N., Ou, W., Zhang, Z. et al. (2021). Recent advances in detoxification strategies for zearalenone contamination in food and feed. *Chin. J. Chem. Eng.* 30 (2): 168–177.

Xu, Y., Wang, Y., Ji, J. et al. (2019). Chemical and toxicological alterations of zearalenone under ozone treatment. *Food Addit. Contam. Part A Chem. Anal. Control. Expo. Risk Assess.* 36 (1): 163–174.

Yang, K., Li, K., Pan, L. et al. (2020). Effect of ozone and electron beam irradiation on degradation of zearalenone and ochratoxin A. *Toxins* 12 (2): 138–148.

Yooussef, M.M., Pham, Q., Achar, P.N., and Sreenivasa, M.Y. (2016). Antifungal activity of essential oils on *Aspergillus parasiticus* isolated from peanuts. *J. Plant Protect. Res.* 56 (2): 139–142. https://doi.org/10.1515/jppr-2016-0021.

Yu, Z., Zhang, L., Wu, D., and Liu, F. (2005). Anti-apoptotic action of zearalenone in MCF-7 cells. *Ecotoxicol. Environ. Saf.* 62 (3): 441–446.

Zhang, G.-L., Feng, Y.-L., Song, J.-L., and Zhou, X.-S. (2018). Zearalenone: a mycotoxin with different toxic effect in domestic and laboratory animals' granulosa cells. *Front. Genet.* 9: 1–8.

Zheng, Y., Hossen, S.M., Sago, Y. et al. (2014). Effect of milling on the content of deoxynivalenol, nivalenol, and zearalenone in Japanese wheat. *Food Control* 40: 193–197.

Zinedine, A., Brera, C., Elakhdari, S. et al. (2006). Natural occurrence of mycotoxins in cereals and spices commercialized in morocco. *Food Control* 17: 868–874.

Zinedine, A., Soriano, J.M., Moltó, J.C., and Mañes, J. (2007). Review on the toxicity, occurrence, metabolism, detoxification, regulations and intake of zearalenone: an oestrogenic mycotoxin. *Food Chem. Toxicol. Int. J. Publ. Br. Ind. Biol. Res. Assoc.* 45 (1): 1–18.

Further Reading

González Pereyra, M.L., Di Giacomo, A.L., Lara, A.L. et al. (2020). Aflatoxin-degrading *Bacillus* sp. strains degrade zearalenone and produce proteases, amylases and cellulases of agro-industrial interest. *Toxicon* 180: 43–48.

Nahle, S., El Khoury, A., Savvaidis, I. et al. (2022). Detoxification approaches of mycotoxins: by microorganisms, biofilms and enzymes. *Int. J. Food Contam.* 9: 3–17.

8

Decontamination and Detoxification of Deoxynivalenol – An Emetic Toxin of Food and Feed

Prakash Sumalatha and Pavagada K. Maheshwar

Department of Microbiology, Yuvaraja's College, University of Mysore, Mysore, Karnataka, India

CONTENTS

Abstract

Deoxynivalenol or vomitoxin belongs to the group of trichothecenes, produced primarily by *Fusarium* species and is a well-known contaminant of cereals and cereal products. Deoxynivalenol is majorly responsible for vomiting, diarrhea, gastrointestinal inflammation, and decreased immunity. Deoxynivalenol also affects reproduction in both animals and humans. Deoxynivalenol has attracted attention on a global scale because of its widespread

Anti-Mycotoxin Strategies for Food and Feed, First Edition. Edited by Deepa Nagaraju, Sreenivasa Marikunte Yanjarappa, Premila N. Achar, and Angel Medina Vaya.

occurrence and severe impacts on both human and animal health. As a result, control measures have been developed to prevent, exclude, or inactivate deoxynivalenol in food and feeds. Both pre-harvest and post-harvest strategies aim to minimize or eliminate deoxynivalenol contamination from foods and feeds. Biological methods proved to be more specialized and effective, as well as eco-friendly and without any nutrient loss in comparison with physical and chemical processes. The present data suggests the appropriate control measures prevent spoilage and good storage practices (GSPs) to be followed for the prevention of deoxynivalenol from affecting the food chain.

Keywords *Fusarium graminearum, deoxynivalenol, trichothecenes, vomitoxin, mycotoxigenic fungi, biocontrol agent, detoxification.*

8.1 Introduction

Mycotoxins are secondary metabolites with low molecular weight, produced by *Fusarium*, *Penicillium*, *Aspergillus*, *Alternaria*, and *Claviceps*. Historical evidence of mycotoxicological risks has existed since the very first period of organized agricultural production. Severe diseases in humans and livestock are caused by the ingestion of mycotoxin-contaminated food or feed (Smith et al. 1995). Mycotoxicity is known to induce mutagenic, carcinogenic, teratogenic, immunosuppressive, and endocrine disorders (Calado et al. 2014). The Food and Agriculture Organization (FAO) of the United Nations has estimated that approximately 25–50% of cereal products produced globally are highly contaminated with mycotoxins, resulting in significant economic losses, increased mortality rates of humans and animals, and the added burden of decreased agricultural productivity. Mycotoxicity also leads to rejection of commodities by national or international markets (Sreenivasa et al. 2008; Pitt and Miller 2016). The major mycotoxins influencing human as well as animal health are aflatoxins, trichothecenes, fumonisins, zearalenone, ochratoxins, patulin, citrinin, and ergot alkaloids (Calado et al. 2014).

8.2 Deoxynivalenol

Deoxynivalenol (DON) is the most widely studied mycotoxin that belongs to the type-B trichothecenes produced by *Fusarium graminearum* and *Fusarium culmorum*. These fungi are known to frequently infect barley, maize, wheat, paddy, oats, rye, sorghum, and other grains in the field or during storage (Castillo et al. 2008; Sreenivasa et al. 2011b; Deepa et al. 2016a, b). DON was isolated in the 1970s, which caused vomiting and other gastrointestinal disorders in Japanese men and American swine on consumption of moldy grain and maize, respectively (Vesonder et al. 1973; Ueno 1985). Vomiting and feed refusal are

Graphical Representation

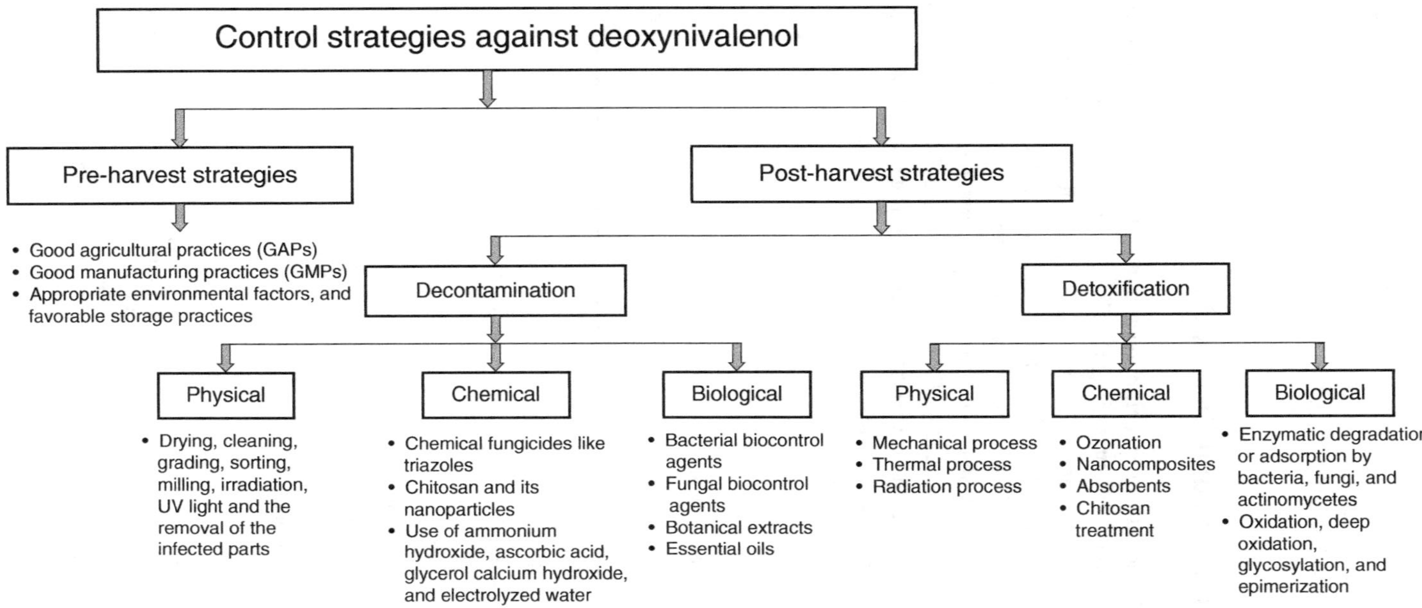

two of the most common toxic symptoms which give DON its alternative name of vomitoxin (WHO 1990). Type B trichothecenes also include nivalenol (NIV) and acetylated derivatives of DON (3-ADON and 15-ADON). Structurally, DON is a polar organic compound, and its chemical name is 3,7,15-trihydroxy-12,13-epoxytrichothec-9-en-8-1. The three free hydroxyl groups (–OH) in the DON molecule are responsible for the toxicity (Sobrova et al. 2010) (Table 8.1).

8.3 Occurrence and Distribution

DON is produced during *Fusarium* head blight (FHB) infections particularly during flowering and, to a lesser extent, during harvest. Local temperature, precipitation, and humidity are some of the key factors leading to infections during flowering. The timing of rainfall is the most critical factor than the amount of rainfall for DON contamination (CODEX 2002). Several species, including *Fusarium verticillioides*, *Fusarium poae*, *Fusarium subglutinans*, *Fusarium temperatum*, and *Fusarium proliferatum* have been identified to cause such infections (Pfordt et al. 2020). FHB incidence and DON contamination in cereal are influenced by many climatic variables, such as spring rainfall, warm temperatures, a_W, and incubation periods. The ideal conditions of incubation are 20–30 °C, 0.95–0.98 a_W, and 7–28 days (Han et al. 2018).

Table 8.1 Physicochemical properties of DON.

S. No.	Parameters	Properties
1.	Name	DON, vomitoxin
2.	IUPAC name	3,7,15-trihydroxy-12,13-epoxytrichothec-9-en-8-one
3.	Molecular formula	$H_{15}O_{20}O_6$
4.	Molar mass	296.32 g/mol
5.	Physical state	Colorless fine needles
6.	Boiling point (°C)	543.9 ± 50.0 °C
7.	Melting point (°C)	151–153 °C
8.	Flashpoint (°C)	206.9 ± 2.5
9.	Vapor pressure (Torr)	4.26×10^{-14} 25 °C
10.	Solubility	Soluble in polar organic solvents like aqueous methanol, chloroform, acetonitrile, ethanol, ethyl acetate, and water

Source: Sobrova et al. (2010)/Slovak Toxicology Society SETOX/CCBY 2.0.

The Joint FAO/WHO Expert Committee on Food Additives (JECFA) (2001) has evaluated the levels and distribution of DON in food products based on the information obtained from Argentina, Canada, Brazil, China, Finland, Germany, Italy, the Netherlands, Sweden, Norway, the United Kingdom, the United States, and Uruguay. The data revealed that DON is most frequently associated with cereal grains such as oats (68%), barley (59%), wheat (57%), maize (41%), rye (49%), and rice (27%). Further, it was also reported in buckwheat, sorghum, popcorn, triticale, and in various processed food items such as bread, noodles, wheat flour, breakfast cereals, baby and infant foods, fried pancakes, malt, and beer (JECFA 2001; Sreenivasa et al. 2011a; Nagaraja et al. 2016).

8.3.1 Deoxynivalenol in Food and Feed

The primary source of DON across all age groups was found to be bread and derived foodstuffs (Narvaez et al. 2022). Meta-analysis was carried out to examine the incidence and DON levels in cereals and their products intended for human consumption in Spanish markets. The findings demonstrated that DON has a significant impact on bread, breakfast cereals, and bread-derived foodstuffs. DON exposure was found to be high, particularly in newborns and young children under the age of three, according to the exposure assessment. DON and NIV toxins were detected in more than 90% of the oat samples from Sweden, contaminated with *F. culmorum*, *Fusarium sporotrichioides*, *F. poae*, *Fusarium tricinctum*, *F. graminearum*, and *Fusarium avenaceum* (Fredlund et al. 2013; Deepa and Sreenivasa 2017a, b). *F. culmorum* has been reported from fresh samples of maize harvested from places in south India. Ninety-four isolates were found to produce DON/NIV by mPCR assay (Venkataramana et al. 2013). The most recent survey of 21 709 samples of maize and wheat from seven continents showed a significant occurrence of DON in the samples, viz. the Asia-Pacific region (86%), the Middle East (78%), and Central America (76%) (Biomin 2021). The average concentration of DON in wheat samples from South America was $\geq 1.5\,\mu g/g$, which represented a significant risk for animals, particularly swine.

8.4 Toxicological Effects of Deoxynivalenol

Humans are vulnerable to significant health risks by directly consuming foods like cereals, flour, and bread contaminated with DON or indirectly through the consumption of foods of animal origin (Krieger et al. 2010). The main symptoms of DON poisoning are acute temporary nausea, vomiting, headache, abdominal pain, dizziness, and diarrhea (Ji et al. 2015). DON inhibits protein synthesis and interferes with proper cell function as it binds to the 60S ribosomal subunit and activates vital cellular kinases responsible for signal transduction (Wollenhaupt et al. 2007; Abd El-Twab et al. 2009). The sublethal level of trichothecenes depends on the exposure frequency and duration, which can stimulate or suppress immune parameters like lymphocyte proliferation, host resistance, and cell-mediated immunity (Pestka and Bondy 1994). Bensassi et al. (2009) examined the toxic effects of DON in the colon cancer cells of humans (HT 29) and observed that the toxin led to DNA damage and activation of p53 and caspase 3. The research claims that DON directly damages DNA and may be classified as a genotoxic substance that might lead to apoptotic cell death (Figure 8.1).

Animals of different species, sex, and age groups have variable levels of DON sensitivity. Swine, cats, dogs, ruminants, poultry, and rodents are most susceptible to DON contamination (Mishra et al. 2020). DON intoxication decreases the production rates of milk, eggs, and meat, and increases the rate of embryonic deformity and chromosomal aberration in chickens. DON contamination also induces weak progeny, stillbirths, stiff hogs, female pig abortions, as well as impaired performance in cattle production (Bracarense et al. 2012; Feizollahi and Roopesh 2021). DON concentration of 12 mg/kg induces an emetic response in animals. Chickens are less susceptible to DON but the concentration ranging from 16 to 20 mg/kg in the feed results in feed rejection and lowered weight gain (Eriksen and Pettersson 2004) (Table 8.2).

8.5 Prevention Strategies Against Deoxynivalenol

Mycotoxigenic fungi-contaminated agricultural commodities might result in poor quality, yield, and mycotoxicosis in human beings and livestock. DON has gained international attention due to its prevalence and negative impacts on both human and animal health. Hence, control measures for preventing, eliminating, or inactivating DON content in food and feeds have been developed. All pre-harvest techniques strive to minimize DON accumulation, whereas post-harvest practices target to eliminate or degrade DON from contaminated foods and feeds (Guo et al. 2020) (Figure 8.2). The prevention strategies include pre-harvest, post-harvest strategies, physical, chemical, and biocontrol methods to manage the effects of toxins (Deepa and Sreenivasa 2019a, b).

8.5.1 Pre-harvest Strategies

The presence of mycotoxins in foods poses a high health threat for the consumers. The prevention of fungal contamination and breeding crops to be resistant to mold infections should be the best strategy. The pre-harvest prevention includes good agricultural practices (GAPs), good manufacturing practices (GMPs), and favorable storage practices (Luo et al. 2018). Implementation of crop rotation, use of fungicides, herbicides, and insecticides, proper treatment of the seed bed, soil analysis, and suppression of mycotoxin production by enhancement of genetic synthesis are GAPs (Alberts et al. 2017; Adebiyi et al. 2019).

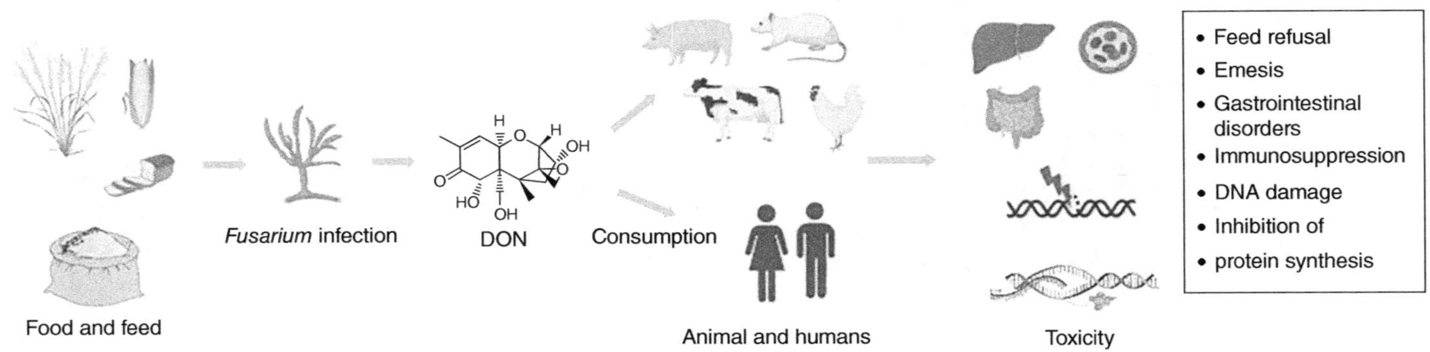

Figure 8.1 Toxicological effects of DON.

Table 8.2 Acceptable limits of DON content in different foods and feeds.

Governing organizations	Food/feed type	Acceptable limit (μg/kg)
European Commission	Cereals and cereal-based products (except for maize byproducts)	8000
	Maize byproducts	12 000
	Complete feeding stuffs and complementary for pigs	900
	Complete feeding stuffs and complementary for calves (<4 mo), lambs, and kids	2000
United States Food and Drug Administration (USFDA)	Wheat products for human consumption	1000
Food and Agricultural Organization (FAO) of the United States/Codex Alimentarius	Maize, barley, and raw wheat	2000
	Maize- or barley-derived flour, semolina, meal, flakes, and wheat	1000
	Cereal-based infant foods	500

Source: Kamle et al. (2022)/MDPI/CC BY 4.0.

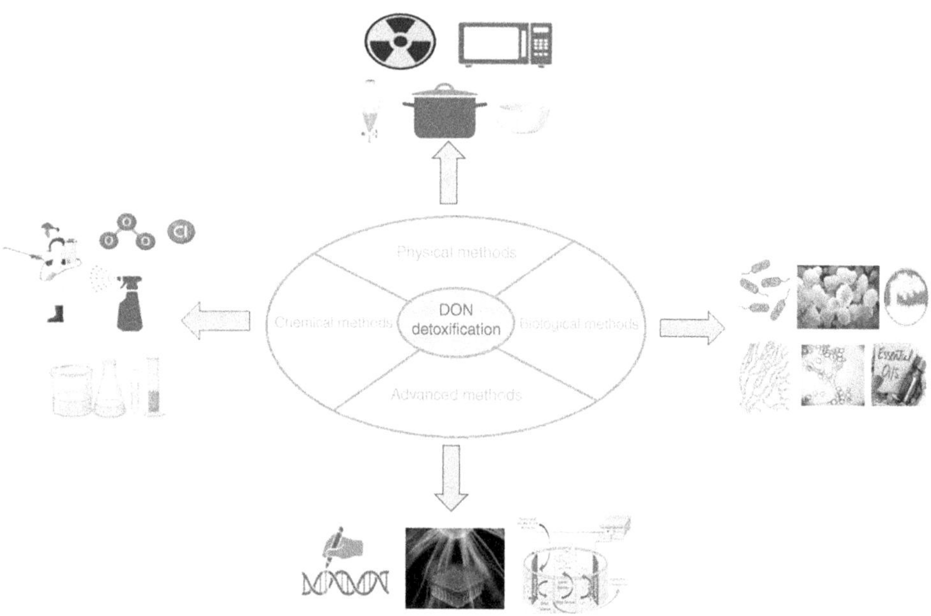

Figure 8.2 Detoxification strategies of DON.

8.5.2 Post-harvest Strategies

Post-harvest strategies aim at decontamination and/or detoxification of mycotoxins from numerous agricultural commodities. Mycotoxins can be removed by physical, chemical, and biological methods (Lyagin and Efremenko 2019). Temperature, humidity, and moisture content of warehouses are critical for growth of mycotoxigenic fungi and mycotoxin production when it pertains to effective storage methods (Luo et al. 2018). Selecting *Fusarium*-resistant wheat varieties, lowering plant stress, and proper drying followed by harvest are the crucial steps in preventing the DON contamination of cereals (CODEX 2002).

8.5.3 Strategies for the Prevention of DON in Food and Feed

Drying, cleaning, grading, sorting, sieving, grinding, radiation treatment, and the elimination of the contaminated parts are the major physical methods primarily used for the prevention of DON (Yi-gang et al. 2016; Sarrocco and Vannacci 2018). Chemical control includes the application of different chemicals to control fungi and its mycotoxin in agricultural commodities. FHB and DON contamination in field conditions can be significantly reduced with good management practices (GMPs) and proper fungicide application (Lehoczki-Krsjak et al. 2010).

8.5.4 Fungicides for the Management of DON

The most effective chemical fungicides applied to wheat and grains are triazoles, which include tebuconazole, prothioconazole, metconazole, and benzimidazole. These agents suppress sterol biosynthesis of fungal pathogens. The combination of tebuconazole, prothioconazole, and metconazole was most effective when administered shortly after anthesis (D'Angelo et al. 2014). Prochloraz, an imidazole derivate, effectively inhibits the mycelial growth of *F. culmorum*, *F. graminearum*, and *F. avenaceum* in grains. In contrast, these fungi developed resistance to carbendazim, a well-known benzimidazole fungicide that has been proven most effective in reducing contamination of wheat heads by around 70%. Chitosan (CS) and CS nanoparticles (CS NPs) can be applied as an alternative to synthetic fungicides to control *F. graminearum* owing to their biocompatibility and antimicrobial properties. The highest growth reduction of 68.18% and 77.5% was recorded with CS and its nanoparticles at 1000 and 5000 ppm concentrations, respectively (Kheiri et al. 2017). Application of CS to infected maize and wheat reduces the accumulation of Fumonisin B (FBs) and DON by *F. proliferatum*, *F. verticillioides*, and *F. graminearum* (Zachetti et al. 2019). Khan and Doohan (2009) demonstrated that the combination of CS and *Pseudomonas fluorescens* effectively reduced the growth of *F. culmorum* responsible for FHB infection and DON accumulation in barley and wheat grains (Gunupuru et al. 2019).

8.6 Biological Control Agents (BCA)

Biological control aims at utilizing microorganisms, and naturally occurring compounds such as enzymes, botanical extracts, and essential oils (EOs) that possess the ability to inhibit microorganisms causing plant diseases. Antagonistic microorganisms like bacteria, yeast, and nonpathogenic fungi are used as biofungicides (Pal and Gardener 2006). BCAs are highly beneficial when fungicides cannot be used on organic crops. Bacterial and fungal biological control agents (BCAs) can be applied directly to residues or wheat spikes to inhibit the growth of perithecia or to reduce the severity of the disease (Prasad et al. 2010; Shah et al. 2018). BCAs that are extensively exploited against FHB-causing *Fusarium* spp. are the species of *Bacillus* and *Pseudomonas* (Yoshida et al. 2012). *Bacillus amyloliquefaciens* FLN13, *Streptomyces* spp. *Lactobacillus plantarum* SLG17 have been employed against *F. graminearum* and *F. culmorum* (Rosello et al. 2013; Baffoni et al. 2015). Fungal BCAs include *Trichoderma* spp., *Cryptococcus* spp., and *Aureobasidium pullulans* (Shah et al. 2018). The inhibitory effect of *Trichoderma* spp. is attributed to chitinases and chitinolytic enzymes (Matarese et al. 2012). *Cladosporium cladosporioides* exhibited broad-spectrum inhibition against *F. graminearum* (Schoneberg et al. 2015). The action mechanism of BCAs includes the synthesis of antifungal metabolites (*Bacillus*), competition for resources and establishment of localized resistance (*Lysobacter*) (McMullen et al. 1997).

8.6.1 Essential Oils

Plant-derived EOs are natural fungicides proven to be beneficial over biological and environmental complications caused by synthetic fungicides (Yooussef et al. 2016; Sumalatha and Maheshwar 2021). Amini et al. (2012) reported that EOs extracted from *Thymus vulgaris*, *Thymus kotschyanus*, and *Zataria multiflora*, effectively inhibited *F. graminearum*. Clove oil and *Ocimum tenuiflorum* have an inhibitory effect on DON accumulation in grains infested with *F. graminearum* (Gurjar et al. 2012; Kalagatur et al. 2015; Achar et al. 2020). Ginger EO inhibited the synthesis of DON *by F. graminearum in vitro* at a concentration of 500 μg/mL (Dias Ferreira et al. 2018). Similar results were observed with ginger and thyme EOs at the concentrations of 11.25 and 364 μg/mL, respectively (Pandey et al. 2022) (Figure 8.2).

8.7 Detoxification of Deoxynivalenol

8.7.1 Physical Methods

Cleaning, washing, dehulling, sieving, grinding, heat treatment, and radiation process are the physical methods employed for eliminating DON from contaminated grains. The effectiveness of these methods depends on the degree of contamination and toxin distribution (Charmley and Prelusky 1994) (Table 8.3).

8.7.1.1 Sieving and Grinding

Bran and germ of the grains tend to acquire mycotoxins. DON contamination can be eliminated in grains through mechanical peeling in the early phases (Brera et al. 2004). Trenholm

Table 8.3 Strategies on detoxification of DON.

S. No.	Anti-DON strategy	Treatment	Methodology	Percent of reduction (%)	References
1.	Physical	Sieving and grinding	Coarse grinding and filtering	16	Trenholm et al. (1991)
		Heat treatment	Boiling, frying, and microwave	10–63	Vidal et al. (2016)
		Irradiation	2–20 KGy (Gamma)	2.4–83	Li et al. (2019) and Feizollahi and Roopesh (2021)
			UV-C	21–66	Murata et al. (2011)
			Pulsed light treatment	14.3–72.5	–
2.	Chemical	Chemical agents	Na_2SO_3, $Na_2S_2O_5$, Na_2CO_3	66–100	Danicke et al. (2005), Abramson et al. (2005)
			Chlorine gas	100	–
			Ozone	26–55	Wang et al. (2016) and Piemontese et al. (2018)
3.	Biological	Biosorption	*Streptomyces albidoflavus* RC 87B and *Bacillus velezensis* RC 218	51	Palazzini et al. (2018)
			B. subtilis ASAG 216	81.1	Jia et al. (2020)
			B. subtilis and *L. plantarum*	74.9	Li et al. (2020)
		Essential oils	Natural essential oils	52.3–100	Perczak et al. (2019a,b)
		Photocatalytic degradation	UCNP@TiO_2 upconversion nanoparticle	100	Zhou et al. (2020)
			Nanocomposites	87	Gonzalez-Jartin et al. (2019)
		Electrochemical oxidation	First-order kinetics	86.4	Xiong et al. (2019)
		ACP	34 kV, 2 mm for 6 min	48.9	Feizollahi et al. (2020)
		Enzymatic treatment	Amylolytic enzymes and β-xylanase	41	Juodeikiene et al. (2011)

et al. (1991) decreased the DON concentration to 16% by eliminating the fungal chitin using coarse grinding and filtering of barley. However, there was a 69% and 40% drop in mass and protein content, respectively. Additionally, cereal grains are more prone to fungal invasion due to mechanical damage.

8.7.1.2 Solvent Extraction

DON can be extracted, separated, and detoxified using a combination of water and organic solvents because it is soluble in both polar and nonpolar solvents. Distilled water, 30% sucrose solution, saturated sodium chloride solution, sodium hydroxide, and sodium carbonate are the major extraction solvents mentioned in the literature. Application of this procedure is limited due to its high cost and the formation of a residual byproduct, which leads to secondary contamination. Additionally, this procedure reduces the nutritional content of the grains (Yener and Köksel 2013).

8.7.1.3 Heat Treatment

Heat treatment including wet methods like boiling and steaming as well as dry methods like baking, roasting, frying, and microwave heating is considered most efficient in reducing DON content in foods (Schaarschmidt and Fauhl-Hassek 2021). DON significantly decreased in cereals with increased temperature at 180–220 °C and baking for 30 minutes, respectively (Pleadin et al. 2019; Stadler et al. 2019). DON in boiled wheat spaghetti was decreased by more than 40% due to the leaching of DON content into the broth (Vidal et al. 2016). Microwave heating of the contaminated corn at 75 °C and 175 °C reduced DON concentration by 10% and 40%, respectively (Young 1986). Frying the turnover pie at 169, 205, and 243 °C reduced DON concentration by >66%, 43%, and 38%, respectively. However, high temperatures deplete the nutrient content in foods and may result in harmful or undesirable byproducts that alter the taste (Bretz et al. 2006).

8.7.1.4 Radiation Process

Several research have also documented the degeneration of DON using UV and gamma radiation without altering the food composition. Gamma irradiation (with Cobalt 60) has a strong penetration and inhibitory effect on microbes; hence, it is extensively used in the food industries (Calado et al. 2014). Gamma radiation between 5 and 8 kGy has significantly reduced DON content in wheat, bread, and flour, inhibiting the growth of *Fusarium* species. DON concentrations were reduced to 85 μg/kg for wheat and 125 μg/kg for flour at 4 kGy irradiation (Aziz et al. 1997). Li et al. (2019) observed that 20 kGy irradiation results in 83% degradation of DON content in acetonitrile water. DON concentration in wheat and soybeans was reduced by 41% and 2.4% at 2 and 5 kGy irradiation, respectively (Feizollahi and Roopesh 2021). Dried DON was exposed to ultraviolet-C (UV-C) treatment (intensity = 0.1 mW/cm^2) for 60 minutes, which decreased DON concentration from 30 ppm to 0.2 ppm. Murata et al. (2011) reported that DON content was reduced by 22% and 21% with UV-C treatment (1.5 mW/cm^2) at 254 nm on moist maize silage for 30 and 60 minutes, respectively. Gamma irradiation cannot be recommended for practical applications due to the requirement of high irradiation doses for the total elimination of DON content in grains.

8.7.2 Chemical Methods

Chemical detoxification mainly involves the application of specific chemicals and ozone treatment for the detoxification of DON content (Figure 8.2).

8.7.2.1 Chemical Agents

Chemicals such as alkaline, sodium bisulfite (Na_2SO_3), ammonium carbonate ($[NH_4]_2CO_3$), sodium metabisulfite ($Na_2S_2O_5$), sodium carbonate (Na_2CO_3), L-ascorbic acid, chlorine, and L-cysteine are used to disintegrate the chemical structure or remove the active groups of mycotoxins (Wu et al. 2020). Numerous reports have assessed the impact of alkaline treatment on DON reduction. According to Mishra et al. (2014), the peak of standard DON was decreased by 66%, and a new peak was detected at pH = 1. The findings indicated that DON may be degraded to its byproducts in the stomach at pH 1–2. The efficiency of $Na_2S_2O_5$ in regulating DON in grains by hot water treatment was investigated by Danicke et al. (2005) and Young (1986). Ninety-two percent of DON in barley was degraded by 1 M of 20% v/w Na_2CO_3 and heating at 80 °C (Abramson et al. 2005). Depending on the concentration and duration of treatment, DON was degraded completely when maize was exposed to 5–100% chlorinated air (Young 1986). The degradation rate of DON in instant noodles was accelerated by adding L-ascorbic acid, Na_2SO_3, or L-cysteine as food additives (Moazami et al. 2014) (Table 8.3).

8.7.2.2 Ozone Treatment

Ozone is a strong oxidizing agent and is capable of detoxifying DON. Ozone is rapidly transformed into oxygen due to its instability and short half-life (20–50 minutes), leaving no residues behind (Wang et al. 2016). Many reports are available on DON degradation by aqueous, dry, and gaseous ozone (Agriopoulou et al. 2020). Ozone treatment of 55 gO_3/h for six hours showed a 29–32% decrease in DON-3-glucoside (DON-3-Glc), its modified form and DON in durum wheat (Piemontese et al. 2018). Ozone treatment (75 mg/L O_3) for 30 and 90 minutes reduced DON levels by 26.4% and 53.5%, respectively, in contaminated wheat samples. The rate of DON decomposition can be enhanced by increasing the ozone concentration, duration, and substrate moisture content (Wang et al. 2016). Despite its effectiveness, ozonation is still inappropriate for large-scale applications due to its high cost and need for specialized equipment (Li et al. 2015).

The physical and chemical approaches have several drawbacks, including sophisticated equipment requirements, high cost, limited efficacy, harmful chemical residues, safety issues, and nutrient loss. Hence, eco-friendly methods using enzymes and beneficial microorganisms are more convenient (Ji et al. 2016) (Table 8.3).

8.7.3 Biological Detoxification

These are regarded as potential detoxification techniques because of their eco-friendly nature, high specificity, and efficiency. These techniques primarily depend on the adsorption (biosorption) of DON onto cell walls of microorganisms or the enzyme-mediated decomposition of DON (Kamle et al. 2022) (Figure 8.2).

8.7.3.1 Biosorption of DON

Some bacterial cell walls can inherently adsorb mycotoxins because of their unique composition. *Streptomyces albidoflavus* RC 87B and *Bacillus velezensis* RC 218 effectively reduced DON accumulation by up to 51% in durum wheat experimented at field conditions (Palazzini et al. 2018). *Devosia insulae* A16 and *Bacillus licheniformis* were able to detoxify DON at 88% and 82.6%, respectively (Wang et al. 2019a,b; Wang et al. 2020). Probiotic yeast *Saccharomyces cerevisiae* can significantly break down DON and slow down the rate at which lactate dehydrogenase (LDH) is released in DON-stimulated cells (Liu et al. 2019; Chennappa et al. 2014, 2016, 2019). 81.1% DON degradation by *B. subtilis* ASAG 216 was observed at optimum conditions of time (eight hours), temperature (35–50 °C), and pH (6.5–9.0) (Jia et al. 2020). *B. subtilis* and *L. plantarum* showed a synergistic effect in DON detoxification up to 74.9% in 96 hours (Li et al. 2020). Enzymatic methods used for DON degradation are fermentation and malting process. DON reduction is inversely proportional to the concentration of yeast, fermentation time, and temperature (Samar et al. 2001). Examined the impact of the peroxidase (PO) and concluded that H_2O_2 was essential as a co-factor for enzymatic catalysis and DON detoxification (Table 8.3).

8.7.3.2 Essential Oils

The inhibition of *F. culmorum* and *F. graminearum* in maize and wheat seeds and reduction in the amount of DON by five EOs *in vitro* was recorded as 52.38% with pink grapefruit, 54.49% with eucalyptus, 62.73% with lemon, 72.28% with palmarosa. Highest reduction of 93.18% was observed at 5.0 μg/mL concentration with white grapefruit EO (Perczak et al. 2019a,b). The influence of oregano, cinnamon, lemongrass, clove, and palmarose EOs was tested on irradiated maize. DON production was inhibited by all the tested EOs at 30 °C and 0.995 a_w (Velluti et al. 2004). In a study, selected EOs (oregano, cinnamon, palmarosa, orange, spearmint, verbena, fennel, and rosewood) reduced the concentrations of DON in wheat grain by 94.51–100% (Perczak et al. 2019a,b) (Table 8.3).

8.7.4 Advanced Techniques for the Detoxification of DON

8.7.4.1 Photocatalytic Degradation

This technique is low-cost, reusable, eco-friendly, and highly stable. It breaks down the targeted toxin using a TiON@PdO nanoparticle, carbon-supported TiO_2, ZnO@graphene hybrids, upconversion nanoparticles@TiO_2 composite, and dendritic-like-Fe_2O_3 (Feizollahi and Roopesh 2021). UCNP@TiO_2 (upconversion nanoparticle) is an efficient DON degrader in cereal products (Zhou et al. 2020). The results indicated a decrease of DON in cereal products below the permissible limits (1 ppm) after 90 minutes and total degradation after 120 minutes of illumination with slightly toxic or non-toxic degradation products. Nanocomposites comprising mixtures of bentonite, activated carbon, and aluminum oxide removed 87% of mycotoxins (Gonzalez-Jartin et al. 2019).

8.7.4.2 Electrochemical Oxidation (ECO)

ECO has evolved as a novel oxidation technology that degrades DON by various mechanisms. DON was dramatically reduced by graphite electrodes because of high voltage and acidic conditions. The degradation rate of DON in contaminated wet distiller's grain was detected to be 86.4% in 60 minutes. Electrochemical oxidation has many advantages like easy operation, mild reactions, no secondary contamination, and fully automatic (Xiong et al. 2019).

8.7.4.3 Atmospheric Cold Plasma Technology (ACP)

Another innovative non-thermal method for detoxifying DON is referred to as ACP, which uses plasma at low atmospheric pressure. It has higher chemical reactivity and efficacy than ozone and UV treatments. As a result, DON is decontaminated in a matter of seconds with less toxic degradation products (Hojnik et al. 2017). ACP is used to decompose mycotoxins chemically via diverse pathways, generating degradation products with low toxicity levels (Misra et al. 2019). It is important to note that during ACP treatments, the temperature of the samples does not rise to more than 60 °C, and hence no degradation of mycotoxin occurs thermally (Ten Bosch et al. 2017). Feizollahi et al. (2020) performed ACP treatment (34 kV, 2 mm gap) for six minutes, which reduced the DON levels on spiked barley by 48.9%.

8.7.4.4 Enzymatic Treatment

Enzymatic processes like oxidation, epimerization, and glycosylation can also be employed to detoxify DON with the formation of less toxic byproducts like DON-3-glucoside (D3G) 3-keto DON, and 3-epi DON (Tian et al. 2016). Wang et al. (2019a,b) reported that deacetylation of 3-ADON and 15-ADON produces DON which is further degraded into 3-keto-DON. *Pelagibacterium halotolerans* ANSP101 can also convert DON into 3-keto-DON (less toxic) by C3 hydroxyl group oxidation (Zhang et al. 2020). Forty one percent of DON can be degraded by combining traditional amylolytic enzymes and β-xylanase at higher doses (Juodeikiene et al. 2011). Degradation by enzymatic action is considered the most promising technology with the greatest commercial potential due to its advantages like reproducibility, consistency, ease of use, and safety (Table 8.1).

8.8 Summary

The mycotoxins present in foods pose a high health threat to consumers. Prevention of fungal contamination and breeding crops to be resistant to mold infections should be the best strategy. Further cleaning, washing, dehulling, and milling are the physical methods effective in eliminating DON from contaminated grains. Mycotoxins enter the food chain due to contamination of crops by fungi either through direct human consumption or as livestock feed. The FAO has estimated that mycotoxins are present in approximately 25% of the cereals produced globally. This fungus may potentially contaminate other foods like spices, fruits, nuts, and their byproducts. Mycotoxin contamination of agricultural crops can occur at various levels of the food chain, including pre-harvest, harvest, drying, and storage. Mycotoxins like DON pose health hazards when associated with food and feed. They are important contaminants which adversely affect animal and human health, as well as significant economic loss. The presence and prevalence of these toxins are increasing each year. Therefore, systematic surveillance of DON is required in food and fodder around the globe.

8.9 Future Implications

Since food safety is becoming a global concern, management and prevention of DON accumulation in food products need increased attention. DON entry into food supply chain can be controlled by following scientific agricultural interventions such as GAPs,

GMPs, and GSPs. An important strategy to combat mycotoxins and mycotoxin-producing microorganisms is through prevention. Prevention of mycotoxin should be done in the pre-harvest stages by directly inhibiting the infection of mycotoxin-producing fungi. Pre-harvest strategies include soil analysis; removal of weeds and damaged kernels; use of fertilizers; resistant varieties; herbicides, fungicides, and insecticides; crop rotation, and the use of genetically modified plants.

Post-harvest strategies include cleaning, sorting, drying, smoking, and use of insecticides and pesticides in storage rooms. The grains must be dried before storage to lower the moisture content, which otherwise promotes fungal growth. Solar driers can be used in place of sun drying because slow drying enhances mycotoxin levels. Regulation of temperature, moisture, and relative humidity is necessary to prevent microbial contamination and mycotoxin production during storage. Detoxification methods can also be adopted in the post-harvest stages without affecting the physical and chemical characteristics of agricultural commodities. Continuous monitoring of mycotoxins in agricultural commodities can prevent substantial problems in marketing, distribution, and consumption of foods.

Future DON research should focus on molecular mechanisms including neuronal toxicity, sensitivity of neuronal cells or tissues in relation to other species, epidemiological association with chronic gastroenteritis in humans, emetic effects in primates, and vigilance of DON in cereal crops worldwide.

8.10 Study Questions

1) Write the acceptable limits of deoxynivalenol in food and feeds.
2) Give the alternative term for deoxynivalenol.
3) What are some of the important detoxification strategies?
4) What are the biological effects of deoxynivalenol on animal and human health?

Acknowledgments

The authors acknowledge Yuvaraja's College, University of Mysore, India for the support provided for the preparation of this manuscript.

Conflict of Interest

The authors confirm that they have no conflicts of interest.

Author Contributions

Conceptualization and writing S. P., supervision, review, coordinating, and editing P. K. M.

References

Abd El-Twab, M.H., Mahmoud, M.A.H., Helmey, R.K., and Fadl-Allah, E.M. (2009). Molecular cytogenetical effects of some mycotoxins to chromosomes of *Triticum durum* using RAPD-PCR fluorescence in situ hybridization. *Chromosom. Bot.* 4 (1): 13–18.

Abramson, D., House, J.D., and Martin Nyachoti, C. (2005). Reduction of deoxynivalenol in barley by treatment with aqueous sodium carbonate and heat. *Mycopathologia* 160 (4): 297–301.

Achar, P.N., Quyen, P., Adukwu, E.C. et al. (2020). Investigation of the antifungal and anti-aflatoxigenic potential of plant-based essential oils against *Aspergillus flavus* in peanuts. *J. Fungi* 6 (4): 383. https://doi.org/10.3390/jof6040383.

Adebiyi, J.A., Kayitesi, E., Adebo, O.A. et al. (2019). Food fermentation and mycotoxin detoxification: an African perspective. *Food Control* 106: 106731.

Agriopoulou, S., Stamatelopoulou, E., and Varzakas, T. (2020). Advances in occurrence, importance, and mycotoxin control strategies: prevention and detoxification in foods. *Foods* 9 (2): 137.

Alberts, J.F., Lilly, M., Rheeder, J.P. et al. (2017). Technological and community-based methods to reduce mycotoxin exposure. *Food Control* 73: 101–109.

Amini, M., Safaie, N., Salmani, M.J., and Shams-Bakhsh, M. (2012). Antifungal activity of three medicinal plant essential oils against some phytopathogenic fungi. *Trakia J. Sci.* 10: 1–8.

Aziz, N.H., Attia, E.S., and Farag, S.A. (1997). Effect of gamma-irradiation on the natural occurrence of *Fusarium* mycotoxins in wheat, flour, and bread. *Food/Nahrung* 41 (1): 34–37.

Baffoni, L., Gaggia, F., Dalanaj, N. et al. (2015). Microbial inoculants for the biocontrol of *Fusarium* spp. in durum wheat. *BMC Microbiol.* 15: 242.

Bensassi, F., El Golli-Bennour, E., Abid-Essefi, S. et al. (2009). Pathway of deoxynivalenol-induced apoptosis in human colon carcinoma cells. *Toxicology* 264: 104–109.

Biomin. (2021). World mycotoxin survey: impact in 2021. https://www.biomin.net/br/science-hub/pesquisa-mundial-de-micotoxinas-impacto-em-2021 (accessed 29 October 2022).

Bracarense, A.P.F., Lucioli, J., Grenier, B. et al. (2012). Chronic ingestion of deoxynivalenol and fumonisin, alone or in interaction, induces morphological and immunological changes in the intestine of piglets. *Br. J. Nutr.* 107: 1776–1786.

Brera, C., Debegnach, F., Grossi, S., and Miraglia, M. (2004). Effect of industrial processing on the distribution of fumonisin B1 in dry milling corn fractions. *J. Food Protect.* 67: 1261–1266.

Bretz, M., Beyer, M., Cramer, B. et al. (2006). Thermal degradation of the *Fusarium* mycotoxin deoxynivalenol. *J. Agric. Food Chem.* 54: 6445–6451.

Calado, T., Venancio, A., and Abrunhosa, L. (2014). Irradiation for mold and mycotoxin control: a review. *Compr. Rev. Food Sci. Food Saf.* 13 (5): 1049–1061.

Castillo, M.A., Montes, R., Navarro, A. et al. (2008). Occurrence of deoxynivalenol and nivalenol in Spanish corn-based food products. *J. Food Compos. Anal.* 21 (5): 423–427.

Charmley, L.L. and Prelusky, D.B. (1994). Decontamination of *Fusarium* mycotoxins. In: *Mycotoxins in Grain. Compounds Other than Aflatoxin* (ed. J.D. Miller and H.L. Trenholm), 421–435. St. Paul, MN: Eagen Press.

Chennappa, G., Adkar-Purushothama, C.R., Umdale Suraj, K., and Tamilvendan, M.Y.S. (2014). Impact of pesticides on PGPR activity of *Azotobacter* sp. isolated from pesticide flooded paddy soils. *Greener J. Agric. Sci.* 4 (4): 117–129.

Chennappa, G., Naik, M.K., Adkar-Purushothama, C.R. et al. (2016). PGP, abiotic stress tolerant and antifungal activity of *Azotobacter* sp. isolated from paddy soils. *Indian J. Exp. Biol.* 54 (5): 322–331.

Chennappa, G., Udaykumar, N., Vidya, M. et al. (2019). *Azotobacter*—a natural resource for bioremediation of toxic pesticides in soil ecosystems. In: *New and Future Developments in Microbial Biotechnology and Bioengineering* (ed. J.S. Singh and D.P. Singh), 267–279. Elsevier. ISBN: 9780444641915.

CODEX. (2002). Codex committee on food additives and contaminants (CX/FAC 02/29). Discussion paper on deoxynivalenol. Codex alimentarius commission/FAO/WHO, Rotterdam, The Netherlands.

D'Angelo, D.L., Bradley, C.A., Ames, K.A. et al. (2014). Efficacy of fungicide applications during and after anthesis against *Fusarium* head blight and deoxynivalenol in soft red winter wheat. *Plant Dis.* 98: 1387–1397.

Danicke, S., Valenta, H., Gareis, M. et al. (2005). On the effects of a hydrothermal treatment of deoxynivalenol (DON)-contaminated wheat in the presence of sodium metabisulphite ($Na_2S_2O_5$) on DON reduction and on piglet performance. *Anim. Feed Sci. Technol.* 118: 93–108.

Deepa, N. and Sreenivasa, M.Y. (2017a). *Fusarium verticillioides*, a globally important pathogen of agriculture and livestock: a review. *J. Vet. Med. Res.* 4 (4): 1084.

Deepa, N. and Sreenivasa, M.Y. (2017b). Fumonisins: a review on its global occurrence, epidemiology, toxicity and detection. *J. Vet. Med. Res.* 4 (6): 1093.

Deepa, N. and Sreenivasa, M.Y. (2019a). Biocontrol strategies for effective management of phytopathogenic fungi associated with cereals. In: *New and Future Developments in Microbial Biotechnology and Bioengineering* (ed. J.S. Singh and D.P. Singh), 177–189. Elsevier. ISBN: 9780444641915 10.1016/B978-0-444-64191-5.00013-4.

Deepa, N. and Sreenivasa, M.Y. (2019b). Molecular methods and key genes targeted for the detection of fumonisin producing *Fusarium verticillioides* - an updated review. *Food Biosci.* 32: 100473. https://doi.org/10.1016/j.fbio.2019.100473.

Deepa, N., Nagaraja, H., and Sreenivasa, M.Y. (2016a). Prevalence of fumonisin producing *Fusarium verticillioides* associated with cereals grown in Karnataka (India). *Food Sci. Human Well.* 5: 156–162. https://doi.org/10.1016/j.fshw.2016.07.001.

Deepa, N., Charith Raj, A.P., and Sreenivasa, M.Y. (2016b). Multiplex PCR method for the early detection of fumonisin producing *Fusarium verticillioides*. *Food Biosci.* 13: 84–88.

Dias Ferreira, F.M., Hirooka, E.Y., Dias Ferreira, F. et al. (2018). Effect of *Zingiber officinale* Roscoe essential oil in fungus control and deoxynivalenol production of *Fusarium graminearum* Schwabe *in vitro*. *Food Addit. Contam. Part A* 35 (11): 2168–2174.

Eriksen, G.S. and Pettersson, H. (2004). Toxicological evaluation of trichothecenes in animal feed. *Anim. Feed Sci. Technol.* 114: 205–239.

Feizollahi, E. and Roopesh, M.S. (2021). Mechanisms of deoxynivalenol (DON) degradation during different treatments: a review. *Crit. Rev. Food Sci. Nutr.* 1–22.

Feizollahi, E., Iqdiam, B., Vasanthan, T. et al. (2020). Effects of atmospheric-pressure cold plasma treatment on deoxynivalenol degradation, quality parameters, and germination of barley grains. *Appl. Sci.* 10: 3530.

Fredlund, E., Gidlund, A., Sulyok, M. et al. (2013). Deoxynivalenol and other selected *Fusarium* toxins in Swedish oats-occurrence and correlation to specific *Fusarium* species. *Int. J. Food Microbiol.* 167 (2): 276–283.

Gonzalez-Jartin, J.M., de Castro Alves, L., Alfonso, A. et al. (2019). Detoxification agents based on magnetic nanostructured particles as a novel strategy for mycotoxin mitigation in food. *Food Chem.* 294: 60–66.

Gunupuru, L.R., Patel, J.S., Sumarah, M.W. et al. (2019). A plant biostimulant made from the marine brown algae *Ascophyllum nodosum* and chitosan reduce *Fusarium* head blight and mycotoxin contamination in wheat. *PLoS One* 14: e0220562.

Guo, H., Ji, J., Wang, J.S., and Sun, X. (2020). Deoxynivalenol: masked forms, fate during food processing, and potential biological remedies. *Compr. Rev. Food Sci. Food Saf.* 19: 895–926.

Gurjar, M.S., Ali, S., Akhtar, M., and Singh, K.S. (2012). Efficacy of plant extracts in plant disease management. *Agric. Sci.* 3: 425–433.

Han, Z., Shen, Y., Di Mavungu, J.D. et al. (2018). Relationship between environmental conditions, TRI5 gene expression and deoxynivalenol production in stored Lentinula edodes infected with *Fusarium graminearum*. *World Mycotoxin J.* 11: 177–186.

Hojnik, N., Cvelbar, U., Tavčar-Kalcher, G. et al. (2017). Mycotoxin decontamination of food: cold atmospheric pressure plasma versus "classic" decontamination. *Toxins* 9 (5): 151.

Ji, C., Li, L., Li, X., and Liu, S. (2015). Research progress of biodegradation of vomit toxin. *Feed Ind.* 36 (10): 1–5.

Ji, C., Fan, Y., and Zhao, L. (2016). Review on biological degradation of mycotoxins. *Anim. Nutr.* 2: 127–133.

Jia, R., Cao, L., Liu, W., and Shen, Z. (2020). Detoxification of deoxynivalenol by *Bacillus subtilis* ASAG 216 and characterization the degradation process. *Eur. Food Res. Technol.* 247: 67–76.

Joint FAO/WHO Expert Committee on Food Additives. (2001). Fifty sixth meeting. http://www.fao.org/ES/esn/jecfa/jecfa56.pdf (accessed 18 December 2022).

Juodeikiene, G., Basinskiene, L., Vidmantiene, D. et al. (2011). Benefits of β-xylanase for wheat biomass conversion to bioethanol. *J. Sci. Food Agric.* 92 (1): 84–91.

Kalagatur, N.K., Mudili, V., Siddaiah, C. et al. (2015). Antagonistic activity of *Ocimum sanctum* L. essential oil on growth and zearalenone production by *Fusarium graminearum* in maize grains. *Front. Microbiol.* 6: 892.

Kamle, M., Mahato, D.K., Gupta, A. et al. (2022). Deoxynivalenol: an overview on occurrence, chemistry, biosynthesis, health effects and its detection, management, and control strategies in food and feed. *Microbiol. Res.* 13: 292–314.

Khan, M.R. and Doohan, F.M. (2009). Comparison of the efficacy of chitosan with that of a fluorescent pseudomonad for the control of *Fusarium* head blight disease of cereals and associated mycotoxin contamination of grain. *Biol. Control* 48 (48): 54.

Kheiri, A., Moosawi Jorf, S.A., Malihipour, A. et al. (2017). Synthesis and characterization of chitosan nanoparticles and their effect on *Fusarium* head blight and oxidative activity in wheat. *Int. J. Biol. Macromol.* 102: 526–538.

Krieger, J., Jacobs, D.E., Ashley, P.J. et al. (2010). Housing interventions and control of asthma-related indoor biologic agents: a review of the evidence. *J. Public Health Manag. Pract.* 16 (50): S11.

Lehoczki-Krsjak, S., Szabo-Hever, A., Toth, B. et al. (2010). Prevention of *Fusarium* mycotoxin contamination by breeding and fungicide application to wheat. *Food Addit. Contam. Part A Chem.* 27: 616–628.

Li, M.M., Guan, E.Q., and Bian, K. (2015). Effect of ozone treatment on deoxynivalenol and quality evaluation of ozonised wheat. *Food Addit. Contam. Part A Chem. Anal. Control Expo. Risk Assess.* 32: 544–553.

Li, M., Guan, E., and Bian, K. (2019). Detoxification of deoxynivalenol by 60Co γ-ray irradiation and toxicity analyses of radiolysis products. *J. AOAC Int.* 102: 1749–1755.

Li, W., Yu, S.Y., Cheng, P., and Zhang, J.B. (2020). Screening, identification, and application of deoxynivalenol-detoxifying bacteria from mildewed alfalfa silage. *Int. Food Res. J.* 27: 350–356.

Liu, Y., Chang, J., Wang, P. et al. (2019). Effects of *Saccharomyces cerevisiae* on alleviating cytotoxicity of porcine jejunal epithelia cells induced by deoxynivalenol. *AMB Express.* 9: 137.

Luo, Y., Liu, X., and Li, J. (2018). Updating techniques on controlling mycotoxins-a review. *Food Control* 89: 123–132.

Lyagin, I. and Efremenko, E. (2019). Enzymes for detoxification of various mycotoxins: origins and mechanisms of catalytic action. *Molecules* 24: 2362.

Matarese, F., Sarrocco, S., Gruber, S. et al. (2012). Biocontrol of *Fusarium* head blight: interactions between trichoderma and mycotoxigenic *Fusarium*. *Microbiology* 158: 98–106.

McMullen, M., Jones, R., and Gallenberg, D. (1997). Scab of wheat and barley: a re-emerging disease of devasting impact. *Plant Dis.* 81: 1340–1348.

Mishra, S., Dixit, S., Dwivedi, P.D. et al. (2014). Influence of temperature and pH on the degradation of deoxynivalenol (DON) in aqueous medium: comparative cytotoxicity of DON and degraded product. *Food Addit. Contam. Part A* 31 (1): 121–131.

Mishra, S., Srivastava, S., Dewangan, J. et al. (2020). Global occurrence of deoxynivalenol in food commodities and exposure risk assessment in humans in the last decade: a survey. *Crit. Rev. Food Sci. Nutr.* 60: 1346–1374.

Misra, N.N., Yadav, B., Roopesh, M.S., and Jo, C. (2019). Cold plasma for effective fungal and mycotoxin control in foods: mechanisms, inactivation effects, and applications. *Compr. Rev. Food Sci. Food Saf.* 18: 106–120.

Moazami, F.E., Jinap, S., Mousa, W., and Hajeb, P. (2014). Effect of food additives on deoxynivalenol (DON) reduction and quality attributes in steamed-and-fried instant noodles. *Cereal Chem.* 91 (1): 88–94.

Murata, H., Yamaguchi, D., Nagai, A., and Shimada, N. (2011). Reduction of deoxynivalenol contaminating corn silage by short-term ultraviolet irradiation: a pilot study. *J. Vet. Med. Sci.* 73: 1059–1060.

Nagaraja, H., Chennappa, G., Poorna Chandra Rao, K. et al. (2016). Diversity of toxic and phytopathogenic *Fusarium* species occurring on cereals grown in Karnataka state, India. *3 Biotech* 6: 57.

Narvaez, A., Castaldo, L., Izzo, L. et al. (2022). Deoxynivalenol contamination in cereal-based foodstuffs from Spain: systematic review and meta-analysis approach for exposure assessment. *Food Control* 132: 108521.

Pal, K.K. and Gardener, B.M. (2006). Biological control of plant pathogens. *Plant Health Instr.* 2006: 1–25.

Palazzini, J., Roncallo, P., Cantoro, R. et al. (2018). Biocontrol of *Fusarium graminearum* sensu stricto, reduction of deoxynivalenol accumulation and phytohormone induction by two selected antagonists. *Toxins* 10: 88.

Pandey, A.K., Silva, A.S., Chávez-González, M.L., and Singh, P. (2022). Recent advances in delivering free or nanoencapsulated curcuma byproducts as antimicrobial food additives. *Crit. Rev. Biotechnol.* 1–27.

Perczak, A., Jus, K., Gwiazdowska, D. et al. (2019a). The efficiency of deoxynivalenol degradation by essential oils under *in vitro* conditions. *Foods* 8: 403.

Perczak, A., Gwiazdowska, D., Marchwińska, K. et al. (2019b). Antifungal activity of selected essential oils against *Fusarium culmorum* and *F. graminearum* and their secondary metabolites in wheat seeds. *Arch. Microbiol.* 201: 1085–1097.

Pestka, J.J. and Bondy, G.S. (1994). Mycotoxin-induced immune modulation. In: *Immunopharmacology and Immunotoxicology* (ed. J.H. Dean, M.I. Luster, and I. Kimber), 163–182. New York: Raveen Press.

Pfordt, A., Schiwek, S., Rathgeb, A. et al. (2020). Occurrence, pathogenicity, and mycotoxin production of *Fusarium temperatum* in relation to other *Fusarium* species on maize in Germany. *Pathogens* 9: 864.

Piemontese, L., Messia, M.C., Marconi, E. et al. (2018). Effect of gaseous ozone treatments on DON, microbial contaminants and technological parameters of wheat and semolina. *Food Addit. Contam. Part A Chem. Anal. Control Expo. Risk Assess.* 35: 760–771.

Pitt, J.I. and Miller, J.D. (2016). A concise history of mycotoxin research. *J. Agric. Food Chem.* 65 (33): 7021–7033.

Pleadin, J., Babic, J., Vulic, A. et al. (2019). The effect of thermal processing on the reduction of deoxynivalenol and zearalenone cereal content. *Croat. J. Food Sci. Technol.* 11: 44–51.

Prasad, M.N.N., Shankara Bhat, S., and Sreenivasa, M.Y. (2010). Antifungal activity of essential oils against *Phomopsis azadirachtae*- the causative agent of die-back disease of neem. *J. Agric. Technol.* 6 (1): 127–133.

Rosello, G., Bonaterra, A., Frances, J. et al. (2013). Biological control of fire blight of apple and pear with antagonistic *Lactobacillus plantarum*. *Eur. J. Plant Pathol.* 137: 621–633.

Samar, M.M., Neira, M.S., Resnik, S.L., and Pacin, A. (2001). Effect of fermentation on naturally occurring deoxynivalenol (DON) in Argentinean bread processing technology. *Food Addit. Contam.* 18 (11): 1004–1010.

Sarrocco, S. and Vannacci, G. (2018). Preharvest application of beneficial fungi as a strategy to prevent postharvest mycotoxin contamination: a review. *J. Crop Protect.* 110: 160–170.

Schaarschmidt, S. and Fauhl-Hassek, C. (2021). The fate of mycotoxins during secondary food processing of maize for human consumption. *Compr. Rev. Food Sci. Food Saf.* 20: 91–148.

Schoneberg, A., Musa, T., Voegele, R.T., and Vogelgsang, S. (2015). The potential of antagonistic fungi for control of *Fusarium graminearum* and *Fusarium crookwellense* varies depending on the experimental approach. *J. Appl. Microbiol.* 118: 1165–1179.

Shah, L., Ali, A., Yahya, M. et al. (2018). Integrated control of *Fusarium* head blight and deoxynivalenol mycotoxin in wheat. *Plant Pathol.* 67 (3): 532–548.

Smith, J.E., Solomons, G., Lewis, C., and Anderson, J.G. (1995). Role of mycotoxins in human and animal nutrition and health. *Nat. Toxins* 3 (4): 187–192.

Sobrova, P., Adam, V., Vasatkova, A. et al. (2010). Deoxynivalenol and its toxicity. *Interdiscip. Toxicol.* 3 (3): 94–99.

Sreenivasa, M.Y., Dass, R.S., Charith Raj, A.P., and Janardhana, G.R. (2008). PCR-based detection of genus *Fusarium* and Fumonisin-producing isolates from freshly harvested sorghum grains grown in Karnataka, India. *J. Food Saf.* 28: 236–237.

Sreenivasa, M.Y., Dass, R.S., Raj, A.-P.C. et al. (2011a). Assessment of the growth inhibiting effect of some plant essential oils on different *Fusarium* species isolated from sorghum and maize grains. *J. Plant Dis. Protect.* 118 (6): 208–213.

Sreenivasa, M.Y., Dass, R.S., Charith Raj, A.P., and Janardhana, G.R. (2011b). Mycological evaluation of maize grains produced in Karnataka (India) for the post-harvest fungal contamination. *World Appl. Sci. J.* 13 (4): 688–692.

Stadler, D., Lambertini, F., Woelflingseder, L. et al. (2019). The influence of processing parameters on the mitigation of deoxynivalenol during industrial baking. *Toxins* 11: 317.

Sumalatha, P. and Maheshwar, P.K. (2021). Management of *Fusarium* species isolated from *Zingiber officinale* (ginger) by essential oils. *Plant Arch.* 21 (1): 306–310.

Ten Bosch, L., Pfohl, K., Avramidis, G. et al. (2017). Plasma-based degradation of mycotoxins produced by *Fusarium*, *Aspergillus* and *Alternaria* species. *Toxins* 9: 97.

Tian, Y., Tan, Y., Liu, N. et al. (2016). Detoxification of deoxynivalenol via glycosylation represents novel insights on antagonistic activities of trichoderma when confronted with *Fusarium graminearum*. *Toxins* 8: 335.

Trenholm, H.L.C., Lynne, L., Prelusky, D.B., and Warner, R.M. (1991). Two physical methods for the decontamination of four cereals contaminated with deoxynivalenol and zearalenone. *J. Agric. Food Chem.* 39: 356–360.

Ueno, Y. (1985). The toxicology of mycotoxins. *Crit. Rev. Toxicol.* 14: 99–132.

Velluti, A., Sanchis, V., Ramos, A.J. et al. (2004). Impact of essential oils on growth rate, zearalenone and deoxynivalenol production by *Fusarium graminearum* under different temperature and water activity conditions in maize grain. *J. Appl. Microbiol.* 96: 716–724.

Venkataramana, M., Shilpa, P., Balakrishna, K. et al. (2013). Incidence and multiplex PCR based detection of trichothecenes chemotypes of *Fusarium culmorum* isolates collected from freshly harvested maize kernels in Southern India. *Braz. J. Microbiol.* 44 (2): 401–406.

Vesonder, R.F., Cigler, A., and Jensen, A.H. (1973). Isolation of the emetic principle from *Fusarium*-infected corn. *Appl. Microbiol.* 26: 1008–1010.

Vidal, A., Bendicho, J., Sanchis, V. et al. (2016). Stability and kinetics of leaching of deoxynivalenol, deoxynivalenol-3- glucoside and ochratoxin A during boiling of wheat spaghettis. *Food Res. Int.* 85: 182–190.

Wang, L., Shao, H., Luo, X. et al. (2016). Effect of ozone treatment on deoxynivalenol and wheat quality. *PLoS One* 11 (1): e0147613.

Wang, G., Wang, Y., Ji, F. et al. (2019a). Biodegradation of deoxynivalenol and its derivatives by *Devosia insulae* A16. *Food Chem.* 276: 436–442.

Wang, N., Wu, W., Pan, J., and Long, M. (2019b). Detoxification strategies for zearalenone using microorganisms: a review. *Microorganisms* 7: 208.

Wang, S., Hou, Q., Guo, Q. et al. (2020). Isolation, and characterization of a deoxynivalenol-degrading bacterium *Bacillus licheniformis* YB9 with the capability of modulating intestinal microbial flora of mice. *Toxins* 12: 184.

Wollenhaupt, K., Tomek, W., and Tiemann, U. (2007). Comparison of the molecular effects of the mycotoxins β-zearalenol and deoxynivalenol in porcine endometrial cells-a review. *Acta Vet. Hung.* 55 (1): 123–133.

World Health Organization. (1990). Selected mycotoxins: ochratoxins, trichothecenes, ergot. International Programme on Chemical Safety and World Health Organization. https://apps.who.int/iris/handle/10665/39552 (accessed 25 December 2022).

Wu, N., Ou, W., Zhang, Z. et al. (2020). Recent advances in detoxification strategies for zearalenone contamination in food and feed. *Chin. J. Chem. Eng.* 30: 168–177.

Xiong, S., Li, X., Zhao, C. et al. (2019). The degradation of deoxynivalenol by using electrochemical oxidation with graphite electrodes and the toxicity assessment of degradation products. *Toxins* 11: 478.

Yener, S. and Köksel, H. (2013). Effects of washing and drying applications on deoxynivalenol and zearalenone levels in wheat. *World Mycotoxin J.* 6: 335–341.

Yi-gang, Y., Han-ruo, M., Rui, H. et al. (2016). Degradation of deoxynivalenol in flour by ozone and ultraviolet light and their effects on flour quality. *Mod. Food Sci. Technol.* 32: 196–202.

Yooussef, M.M., Pham, Q., Achar, P.N., and Sreenivasa, M.Y. (2016). Antifungal activity of essential oils on *Aspergillus parasiticus* isolated from peanuts. *J. Plant Protect. Res.* 56 (2): 139–142. https://doi.org/10.1515/jppr-2016-0021.

Yoshida, S., Ohba, A., Liang, Y.M. et al. (2012). Specificity of *Pseudomonas* isolates on healthy and *Fusarium* head blight-infected spikelets of wheat heads. *Microb. Ecol.* 64: 214–225.

Young, J.C. (1986). Reduction in levels of deoxynivalenol in contaminated corn by chemical and physical treatment. *J. Agric. Food Chem.* 34: 465–467.

Zachetti, V.G.L., Cendoya, E., Nichea, M.J. et al. (2019). Preliminary study on the use of chitosan as an eco-friendly alternative to control *Fusarium* growth and mycotoxin production on maize and wheat. *Pathogens* 8: 8010029.

Zhang, J., Qin, X., Guo, Y. et al. (2020). Enzymatic degradation of deoxynivalenol by a novel bacterium, *Pelagibacterium halotolerans* ANSP101. *Food Chem. Toxicol.* 140: 111276.

Zhou, Y., Wu, S., Wang, F. et al. (2020). Assessing the toxicity *in vitro* of degradation products from deoxynivalenol photocatalytic degradation by using upconversion nanoparticles@ TiO_2 composite. *Chemosphere* 238: 124648.

Further Reading

Kamle, M., Mahato, D.K., Gupta, A. et al. (2022). Deoxynivalenol: an overview on occurrence, chemistry, biosynthesis, health effects and its detection, management, and control strategies in food and feed. *Microbiol. Res.* 13: 292–314. https://doi.org/10.3390/microbiolres13020023.

Pestka, J.J. (2010). Deoxynivalenol: mechanisms of action, human exposure, and toxicological relevance. *Arch. Toxicol.* 84 (9): 663–679. https://doi.org/10.1007/s00204-010-0579-8.

Rod, K.S., Bradley, C.A., Sanford, D.A., and Knott, C.A. (2020). Integrating management practices to decrease deoxynivalenol contamination in soft red winter wheat. *Front. Plant Sci.* 11: 1158. https://doi.org/10.3389/fpls.2020.01158.

9

Strategies for the Management and Mitigation of Nivalenol Contamination in Food and Feed

Theresa S.R. Mahadevarao and Raghavendra M. Puttaswamy

Postgraduate Department of Microbiology, Maharani's Science College for Women (Autonomous), JLB Road, Mysuru, Karnataka, India

CONTENTS

Abstract

Nivalenol (NIV) is one of the type B trichothecene mycotoxins produced by *Fusarium* spp., which contaminates various foods such as wheat, barley, maize, rye, and oats in the field as well as during post-harvest handling and management. It has also been detected in grain-based bread, beer, and malt food products and is currently a global health concern due to its cytotoxic

Anti-Mycotoxin Strategies for Food and Feed, First Edition. Edited by Deepa Nagaraju, Sreenivasa Marikunte Yanjarappa, Premila N. Achar, and Angel Medina Vaya.

and protein-inhibitory activity. This chapter briefly examined the incidence and biochemistry of NIV. Furthermore, a concise review of sophisticated detection methods and management strategies with the implications of processing and environmental factors on NIV susceptibility is highlighted. Overall, the chapter aimed at providing reliable current information on NIV as a mycotoxin of concern in food and feed with possible mitigation methods to assure food safety and security.

Keywords *Nivalenol, mycotoxin, food and feed, contamination, toxicology, detection, detoxification and management strategies*

Graphical Representation

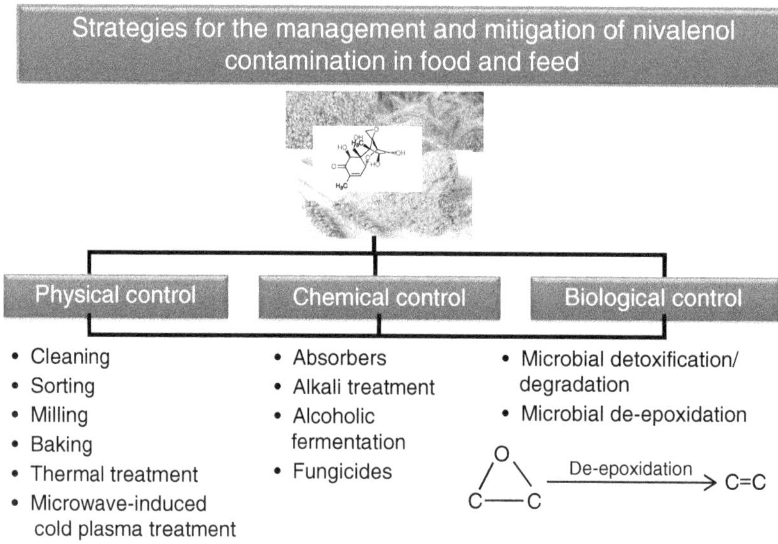

9.1 Introduction

Mycotoxins are secondary metabolites produced by fungi that may be harmful to humans and animals upon ingestion, inhalation, or skin contact, and diseases they cause is termed as mycotoxicosis, which need not involve the toxin-producing fungus (Marin et al. 2013). Asia is one the largest cereal crops producers and consumers in the world and 708.86 Mt of rice, 340.46 Mt of wheat, 18.19 Mt of barley, 17 Mt of millets, 1.58 Mt of maize, and 1.18 Mt of oats were produced annually (FAO, 2021). Approximately, 1 billion tonnes of annual food loss occurs due to mycotoxin contamination of cereal crops in Asia and this adversely affects the economy of several Asian countries (Sun et al. 2023). The *Fusarium* species are associated with *Fusarium* head blight (FHB) disease and most toxigenic strains produce various trichothecene mycotoxins such as T-2 toxin, HT-2, nivalenol (NIV), and deoxynivalenol (DON) in various forms that contaminate cereal-based foods and feeds (Schollenberger et al. 2006; Sreenivasa et al. 2008; Deepa et al. 2016a). These toxins are also produced by species of *Trichoderma*, *Trichothecium*, *Stachybotrys*, *Cephalosporium*, *Verticimonosporium*, and *Myrothecium* (Aupanun et al. 2019). These fungal pathogens release mycotoxins in cereal grains during progression of disease in the crop field and during post-harvest storage (Homdork and Beck 2000; Bianchini et al. 2015). Particularly, the fungal toxins get into the food chain (Bryden 2007) and consumption of such contaminated foods and feeds may cause severe mycotoxicosis in humans and animals (Pestka and Smolinski 2005; Sherif et al. 2009; Miller et al. 2013; Streit et al. 2013).

The trichothecenes are tricyclic sesquiterpenes categorized by a double bond next to C9, 10, and 12 positions and C13 epoxy functional group is the chief moiety for fungal secondary metabolites which elicit toxicity in eukaryotic organisms (Desjardins 2006). Four groups of trichothecene mycotoxins are classified based on their chemical structure and include: A, B, C, and D types. The A and B types are the most generally found mycotoxins and commonly cause toxicity to cattle and humans (McCormick et al. 2011; Lee and Ryu 2017; Foroud et al. 2019). Binary types of trichothecenes are categorized by the existence of a ketone at C8 position in type B which include DON, NIV, Fusarenone X (FUS), 3-Acetyl DON (3-ADON), and 15-Acetyl DON (15-ADON) and is deficient in type A trichothecenes such as T2-toxin, HT-2 toxin, and neosolaniol (NEO) (Omurtag 2008). These trichothecenes are produced on cereal crops such as maize, rye, oats, barley, or wheat in the field by FHB (scab) pathogens such as *Fusarium graminearum*, *Fusarium culmorum*, and *Fusarium cerealis*, and end up in the food or feed chains (Sreenivasa et al. 2011b; Ferrigo et al. 2016; Foroud et al. 2019). DON, NIV, and their acetylated derivatives are the most common trichothecene mycotoxins found in grains and cereal-based foods (Foroud and Francois 2009; Zhang et al. 2013).

9.2 Biochemistry and Occurrence

NIV is a type B trichothecene mycotoxin produced by several *Fusarium* spp. and a biologically active metabolite of DON, present in agricultural products (Tanaka et al. 2004; Schollenberger et al. 2005). Both NIV and DON mycotoxins are structurally alike; however, NIV differs from DON only at C4 position with respect to an oxygen atom (Figure 9.1). An extensive data survey has reported that DON and NIV were present in 57% and 16%, respectively, of food samples collected in European countries as a natural contaminant (Schothorst and van Egmond 2004). Incidences of DON and NIV were at 13% and 12%, respectively, from Korean market foods (Lee et al. 2020). Also, Egyptian cereal-derived product analysis reported DON and NIV at 70.2% and 54.8% correspondingly (Gab-Allah et al. 2022). NIV is more lethal than DON to humans and cattle with permissible restricted daily intake of NIV as 0.7 μg/kg body weight and 1 μg/kg for DON by the European Scientific Committee for Food (SCF) (Schothorst and van Egmond 2004; EFSA 2013). Worldwide, NIV is commonly found in various foodstuffs as contaminant and cereal crops generally contaminated include barley, corn, and wheat (Eckard et al. 2011; Schollenberger et al. 2012; De Boevre et al. 2013). However, the intensity of contamination varies with the crop type and environmental factors. NIV contamination mainly depends on environmental factors that include temperature and humidity as well as farm practices such as treatment, storage, processing, and supply of food crops (Magan et al. 2010). Hence, understanding the effect of weather

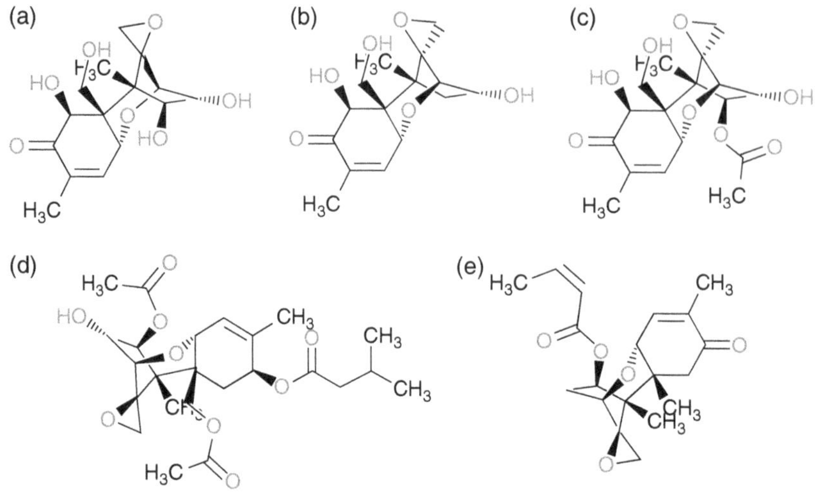

Figure 9.1 Chemical structure of (a) nivalenol, (b) deoxynivalenol, (c) fusarenon-X, (d) T-2 toxin, and (e) trichothecin.

conditions on growth patterns and mycotoxin production in *Fusarium* spp. is crucial to managing the threat of NIV in foodstuff and fodder (Shen et al. 2012) (Figure 9.1). Moreover, NIV is resistant to food processing methods due to presence of an epoxide moiety in the molecule, causing NIV-induced mycotoxicosis in cattle and humans (Nagashima 2018). A 90 days' study in rats fed with diets containing NIV reported hematological disorders such as anemia, leukopenia, neutropenia, and thrombocytopenia (EFSA 2013). Chronic consumption of NIV-contaminated foods subsequently leads to immunotoxicity and hemotoxicity in mammals. Hence, managing NIV exposure is critical (Zingales et al. 2021). Most of the toxicity associated with NIV has been attributed to its ability to inhibit eukaryotic translation process by disrupting the peptidyltransferase and cell proliferation (Rocha et al. 2005; Pestka 2010), induce CXCL8/interleukin (IL)-8 secretions, apoptosis, anemia, and initiate stress-activated mitogen-activated protein kinases (Thuvander et al. 1999; Sugita-Konishi and Pestka 2001; Nagashima et al. 2006).

Toxicity of NIV and DON varies greatly from each other (Aupanun et al. 2019). For instance, *in vitro* studies in cultured cells revealed NIV induced higher levels of redox imbalance and toxicity than DON, due to presence of an oxygen atom at C-4 position in trichothecene structure (Nagashima 2018).

9.3 Distribution of NIV Contamination in Food and Feed

Many *Fusarium* spp. comprising *Fusarium asiaticum*, *Fusarium cortaderae*, *Fusarium crookwellense*, *F. culmorum*, *F. graminearum*, *Fusarium nivale*, and *Fusarium poae* are primarily responsible for the production of NIV and its acetyl derivatives in foodstuff and feeds (Pasquali et al. 2010; Umpiérrez-Failache et al. 2013; Gomes et al. 2015; Vandicke et al. 2019). The *Fusarium* spp. rapidly grow on cereal grains to produce FHB disease under favorable environmental conditions including temperate and moisture, which are ideal for fungal proliferation and mycotoxin production and subsequent contamination of agricultural commodities (Deepa and Sreenivasa 2017a, b). In some cases, the weather and environmental conditions encouraging the growth of different *Fusarium* spp. may differ. It has been demonstrated that *F. graminearum* is commonly found in hot and moistened regions like Eastern Europe, North America, Australia, and South China whereas cold regions of Western Europe favor the proliferation of *F. culmorum* (Bryła et al. 2018). Incidence of periodic FHB disease caused by *F. graminearum* in North India was favored by hot and moistened climatic conditions during March/April on wheat and barley crops, which was reported from several areas of Punjab and Himachal Pradesh (Saharan et al. 2004).

F. graminearum is the main FHB constituent in wheat, barley, and maize in Europe (Nielsen et al. 2011, 2012). *F. asiaticum*, widespread in rice-grown areas of Southern United States, produced NIV chemotypes (Gale et al. 2011) and presence of *F. graminearum* 3-ADON producers was observed in barley fields (Burlakoti et al. 2011). In Latin America, *F. asiaticum* NIV producers were predominant in wheat besides rice-producing regions (Umpiérrez-Failache et al. 2013). In Japan, *Fusarium* spp. was distributed across the wheat and barley fields with the northern region mainly contaminated with either 3-ADON or 15-ADON producing *F. graminearum* while the southern region was contaminated with NIV-producing *F. asiaticum* (Suga et al. 2008). In addition, *F. asiaticum* was observed in wheat-/rice-grown regions of Southern China, whereas, in the North of China, *F. graminearum* was prevalent in wheat-/maize-cultivated areas (Zhang et al. 2012; Deepa et al. 2016b). Similarly, NIV-producing *F. asiaticum* was widespread in rice fields in South Korea, while DON-producing *F. graminearum* was predominant species on maize (Lee et al. 2010). FHB constituents revealed host preferences that consist of *F. asiaticum* on rice, *F. boothii* and *F. meridionale* on maize, whereas *F. graminearum* was widespread on barley, maize, and wheat (Maier et al. 2006).

9.4 Nivalenol Biogenesis

Trichothecenes with core tricyclic sesquiterpenoid frame consist of an epoxide functional group and a flexible arrangement of oxygen and ester groups is called 12,13-epoxytrichothec-9-ene (EPT) (Wu et al. 2013). Several fungal taxa produce diverse trichothecenes that have been grouped based on changeover arrangement in the EPT core into four classes: A, B, C, and D types (Alexander et al. 2009; McCormick et al. 2011). The adverse effects associated with trichothecenes have led to the worldwide search to further understand the numerous effects of trichothecenes and their principal mechanisms in order to alleviate the immense losses instigated by *Fusarium* diseases which threaten the sustainability of farms and rural populations (Pestka and Smolinski 2005; Burlakoti et al. 2008; Xu and Nicholson 2009; Escriva et al. 2015). Trichothecenes producing *Fusarium* spp. can be grouped into two prime chemotypes based on the development of 8-ketotrichothecenes to produce either DON or NIV (Miller et al. 1991). The expression of *TRI13* (encodes 15-O-acetyltransferase) and *TRI7* (encodes 3-acetyltrichothececene 4-O-acetyltransferase) was the major genetic variation in the middle of NIV and DON chemotypes (Lee et al. 2002). In DON-producing *Fusarium* chemotypes, both genes were inactive (Brown et al. 2001). DON and NIV are the most abundant type B trichothecene contaminants of cereal grains in Asia and cause extreme toxicities (Ji et al. 2019).

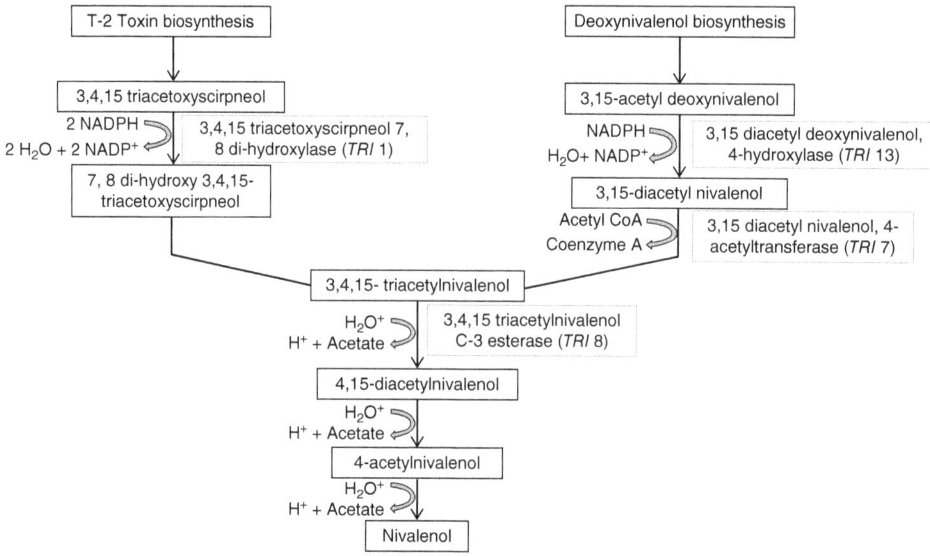

Figure 9.2 Nivalenol biosynthetic pathway.

TRI cluster in *F. graminearum* and *F. sporotrichioides* has been reported to be 26 000 bp of DNA that comprises three loci: a single gene *TRI101* locus, a two-gene *TRI1–TRI16* locus and a 12 gene core TRI cluster (Proctor et al. 2018). TRI cluster genes aid in the biogenesis, control and passage of mycotoxins through the plasmalemma (McCormick et al. 2011, 2013). Report shows that *TRI3*, *TRI4*, *TRI5*, *TRI7*, *TRI8*, *TRI11*, and *TRI13* genes encode enzymes that catalyze 10 reactions in the trichothecene biosynthesis (Cardoza et al. 2011). *TRI6* is a zinc finger transcriptional regulatory protein, while *TRI10* is a positive transcriptional regulator (Tag et al. 2001; Peplow et al. 2003; Nasmith et al. 2011). *TRI5* encodes trichodiene synthase (Tijerino et al. 2011) and *TRI101* encodes 3-O-acetyltransferase suggested to execute resistance mechanism during biosynthesis (Wuchiyama et al. 2000; McCormick and Alexander 2002). The occurrence of a free C-3 –OH group is a crucial aspect of *Fusarium* trichothecene toxicity. *TRI8,* an esterase, removes the C-3 protecting group and, hence, *TRI8* may be considered a toxicity factor. Interference of *TRI7* and *TRI13* genes effects in 3-ADON or 15-ADON mycotoxin production (Brown et al. 2001; Kimura et al. 2003; Rep and Kistler 2010). Noteworthy, the *TRI13* (a cytochrome P450 monooxygenase) encodes trichothecene-15-O-acetyltransferase (15-ADON) present in NIV-producing *Fusarium* chemotypes and interference of *TRI13* results in DON-producing chemotypes (Lee et al. 2002). NIV biosynthetic pathway in *F. graminearum* was elucidated (Figure 9.2) (Kimura et al. 2003; Cardoza et al. 2011; Lee et al. 2010; Alexander et al. 2011; Caspi et al. 2016).

9.5 Effects of Ecological Factors on Nivalenol Production

Ecological factors involving meteorological conditions and agricultural practices including handling, storage, treatment, and shipping of cereal crops contribute to NIV contamination (Magan et al. 2010). For example, NIV production in durum wheat was observed at temperatures ≤10 °C (Nazari et al. 2018). On the contrary, NIV generation in wheat was reported at temperature of 24.7 °C (Shen et al. 2012). A factorial design study in corn kernel cultures indicated no NIV production at 32 °C or above (Llorens et al. 2004). Apart from temperature, water activity (a_W) and substrate also effect NIV production by numerous fungal species. According to Hope and Magan (2003), the maximum NIV production was reported at 0.981 a_W in *F. culmorum*, whereas at 0.9 a_W, its production was not observed (Neme and Mohammed 2017). In terms of substrate, few substrate preferences for NIV production include wholemeal wheat flour in *in vitro* settings (Nazari et al. 2018), maize kernels, followed by wheat, oat, and rice (Vogelgsang et al. 2008), and barley (Pettersson 1991). NIV contamination in oats was observed at 10 °C and 99% relative humidity over an incubation period of 12 hours (Schöneberg et al. 2019).

9.6 Nivalenol Tolerance Limits

To secure the well-being of humans and animals from contaminated agricultural produce, the utmost restriction for various mycotoxins was recognized for various food products. As such, specific guidelines for utmost NIV prevalence in foodstuff and forage are needed. NIV contamination was found highest in grains and their based products (107.2 μg/kg), followed by pulses and their based products (31.7 μg/kg) in Algeria, Brazil, China, and Luxembourg (Zingales et al. 2021). At present, there is scarcity of knowledge about the predominance of NIV and its toxicological consequences. China has no regulations on NIV limit in meals and feeds, and quite a lot of countries consent to insignificant levels of NIV in crops (Ji et al. 2019). NIV tolerance limits are listed in Table 9.1.

9.7 Detection Methods of Nivalenol

Detection systems are crucial for studying the incidence and possible restriction of NIV. Due to co-existence of DON and NIV mycotoxins in the food, NIV analysis in food samples is critical. NIV detection methods are generally classified as immunological and chromatographic methods (Iqbal 2021). Immunoassays assist in screening and analysis of NIV to ensure food safety (Pereira et al. 2019). Antigen-antibody reaction is the basis of immunoassays. Moreover, immunoassays are simple, affordable, sensitive, selective, quick, portable, and handy; hence, they are used for preliminary screening of NIV in foodstuff and

Table 9.1 Nivalenol tolerance limits by different organizations.

Organization	Limit	References
European Scientific Committee for Food	0.7 μg/kg body weight per day	Schothorst and van Egmond (2004)
European Food Safety Authority	1.2 μg/kg body weight per day	EFSA (2013)
Food Safety Commission of Japan	0.4 μg/kg body weight per day	Food Safety Commission of Japan (2020)

fodder (Wang et al. 2022). Commercial enzyme-linked immunosorbent assay (ELISA) sets are available for NIV detection in food quality analysis across the food chain (Pereira et al. 2014). ELISA method developed for sensing NIV in wheat kernels can detect up to 80 ng/g (Yoshizawa et al. 2004). Accompanied by ELISA, immunochromatographic test (ICT) is also frequently used for optical finding and semi-quantitative NIV analysis (Dzantiev et al. 2014). Other rapid immunological NIV detection methods include lateral flow immunoassay (Zhang et al. 2017) and surface plasmon resonance (SPR) immunoassays (Kadota et al. 2010). In lateral flow immunoassay, the target toxin is measured by intensity and stretch of the color label which can be visualized using smartphones (Wang et al. 2022). SPR technology provides accurate and quick non-destructive target analyte detection with increased sensitivity, and finds its applications in sensor-based devices. Along with analytical detection of NIV, SPR also contributes details with respect to affinity, specificity, and kinetic characteristics of biomolecular interactions (Mohammadzadeh-Asl et al. 2019). Limitations of immunoassays include scarcity of specific antibodies for NIV detection to be sold as marketable test kits. Also, immunoassays need to be validated in laboratory validation studies with certified reference matrix materials (EFSA 2013).

Chromatographic techniques are harnessed for quantitative detection of NIV by using consistent methodical devices, such as liquid chromatography (LC), gas chromatography (GC), and ultra-performing LC combined with photodiode array (UPLC-PDA) (Pascale et al. 2014; Bryła et al. 2018; Mahmoudpour et al. 2019). Chromatographic methods coupled with detectors such as ultra-violet (UV) or fluorescence (FLD) or high-resolution mass spectrometry (HRMS) and tandem mass spectrometry (MS/MS) are mostly designed for validatory studies, especially in low-middle-income countries to confirm the formerly determined screening tests in compliance with regulations. The techniques also aid in validation and standardization for immunoassays. LC-MS/MS techniques have been extensively used for NIV detection due to its high sensitivity, selectivity, accuracy, and productivity with minimal or no sample purification (Anfossi et al. 2016). Instrumental techniques including high-performance liquid chromatography (HPLC/UV) (Ok et al. 2018), thin-layer chromatography (TLC) (Saini et al. 2021), HPLC (Lee et al. 2020), and LC-MS/MS (Tahoun et al. 2021) are often used conventional methods for NIV detection. LC-MS/MS has been extensively used for NIV detection without derivatization (Gab-Allah et al. 2022). TLC is cost-effective analytical method for NIV identification (Turner et al. 2009; Saini et al. 2021). NIV was identified in agricultural produce and feed by using TLC method (Al-Julaifi and Al-Falih 2001). For NIV detection in human urine samples obtained from Cameroon, LC-electron spray ionization-MS/MS quantitative technique has been designed using quick and simple "dilute and shoot" method (Warth et al. 2012).

9.8 Recent Management and Mitigation Strategies against Nivalenol

Recent strategies to mitigate NIV contamination include physical methods (grading, refining, grinding) (Karlovsky et al. 2016; Schaarschmidt and Fauhl-Hassek 2018), heat treatment (cooking, baking, extrusion, per-boiling, roasting) (Cazzaniga et al. 2001; Stadler

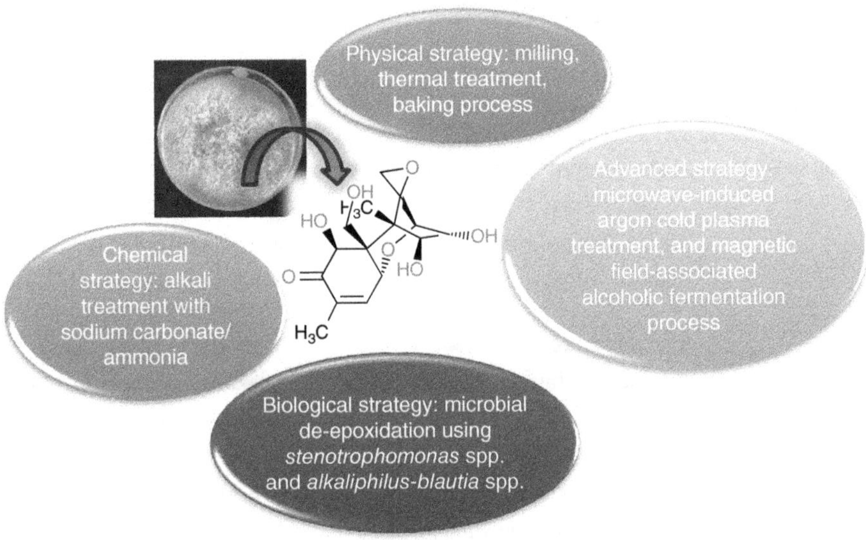

Figure 9.3 Strategies for detoxification of nivalenol.

et al. 2019), chemical treatments, fermentation processes (Stadler et al. 2020), biological detoxification, and advanced methods (Figure 9.3).

Good farming, management, and storage practices should be adapted to minimize NIV contamination (Mahato et al. 2022). Cultural practices including rotation of crops, tilling, use of fertilizers, noting the planting date and harvest times, selection of resistant varieties and fungicide or bio-control treatments may reduce the *Fusarium* spp. contamination and lessen mycotoxin production in crops (Deepa and Sreenivasa 2019a, b; Leslie et al. 2021). In addition to physical, chemical, and biological methods, diverse plant extracts containing bioactive compounds, essential oils, and phytochemicals have been known as green preservatives to extend storage time of foods (Kumar et al. 2022). At 500 ppm, concentrations of butylated hydroxy anisole, cinnamon, and clove essential oils were found to be the most effective in the inhibition of *F. culmorum* (Hope et al. 2002) (Table 9.2).

9.8.1 Physical Control

Milling is an effective process for NIV content reduction in flour. The process decreased NIV content by 34.8% in grains while the conventional grain cleaner reduced by 15.5% (Lesnik et al. 2008). Milling types and grain fractionation determine the intensity of NIV contamination. For instance, roller-grinder milling of grains reduced 130–200 μg/kg NIV contamination to 64.8–71%, hammer crasher mill caused reduction to 38.1–59.9%, and millstone milling caused reduction to 37–54.4% (Lesnik et al. 2008). Also, NIV contamination was higher in wheat's outer kernel and lesser in the endosperm portion. Manual separation of undesirable kernels (such as split and poor-quality kernels, cob pieces) followed by industrial refining, floatation, and washing facilitated 50% NIV contamination reduction (Schaarschmidt and Fauhl-Hassek 2018). Primary processes such as sorting, cleaning, and grading of wheat, considerably reduced *Fusarium* growth and NIV production in crops

Table 9.2 Strategies for detoxification of nivalenol in food and feedstuff.

S. No.	Anti-nivalenol strategy	Methodology	References
1	Physical	Cleaning, sorting, and grading of crops	Tibola et al. (2016)
		Milling process	Lesnik et al. (2008)
		Dry milling process	Trigo-Stockli (2002)
		Industrial dry cleaning, floatation, and washing	Schaarschmidt and Fauhl-Hassek (2018)
		Cooking process	Hossen et al. (2014)
		Thermal treatment	Sugita-Konishi et al. (2006)
		Baking process	Yumbe-Guevara et al. (2003)
		Extrusion process	Scudamore et al. (2008)
2	Chemical	Alkali treatment with sodium carbonate	Abramson et al. (2005)
		Alkali treatment with ammonia and sodium hydroxide, sodium bisulfite, sodium metabisulfite, and ascorbic acid	Leslie et al. (2021)
3	Biological	Microbial de-epoxidation candidates: *Stenotrophomonas* spp. and *Alkaliphilus-Blautia* spp.	Ahad et al. (2017)
		Desulfitobacterium sp. PGC-3-9	He et al. (2020)
		Candida tropicalis C28 and *Meyerozyma guilliermondii*	Podgórska-Kryszczuk et al. (2022)
4	Advanced	Microwave-induced argon cold plasma treatment	Park et al. (2007)
		Magnetic field-associated alcoholic fermentation process	Boeira et al. (2021)
		Use of essential oils as bio-fungicide	Sreenivasa et al. (2011b)

(Tibola et al. 2016). Interestingly, the water-soluble nature of NIV aids in cleaning wheat grains and subsequent milling processes and this efficiently reduced NIV by 74% in two unlike wheat varieties, namely norin 61 and Chikugoizumi (Zheng et al. 2014). In most of the cases, there was lessened NIV in milled flour compared to contaminated whole grains (Thammawong et al. 2010). Cooking process reduced 50% of NIV content in contaminated noodles prepared from Japanese soft wheat cultivar namely Chikugoizumi (Hossen et al. 2014). Heat treatment on the NIV was limited due to its heat resistance nature (Sugita-Konishi et al. 2006). Baking process at 200 °C for 70 minutes of barley flour reduced 77% of NIV (Yumbe-Guevara et al. 2003). Also, during baking process, NIV in mild alkaline conditions degrades NIV into mixture of four compounds, such as norNIV A, norNIV B, norNIV C, and NIV lactone which were less cytotoxic compared to NIV (Bretz et al. 2005). Extrusion of wheat flour at 140 °C with low moisture lessens NIV content (Scudamore et al. 2008) (Table 9.2).

9.8.2 Chemical Control

Chemical control of mycotoxins strives to abate the threat of contamination or elimination of fungi from food and feeds. Strategy used here is to either prevent or interfere with fungal growth and production of mycotoxins by use of natural or synthetic agents. Chemical agents include use of alkalis and absorbers to manage trichothecene contamination. Absorber-like activated carbon is generally used for mycotoxin decontamination from foodstuff and fodder. Biodegradable microbial cell wall polysaccharides and peptidoglycans can bind to mycotoxins minimizing the contamination by interactions like hydrogen bonds and van der Waals forces (Wambacq et al. 2016). NIV can be trapped at low pH by using lactic acid and propionic acid bacteria fermentation process (Niderkorn et al. 2006). Commonly used chemicals for treatment of mycotoxin-contaminated cereals include sodium carbonate (Abramson et al. 2005), ammonia and sodium hydroxide, sodium bisulfite, sodium metabisulfite, and ascorbic acid which altered potent toxins into less toxic compounds (Leslie et al. 2021). Carbendazim, triazoles, and strobilurins either singly or in combinations of two or more of these fungicides were widely used agrochemicals for the control and management of FHB. Effectiveness of these chemicals depends on dose, intervals, and host sensitivity to fungicide is also an important aspect in defining the effectiveness of the fungicide (McMullen et al. 2012; Leslie et al. 2021) (Table 9.2).

9.8.3 Biological Control

Mycotoxins are primarily found in food or feed. Thus, the gut is the first target for mycotoxin toxicity and a site of mycotoxin absorption. Therefore, understanding of mycotoxin and gut microbiota interactions may possibly guide us to devise more effective biological control of mycotoxins (Deepa et al. 2021). The gut microbiome is able to modify the toxicity of mycotoxins by quite a lot of mechanisms which include altering toxicokinetics of the mycotoxins or biotransformation of mycotoxins by enzymes of microbial cells secreted into the gut. Significance of this biotransformation alters the metabolites formed. In most of the reactions, hydrolysis of mycotoxins occurs and results in the formation of metabolites that are less toxic than the parent compound. Effects of rumen microbiome on NIV revealed formation of de-epoxy-nivalenol (Young et al. 2007). Trichothecenes toxicity is due to presence of an epoxide moiety in the molecule and opening the epoxide ring intensely reduces the toxicity (Sreenivasa et al. 2011a; Nagaraja et al. 2016). Design of biotechnological strategies for trichothecenes elimination from contaminated farm produces identified *Stenotrophomonas* spp. and *Alkaliphilus-Blautia* spp. to be involved in both aerobic and anaerobic de-epoxidation of trichothecenes for improving food or feed quality and safety (Ahad et al. 2017). Plant growth-promoting (PGP) rhizobacteria and essential oils also play a key role as a biocontrol agent against mycotoxins of trichothecenes and fumonisin species due to its PGP attributes (Prasad et al. 2010; Chennappa et al. 2014, 2016, 2019; Yooussef et al. 2016; Achar et al. 2020). HT-2, DON, NIV, and 15-ADON de-epoxidating bacterium, *Desulfitobacterium* sp. PGC-3-9, was isolated from a consortium obtained from soil of wheat field, identified for the occurrence of recurrent FHB epidemics under aerobic conditions (He et al. 2020) (Table 9.2).

Biological processes, for example, redox reactions, hydrolysis, hydration, glycosylation, and isomerization were reported for the alleviation of trichothecenes (Boeira et al. 2021). Yeast strains like *Candida tropicalis* C28 and *Meyerozyma guilliermondii* K2 for degradation of *Fusarium* mycotoxins showed 70.4% and 56.3% reduction in the level of NIV in wheat grains and were suggested as a promising alternative to chemical food additives to mitigate NIV contamination in food (Podgórska-Kryszczuk et al. 2022) (Table 9.2).

9.8.4 Advanced Methods for Detoxification of Nivalenol

Increase in food safety and security awareness, demand for advanced strategies to manage and mitigate NIV contamination in food and feed by adapting microwave-induced cold plasma treatments, magnetic field-associated fermentation process, and by use of natural essential oils.

Microwave-induced argon cold plasma treatment for five seconds reduced NIV content in food products (Park et al. 2007) and this could be due to breakdown of NIV by argon plasma-generated microwaves (Hojnik et al. 2017). Also, NIV reduction during plasma treatments altered the structural features (Niedzwiedz et al. 2019). In a more recent study, it was observed that magnetic field-associated alcoholic fermentation process reduced NIV contamination by 56.5% and is likely to be an effectual method for NIV breakdown (Boeira et al. 2021).

NIV degradation by 56.5% in an alcoholic fermentation process involving *Saccharomyces cerevisiae* US-05 with magnetic field usage in malted cereals has been identified and this was due to production of both glutathione redox molecule and enzyme peroxidase (Boeira et al. 2021).

Essential oils like clove oil, lemongrass oil, citronella oil, and peppermint oil showed inhibitory effects against *Fusarium* spp. and inhibited the growth at 500 ppm and higher minimum inhibitory concentrations (Sreenivasa et al. 2011b) (Table 9.2).

9.9 Summary

Toxigenic *Fusarium* species produces NIV that contaminates agricultural harvests and this is a food safety, food security, and economic concern. Also, consumption of NIV-contaminated foodstuffs by human beings and animals poses serious health threat worldwide. NIV enters food chains by contaminating foodstuffs during the harvest, transport, or storage of agricultural products. Cytotoxic nature of NIV raises the threat to health concerns. Hence, appropriate hazard analysis critical control point techniques and good agricultural and manufacturing practices are required to effectively regulate the NIV during various cultivation and processing phases. In order to determine NIV contamination, suitable rapid, and precise detection methods are essential to find measures and alleviate the same. Slight information is available on the concealed NIV forms of food products and these forms possibly go unnoticed causing alarm for food affluence. Therefore, forthcoming investigation must concentrate on a comprehensive study for establishment of strict regulations and permissible limits of NIV in foodstuff and fodder followed by deciphering molecular basis of NIV pathogenicity.

9.10 Future Perspective

Detection of NIV and its products is still in dormancy in many countries. Considering its deleterious effect on human beings as a food intoxicant at this time is a vital need to standardize the protocol for early detection and quantification of this toxin in food commodities used by animals and humans. In view of this, an overview of its production pathway and environmental factors favoring its production in specific fungi is discussed in this chapter.

9.11 Study Questions

1) Describe the incidence of nivalenol.
2) Elucidate the biosynthesis of nivalenol.
3) Write short notes on detection methods of nivalenol.
4) Describe recent strategies to manage NIV contamination.

Acknowledgments

This research received no external funding.

Conflict of Interest

The authors declare no conflict of interest.

Author Contributions

MPR designed and supervised the script. TSRM wrote and edited the script. MPR and TSRM critically reviewed the script.

References

Abramson, D., House, J.D., and Nyachoti, C.M. (2005). Reduction of deoxynivalenol in barley by treatment with aqueous sodium carbonate and heat. *Mycopathologia* 160: 297–301.

Achar, P.N., Quyen, P., Adukwu, E.C. et al. (2020). Investigation of the antifungal and anti-aflatoxigenic potential of plant-based essential oils against *Aspergillus flavus* in peanuts. *J. Fungi* 6 (4): 383. https://doi.org/10.3390/jof6040383.

Ahad, R., Zhou, T., Lepp, D., and Pauls, K. (2017). Peter microbial detoxification of eleven food and feed contaminating trichothecene mycotoxins. *BMC Biotech.* 17: 30–41.

Alexander, N.J., Proctor, R.H., and McCormick, S.P. (2009). Genes, gene clusters, and biosynthesis of trichothecenes and fumonisins in *Fusarium*. *Toxin Rev.* 28: 198–215.

Alexander, N.J., McCormick, S.P., Waalwijk, C. et al. (2011). The genetic basis for 3-ADON and 15-ADON trichothecene chemotypes in *Fusarium*. *Fungal Genet. Biol.* 48: 485–495.

Al-Julaifi, M.Z. and Al-Falih, A.M. (2001). Detection of trichothecenes in animal feeds and foodstuffs during the years 1997 to 2000 in Saudi Arabia. *J. Food Prot.* 64: 1603–1606.

Anfossi, L., Giovannoli, C., and Baggiani, C. (2016). Mycotoxin detection. *Curr. Opin. Biotechnol.* 37: 120–126.

Aupanun, S., Poapolathep, S., Phuektes, P. et al. (2019). Individual and combined mycotoxins deoxynivalenol, nivalenol, and fusarenon-X induced apoptosis in lymphoid tissues of mice after oral exposure. *Toxicon* 165: 83–94.

Bianchini, A., Horsley, R., Jack, M.M. et al. (2015). DON occurrence in grains: a North American perspective. *Cereal Foods World* 60: 32–56.

Boeira, C.Z., de Carvalho Silvello, M.A., Remedi, R.D. et al. (2021). Mitigation of nivalenol using alcoholic fermentation and magnetic field application. *Food Chem.* 340: 127935.

Bretz, M., Knecht, A., Göckler, S., and Humpf, H.U. (2005). Structural elucidation and analysis of thermal degradation products of the *Fusarium* mycotoxin nivalenol. *Mol. Nutr. Food Res.* 49: 309–316.

Brown, D.W., McCormick, S.P., Alexander, N.J. et al. (2001). A genetic and biochemical approach to study trichothecene diversity in *Fusarium sporotrichioides* and *Fusarium graminearum*. *Fungal Genet. Biol.* 32: 121–133.

Bryden, W.L. (2007). Mycotoxins in the food chain: human health implications. *Asia Pac. J. Clin. Nutr.* 16: 95–101.

Bryła, M., Ksieniewicz-Wozniak, E., Waskiewicz, A. et al. (2018). Natural occurrence of nivalenol, deoxynivalenol, and deoxynivalenol-3-glucoside in polish winter wheat. *Toxins* 10: 81.

Burlakoti, R.R., Ali, S., Secor, G.A. et al. (2008). Comparative mycotoxin profiles of *Gibberella zeae* populations from barley, wheat, potatoes, and sugar beets. *Appl. Environ. Microbiol.* 74: 6513–6520.

Burlakoti, R.R., Neate, S.M., Adhikari, T.B. et al. (2011). Trichothecene profiling and population genetic analysis of *Gibberella zeae* from barley in North Dakota and Minnesota. *Phytopathology* 101: 687–695.

Cardoza, R., Malmierca, M., Hermosa, M. et al. (2011). Identification of loci and functional characterization of trichothecene biosynthetic genes in the filamentous fungus *Trichoderma*. *Appl. Environ. Microbiol.* 77: 4867–4877.

Caspi, R., Billington, R., Ferrer, L. et al. (2016). The MetaCyc database of metabolic pathways and enzymes and the BioCyc collection of pathway/genome databases. *Nucl. Acids Res.* 44: 471–480.

Cazzaniga, D., Basilico, J.C., Gonzalez, R.J. et al. (2001). Mycotoxins inactivation by extrusion cooking of corn flour. *Lett. Appl. Microbiol.* 33: 144–147.

Chennappa, G., Adkar-Purushothama, C.R., Umdale, S. et al. (2014). Impact of pesticides on PGPR activity of *Azotobacter* sp. isolated from pesticide flooded paddy soils. *Greener J. Agri. Sci.* 4 (4): 117–129.

Chennappa, G., Naik, M.K., Adkar-Purushothama, C.R. et al. (2016). PGP, abiotic stress tolerant and antifungal activity of *Azotobacter* sp. isolated from paddy soils. *Indian J. Exp. Biol.* 54 (5): 322–331.

Chennappa, G., Udaykumar, N., Vidya, M. et al. (2019). *Azotobacter*—a natural resource for bioremediation of toxic pesticides in soil ecosystems. In: *New and Future Developments in Microbial Biotechnology and Bioengineering* (ed. J.S. Singh and D.P. Singh), 267–279. Elsevier. ISBN: 9780444641915.

De Boevre, M., Jacxsens, L., Lachat, C. et al. (2013). Human exposure to mycotoxins and their masked forms through cereal-based foods in Belgium. *Toxicol. Lett.* 218: 281–292.

Deepa, N. and Sreenivasa, M.Y. (2017a). *Fusarium verticillioides*, a globally important pathogen of agriculture and livestock: a review. *J. Vet. Med. Res.* 4 (4): 1084.

Deepa, N. and Sreenivasa, M.Y. (2017b). Fumonisins: a review on its global occurrence, epidemiology, toxicity and detection. *J. Vet. Med. Res.* 4 (6): 1093.

Deepa, N. and Sreenivasa, M.Y. (2019a). Biocontrol strategies for effective management of phytopathogenic fungi associated with cereals. In: *New and Future Developments in Microbial Biotechnology and Bioengineering* (ed. J.S. Singh and D.P. Singh), 177–189. Elsevier. ISBN: 9780444641915 10.1016/B978-0-444-64191-5.00013-4.

Deepa, N. and Sreenivasa, M.Y. (2019b). Molecular methods and key genes targeted for the detection of fumonisin producing *Fusarium verticillioides* - an updated review. *Food Biosci.* 32: 100473. https://doi.org/10.1016/j.fbio.2019.100473.

Deepa, N., Nagaraja, H., and Sreenivasa, M.Y. (2016a). Prevalence of fumonisin producing *Fusarium verticillioides* associated with cereals grown in Karnataka (India). *Food Sci. Human Well.* 5: 156–162. https://doi.org/10.1016/j.fshw.2016.07.001.

Deepa, N., Charith Raj, A.P., and Sreenivasa, M.Y. (2016b). Multiplex PCR method for the early detection of fumonisin producing *Fusarium verticillioides*. *Food Biosci.* 13: 84–88.

Deepa, N., Achar, P.N., and Sreenivasa, M.Y. (2021). Current perspectives of biocontrol agents for management of *Fusarium verticillioides* and its Fumonisin in cereals—a review. *J. Fungi* 7: 776. https://doi.org/10.3390/jof7090776.

Desjardins, A.E. (2006). *Fusarium Mycotoxins: Chemistry, Genetics, and Biology*. Minnesota: American Phytopathological Society.

Dzantiev, B.B., Byzova, N.A., Urusov, A.E., and Zherdev, A.V. (2014). Immunochromatographic methods in food analysis. *Trends Anal. Chem.* 55: 81–93.

Eckard, S., Wettstein, F.E., Forrer, H.R., and Vogelgsang, S. (2011). Incidence of *Fusarium* species and mycotoxins in silage maize. *Toxins* 3: 949–967.

EFSA (2013). Panel on contaminants in the food chain. Scientific opinion on risks for animal and public health related to the presence of nivalenol in food and feed. *EFSA J.* 11: 3262.

Escriva, L., Font, G., and Manyes, L. (2015). In vivo toxicity studies of *Fusarium* mycotoxins in the last decade: a review. *Food Chem. Toxicol.* 78: 185–206.

Ferrigo, D., Raiola, A., and Causin, R. (2016). *Fusarium* toxins in cereals: occurrence, legislation, factors promoting the appearance and their management. *Molecules* 21: 627.

Food and Agriculture Organization of the United Nations (FAO). (2021). https://www.fao.org/faostat/en/#data/QCL.

Food Safety Commission of Japan (2020). Deoxynivalenol and nivalenol (2nd edition) [Assuring the maximum level of deoxynivalenol in wheat] (natural toxins and mycotoxins). *Food Saf.* 8 (4): 115–117.

Foroud, N.A. and Francois, E. (2009). Trichothecenes in cereal grains. *Int. J. Mol. Sci.* 10: 147.

Foroud, N.A., Baines, D., Gagkaeva, T.Y. et al. (2019). Trichothecenes in cereal grains—an update. *Toxins* 11: 634.

Gab-Allah, M.A., Tahoun, I.F., Yamani, R.N. et al. (2022). Natural occurrence of deoxynivalenol, nivalenol and deoxynivalenol-3-glucoside in cereal-derived products from Egypt. *Food Control* 137: 108974.

Gale, L.R., Harrison, S.A., Ward, T.J. et al. (2011). Nivalenol-type populations of *Fusarium graminearum* and *F. asiaticum* are prevalent on wheat in southern Louisiana. *Phytopathology* 101: 124–134.

Gomes, L.B., Ward, T.J., Badiale-Furlong, E., and Del Ponte, E.M. (2015). Species composition, toxigenic potential and pathogenicity of *Fusarium graminearum* species complex isolates from southern Brazilian rice. *Plant Pathol.* 64: 980–987.

He, W.J., Shi, M.M., Yang, P. et al. (2020). Novel soil bacterium strain *Desulfitobacterium* sp. PGC-3-9 detoxifies trichothecene mycotoxins in wheat via de-epoxidation under aerobic and anaerobic conditions. *Toxins* 12 (6): 363.

Hojnik, N., Cvelbar, U., Tavcar-Kalcher, G. et al. (2017). Mycotoxin decontamination of food: cold atmospheric pressure plasma versus "classic" decontamination. *Toxins* 9: 151.

Homdork, S. and Beck, R. (2000). Influence of different storage conditions on the mycotoxin production and quality of *Fusarium*-infected wheat grain. *J. Phytopathol.* 148: 7–15.

Hope, R. and Magan, N. (2003). Two-dimensional environmental profiles of growth, deoxynivalenol and nivalenol production by *Fusarium culmorum* on a wheat-based substrate. *Lett. Appl. Microbiol.* 37: 70–74.

Hope, R., Jestoi, M., and Magan, N. (2002). Multitarget environmental approach for control of growth and toxin production by *Fusarium culmorum* using essential oils and antioxidants. *Advances in Stored Product Protection. Proceedings of the 8th International Working Conference on Stored Product Protection*, Elsevier, York, UK (22–26 July 2002). pp. 486–492.

Hossen, M.S., Nakagawa, H., Nagashima, H. et al. (2014). Loss of Nivalenol during cooking of noodles made from *Fusarium*-infected Japanese soft wheat. *J. Food Process. Preserv.* 38: 1113–1118.

Iqbal, S.Z. (2021). Mycotoxins in food, recent development in food analysis and future challenges: a review. *Curr. Opin. Food Sci.* 42: 237–247.

Ji, F., He, D., Olaniran, A.O. et al. (2019). Occurrence, toxicity, production and detection of *Fusarium* mycotoxin: a review. *Food Prod. Process. Nutr.* 1: 6.

Kadota, T., Takezawa, Y., Hirano, S. et al. (2010). Rapid detection of nivalenol and deoxynivalenol in wheat using surface plasmon resonance immunoassay. *Anal. Chim. Acta* 673: 173–178.

Karlovsky, P., Suman, M., Berthiller, F. et al. (2016). Impact of food processing and detoxification treatments on mycotoxin contamination. *Mycotoxin Res.* 32: 179–205.

Kimura, M., Tokai, T., O'Donnell, K. et al. (2003). The trichothecene biosynthesis gene cluster of *Fusarium graminearum* F15 contains a limited number of essential pathway genes and expressed non-essential genes. *FEBS Lett.* 539: 105–110.

Kumar, P., Mahato, D.K., Gupta, A. et al. (2022). Use of essential oils and phytochemicals against the mycotoxins producing fungi for shelf-life enhancement and food preservation. *Int. J. Food Sci. Technol.* 57: 2171–2184.

Lee, H.J. and Ryu, D. (2017). Worldwide occurrence of mycotoxins in cereals and cereal-derived food products: public health perspectives of their co-occurrence. *J. Agric. Food Chem.* 65: 7034–7051.

Lee, T., Han, Y.K., Kim, K.H. et al. (2002). Tri13 and Tri7 determine deoxynivalenol- and nivalenol-producing chemotypes of *Gibberella zeae*. *Appl. Environ. Microbiol.* 68: 2148–2154.

Lee, S.H., Lee, J.K., Nam, Y.J. et al. (2010). Population structure of *Fusarium graminearum* from maize and rice in 2009 in Korea. *Plant Pathol. J.* 26: 321–327.

Lee, S.Y., Woo, S.Y., Tian, F. et al. (2020). Occurrence of deoxynivalenol, nivalenol, and their glucosides in Korean market foods and estimation of their population exposure through food consumption. *Toxins* 12: 89.

Leslie, J.F., Moretti, A., Mesterházy, A. et al. (2021). Key global actions for mycotoxin management in wheat and other small grains. *Toxins* 13: 725.

Lesnik, M., Cencic, A., Vajs, S., and Simoncic, A. (2008). Milling and bread baking techniques significantly affect the mycotoxin (deoxynivalenol and nivalenol) level in bread. *Acta Aliment.* 37: 471–483.

Llorens, A., Mateo, R., Hinojo, M.J. et al. (2004). Influence of environmental factors on the biosynthesis of type B trichothecenes by isolates of *Fusarium* spp. from Spanish crops. *Int. J. Food Microbiol.* 94: 43–54.

Magan, N., Aldred, D., Mylona, K., and Lambert, R.J.W. (2010). Limiting mycotoxins in stored wheat. *Food Addit. Contam.* 27: 644–650.

Mahato, D.K., Pandhi, S., Kamle, M. et al. (2022). Trichothecenes in food and feed: occurrence, impact on human health and their detection and management strategies. *Toxicon* 208: 62–77.

Mahmoudpour, M., Dolatabadi, J.E.N., Torbati, M. et al. (2019). Nanomaterials and new biorecognition molecules-based surface plasmon resonance biosensors for mycotoxin detection. *Biosens. Bioelectron.* 143: 111603.

Maier, F.J., Miedaner, T., Hadeler, B. et al. (2006). Involvement of trichothecenes in fusarioses of wheat, barley and maize evaluated by gene disruption of the trichodiene synthase (Tri5) gene in three field isolates of different chemotype and virulence. *Molec. Plant Pathol.* 7: 449–461.

Marin, S., Ramos, A.J., Cano-Sancho, G., and Sanchis, V. (2013). Mycotoxins: occurrence, toxicology, and exposure assessment. *Food Chem. Toxicol.* 60: 218–237.

McCormick, S.P. and Alexander, N.J. (2002). *Fusarium* Tri8 encodes a trichothecene C-3 esterase. *Appl. Environ. Microbiol.* 68: 2959–2964.

McCormick, S.P., Stanley, A.M., Stover, N.A., and Alexander, N.J. (2011). Trichothecenes: from simple to complex mycotoxins. *Toxins* 3: 802–814.

McCormick, S.P., Alexander, N.J., and Proctor, R.H. (2013). Trichothecene triangle: toxins, genes, and plant disease. In: *Phytochemicals, Plant Growth, and the Environment* (ed. D.R. Gang), 1–17. Berlin: Springer.

McMullen, M., Bergstrom, G., De Wolf, E. et al. (2012). A unified effort to fight an enemy of wheat and barley: *Fusarium* head blight. *Plant Dis.* 96: 1712–1728.

Miller, J.D., Greenhalgh, R., Wang, Y., and Lu, M. (1991). Trichothecene chemotypes of three *fusarium* species. *Mycologia* 83: 121–130.

Miller, J.D., Schaafsma, A.W., Bhatnagar, D. et al. (2013). Mycotoxins that affect the North American agri-food sector: state of the art and directions for the future. *World Mycotoxin J.* 7: 63–82.

Mohammadzadeh-Asl, S., Jafari, A., Aghanejad, A. et al. (2019). Kinetic and thermodynamic studies of sunitinib malate interaction with albumin using surface plasmon resonance and molecular docking methods. *Microchem. J.* 150: 104089.

Nagaraja, H., Chennappa, G., Rao, K.P. et al. (2016). Diversity of toxic and phytopathogenic *Fusarium* species occurring on cereals grown in Karnataka state, India. *3 Biotech* 6: 57.

Nagashima, H. (2018). Deoxynivalenol and nivalenol toxicities in cultured cells: a review of comparative studies. *Food Saf.* 6: 51–57.

Nagashima, H., Nakagawa, H., and Iwashita, K. (2006). Cytotoxic effects of nivalenol on HL60 cells. *Mycotoxins* 56: 65–70.

Nasmith, C.G., Walkowiak, S., Wang, L. et al. (2011). Tri6 is a global transcription regulator in the phytopathogen *Fusarium graminearum*. *PLoS Pathog.* 7: e1002266.

Nazari, L., Pattori, E., Manstretta, V. et al. (2018). Effect of temperature on growth, wheat head infection, and nivalenol production by *Fusarium poae*. *Food Microbiol.* 76: 83–90.

Neme, K. and Mohammed, A. (2017). Mycotoxin occurrence in grains and the role of postharvest management as a mitigation strategy. A review. *Food Control* 78: 412–425.

Niderkorn, V., Boudra, H., and Morgavi, D.P. (2006). Binding of *Fusarium* mycotoxins by fermentative bacteria *in vitro*. *J. Appl. Microbiol.* 101: 849–856.

Niedzwiedz, I., Wasko, A., Pawłat, J., and Polak-Berecka, M. (2019). The state of research on antimicrobial activity of cold plasma. *Pol. J. Microbiol.* 68: 153–164.

Nielsen, L.K., Jensen, J.D., Nielsen, G.C. et al. (2011). *Fusarium* head blight of cereals in Denmark: species complex and related mycotoxins. *Phytopathology* 101: 960–969.

Nielsen, L.K., Jensen, J.D., Rodríguez, A. et al. (2012). TRI12 based quantitative real-time PCR assays reveal the distribution of trichothecene genotypes of *F. graminearum* and *F. culmorum* isolates in Danish small grain cereals. *Int. J. Food Microbiol.* 157: 384–392.

Ok, H.E., Lee, S.Y., and Chun, H.S. (2018). Occurrence and simultaneous determination of nivalenol and deoxynivalenol in rice and bran by HPLC-UV detection and immunoaffinity clean up. *Food Control* 87: 53–59.

Omurtag, G.Z. (2008). Fumonisins, trichothecenes and zearalenone in cereals. *Int. J. Mol. Sci.* 9: 2062–2090.

Park, B.J., Takatori, K., Sugita-Konishi, Y. et al. (2007). Degradation of mycotoxins using microwave-induced argon plasma at atmospheric pressure. *Surf. Coat. Technol.* 201: 5733–5737.

Pascale, M., Panzarini, G., Powers, S., and Visconti, A. (2014). Determination of deoxynivalenol and nivalenol in wheat by ultra-performance liquid chromatography/photodiode-array detector and immunoaffinity column cleanup. *Food Anal. Methods* 7: 555–562.

Pasquali, M., Giraud, F., Brochot, C. et al. (2010). Genetic *Fusarium* chemotyping as a useful tool for predicting nivalenol contamination in winter wheat. *Int. J. Food Microbiol.* 137: 246–253.

Peplow, A.W., Tag, A.G., Garifullina, G.F., and Beremand, M.N. (2003). Identification of new genes positively regulated by Tri10 and a regulatory network for trichothecene mycotoxin production. *Appl. Environ. Microbiol.* 69: 2731–2736.

Pereira, V.L., Fernandes, J.O., and Cunha, S.C. (2014). Mycotoxins in cereals and related foodstuffs: a review on occurrence and recent methods of analysis. *Trends Food Sci. Technol.* 36: 96–136.

Pereira, L.T.P., Putnik, P., Iwase, C.H.T., and de Oliveira Rocha, L. (2019). Deoxynivalenol: insights on genetics, analytical methods and occurrence. *Curr. Opin. Food Sci.* 30: 85–92.

Pestka, J.J. (2010). Deoxynivalenol: mechanisms of action, human exposure, and toxicological relevance. *Arch. Toxicol.* 84: 663–679.

Pestka, J.J. and Smolinski, A.T. (2005). Deoxynivalenol: toxicology and potential effects on humans. *J. Toxicol. Environ. Health* 14 (8): 39–69.

Pettersson, H. (1991). Nivalenol production by *Fusarium poae*. *Mycotoxin Res.* 7: 26–30.

Podgórska-Kryszczuk, I., Solarska, E., and Kordowska-Wiater, M. (2022). Reduction of the *Fusarium* mycotoxins: deoxynivalenol, nivalenol and zearalenone by selected non-conventional yeast strains in wheat grains and bread. *Molecules* 27: 1578.

Prasad, M.N.N., Shankara Bhat, S., and Sreenivasa, M.Y. (2010). Antifungal activity of essential oils against *Phomopsis azadirachtae*- the causative agent of die-back disease of neem. *J. Agri. Technol.* 6 (1): 127–133.

Proctor, R.H., McCormick, S.P., Kim, H.S. et al. (2018). Evolution of structural diversity of trichothecenes, a family of toxins produced by plant pathogenic and entomopathogenic fungi. *PLoS Pathog.* 14: e1006946.

Rep, M. and Kistler, H.C. (2010). The genomic organization of plant pathogenicity in *Fusarium* species. *Curr. Opin. Plant Biol.* 13: 420–426.

Rocha, O., Ansari, K., and Doohan, F.M. (2005). Effects of trichothecene mycotoxins on eukaryotic cells: a review. *Food Addit. Contam.* 22: 369–378.

Saharan, M.S., Kumar, J., Sharma, A.K., and Nagarajan, S. (2004). *Fusarium* head blight (FHB) or head scab of wheat-a review. *Proc. Indian Natl. Sci. Acad.* 70: 255–268.

Saini, A., Parkash, V., Kumar, V. et al. (2021). Detection of mycotoxins from some micro and macro endophytic ascomycetes fungi. *Int. J. Environ. Agric. Biotech.* 6: 216–225.

Schaarschmidt, S. and Fauhl-Hassek, C. (2018). The fate of mycotoxins during the processing of wheat for human consumption. *Compr. Rev. Food Sci. Food Saf.* 17: 556–593.

Schollenberger, M., Müller, H.M., Rüfle, M. et al. (2005). Survey of *Fusarium* toxins in foodstuffs of plant origin marketed in Germany. *Int. J. Food Microbiol.* 97: 317–326.

Schollenberger, M., Müller, H.M., Rüfle, M. et al. (2006). Natural occurrence of 16 *Fusarium* toxins in grains and feedstuffs of plant origin from Germany. *Mycopathologia* 161: 43–52.

Schollenberger, M., Müller, H.M., Ernst, K. et al. (2012). Occurrence and distribution of 13 trichothecene toxins in naturally contaminated maize plants in Germany. *Toxins* 4: 778–787.

Schöneberg, T., Kibler, K., Wettstein, F.E. et al. (2019). Influence of temperature, humidity duration and growth stage on the infection and mycotoxin production by *Fusarium langsethiae* and *Fusarium poae* in oats. *Plant Physiol.* 68: 173–184.

Schothorst, R.C. and van Egmond, H.P. (2004). Report from SCOOP task 3.2.10 "collection of occurrence data of *Fusarium* toxins in food and assessment of dietary intake by the population of EU member states" subtask: trichothecenes. *Toxicol. Lett.* 153: 133–143.

Scudamore, K.A., Guy, R.C.E., Kelleher, B., and MacDonald, S.J. (2008). Fate of the *Fusarium* mycotoxins, deoxynivalenol, nivalenol and zearalenone, during extrusion of wholemeal wheat grain. *Food Addit. Contam.* 25: 331–337.

Shen, C.M., Hu, Y.C., Sun, H.Y. et al. (2012). Geographic distribution of trichothecene chemotypes of the *Fusarium graminearum* species complex in major winter wheat production areas of China. *Plant Dis.* 96: 1172–1178.

Sherif, S.O., Salama, E.E., and Abdel-Wahhab, M.A. (2009). Mycotoxins and child health: the need for health risk assessment. *Int. J. Hyg. Environ. Health* 212: 347–368.

Sreenivasa, M.Y., Dass, R.S., Charith Raj, A.P., and Janardhana, G.R. (2008). PCR-based detection of genus *Fusarium* and Fumonisin-producing isolates from freshly harvested Sorghum grains grown in Karnataka, India. *J. Food Saf.* 28: 236–237.

Sreenivasa, M.Y., Dass, R.S., Adkar-purushothama, C.R., and Janardhana, G.R. (2011a). Mycological evaluation of maize grains produced in Karnataka (India) for the post-harvest fungal contamination. *World Appl. Sci. J.* 13 (4): 688–692.

Sreenivasa, M.Y., Dass, R.S., Charith Raj, A.P. et al. (2011b). Assessment of the growth inhibiting effect of some plant essential oils on different *Fusarium* species isolated from sorghum and maize grains. *J. Plant Dis. Prot.* 118 (6): 208–213.

Stadler, D., Lambertini, F., Bueschl, C. et al. (2019). Untargeted LC–MS based 13C labelling provides a full mass balance of deoxynivalenol and its degradation products formed during baking of crackers, biscuits and bread. *Food Chem.* 279: 303–311.

Stadler, D., Berthiller, F., Suman, M. et al. (2020). Novel analytical methods to study the fate of mycotoxins during thermal food processing. *Anal. Bioanal.Chem.* 412: 9–16.

Streit, E., Naehrer, K., Rodrigues, I., and Schatzmayr, G. (2013). Mycotoxin occurrence in feed and feed raw materials worldwide: long-term analysis with special focus on Europe and Asia. *J. Sci. Food Agric.* 93: 2892–2899.

Suga, H., Karugia, G.W., Ward, T.J. et al. (2008). Molecular characterization of the *Fusarium graminearum* species complex in Japan. *Phytopathology* 98: 159–166.

Sugita-Konishi, Y. and Pestka, J.J. (2001). Differential upregulation of TNF-α, IL-6, and IL-8 production by deoxynivalenol (vomitoxin) and other 8-ketotrichothecenes in a human macrophage model. *J. Toxicol. Environ. Health Part A* 64: 619–636.

Sugita-Konishi, Y., Park, B.J., Kobayashi-Hattori, K. et al. (2006). Effect of cooking process on the deoxynivalenol content and its subsequent cytotoxicity in wheat products. *Biosci. Biotechnol. Biochem.* 70: 1764–1768.

Sun, L., Runyan, L., Bowen, T. et al. (2023). Current status of major mycotoxins contamination in food and feed in Asia—a review. *Food Sci. Technol.* https://doi.org/10.1021/acsfood scitech.2c00331.

Tag, A.G., Garifullina, G.F., Peplow, A.W. et al. (2001). A novel regulatory gene, Tri10, controls trichothecene toxin production and gene expression. *Appl. Environ. Microbiol.* 67: 5294–5302.

Tahoun, I.F., Gab-Allah, M.A., Yamani, R.N., and Shehata, A.B. (2021). Development and validation of a reliable LC-MS/MS method for simultaneous determination of deoxynivalenol and T-2 toxin in maize and oats. *Microchem. J.* 169: 106599.

Tanaka, K., Kobayashi, H., Nagata, T., and Manabe, M. (2004). Natural occurrence of trichothecenes on lodged and water-damaged domestic rice in Japan. *Shokuhin Eiseigaku Zasshi* 45: 63–66.

Thammawong, M., Okabe, M., Kawasaki, T. et al. (2010). Distribution of deoxynivalenol and nivalenol in milling fractions from *Fusarium*-infected Japanese wheat cultivars. *J. Food Prot.* 73: 1817–1823.

Thuvander, A., Wikman, C., and Gadhasson, I. (1999). *In vitro* exposure of human lymphocytes to trichothecenes: individual variation in sensitivity and effects of combined exposure on lymphocyte function. *Food Chem. Toxicol.* 37: 639–648.

Tibola, C.S., Fernandes, J.M.C., and Guarienti, E.M. (2016). Effect of cleaning, sorting and milling processes in wheat mycotoxin content. *Food Control* 60: 174–179.

Tijerino, A., Cardoza, R.E., Moraga, J. et al. (2011). Overexpression of the trichodiene synthase gene tri5 increases trichodermin production and antimicrobial activity in *Trichoderma brevicompactum*. *Fungal Genet. Biol.* 48: 285–296.

Trigo-Stockli, D. (2002). Effect of processing on deoxynivalenol and other trichothecenes. *Adv. Exp. Med. Biol.* 504: 181–188.

Turner, W.N., Subrahmanyam, S., and Piletsky, A.S. (2009). Analytical methods for determination of mycotoxins: a review. *Anal. Chim. Acta* 632: 168–180.

Umpiérrez-Failache, M., Garmendia, G., Pereyra, S. et al. (2013). Regional differences in species composition and toxigenic potential among *Fusarium* head blight isolates from Uruguay indicate a risk of nivalenol contamination in new wheat production areas. *Int. J. Food Microbiol.* 166: 135–140.

Vandicke, J., De Visschere, K., Croubels, S. et al. (2019). Mycotoxins in Flanders' fields: occurrence and correlations with *Fusarium* species in whole-plant harvested maize. *Microorganisms* 7: 571.

Vogelgsang, S., Sulyok, M., Bänziger, I. et al. (2008). Effect of fungal strain and cereal substrate on in vitro mycotoxin production by *Fusarium poae* and *Fusarium avenaceum*. *Food Addit. Contam.* 25: 745–757.

Wambacq, E., Vanhoutte, I., Audenaert, K. et al. (2016). Occurrence, prevention and remediation of toxigenic fungi and mycotoxins in silage: a review. *J. Sci. Food Agric.* 96: 2284–2302.

Wang, Y., Zhang, C., Wang, J., and Knopp, D. (2022). Recent progress in rapid determination of mycotoxins based on emerging biorecognition molecules: a review. *Toxins* 14: 73.

Warth, B., Sulyok, M., Fruhmann, P. et al. (2012). Development and validation of a rapid multi-biomarker liquid chromatography/ tandem mass spectrometry method to assess human exposure to mycotoxins. *Rapid Commun. Mass Spectrom.* 26: 1533–1540.

Wu, Q., Dohnal, V., Kuca, K., and Yuan, Z. (2013). Trichothecenes: structure-toxic activity relationships. *Curr. Drug Metab.* 14: 641–660.

Wuchiyama, J., Kimura, M., and Yamaguchi, I. (2000). A trichothecene efflux pump encoded by Tri102 in the biosynthesis gene cluster of *Fusarium graminearum*. *J. Antibiot.* 53: 196–200.

Xu, X. and Nicholson, P. (2009). Community ecology of fungal pathogens causing wheat head blight. *Annu. Rev. Phytopathol.* 47: 83–103.

Yooussef, M.M., Pham, Q., Achar, P.N., and Sreenivasa, M.Y. (2016). Antifungal activity of essential oils on *Aspergillus parasiticus* isolated from peanuts. *J. Plant Prot. Res.* 56 (2): 139–142. https://doi.org/10.1515/jppr-2016-0021.

Yoshizawa, T., Kohno, H., Ikeda, K. et al. (2004). A practical method for measuring deoxynivalenol, nivalenol, and T-2+ HT-2 toxin in foods by an enzyme-linked immunosorbent assay using monoclonal antibodies. *Biosci. Biotechnol. Biochem.* 68: 2076–2085.

Young, J.C., Zhou, T., Yu, H. et al. (2007). Degradation of trichothecene mycotoxins by chicken intestinal microbes. *Food Chem. Toxicol.* 45: 136–143.

Yumbe-Guevara, B.E., Imoto, T., and Yoshizawa, T. (2003). Effects of heating procedures on deoxynivalenol, nivalenol and zearalenone levels in naturally contaminated barley and wheat. *Food Addit. Contam.* 20: 1132–1140.

Zhang, H., van der Lee, T., Waalwijk, C. et al. (2012). Population analysis of the *Fusarium graminearum* species complex from wheat in China show a shift to more aggressive isolates. *PLoS One* 7: 31722.

Zhang, J.B., Wang, J.H., Gong, A.D. et al. (2013). Natural occurrence of *Fusarium* head blight, mycotoxins and mycotoxin-producing isolates of *Fusarium* in commercial fields of wheat in Hubei. *Plant Pathol.* 62: 92–102.

Zhang, X., Yu, X., Wen, K. et al. (2017). Multiplex lateral flow immunoassays based on amorphous carbon nanoparticles for detecting three *Fusarium* mycotoxins in maize. *J. Agric. Food Chem.* 65: 8063–8071.

Zheng, Y., Hossen, S.M., Sago, Y. et al. (2014). Effect of milling on the content of deoxynivalenol, nivalenol, and zearalenone in Japanese wheat. *Food Control* 40: 193–197.

Zingales, V., Fernández-Franzón, M., and Ruiz, M.J. (2021). Occurrence, mitigation and in vitro cytotoxicity of nivalenol, a type B trichothecene mycotoxin–updates from the last decade (2010–2020). *Food Chem. Toxicol.* 152: 1121.

Further Reading

Lauren, D.R. and Smith, W.A. (2001). Stability of the *Fusarium* mycotoxins nivalenol, deoxynivalenol and zearalenone in ground maize under typical cooking environments. *Food Addit. Contam.* 18 (11): 1011–1016.

Sundstol, G.E., Pettersson, H., and Lundh, T. (2004). Comparative cytotoxicity of deoxynivalenol, nivalenol, their acetylated derivatives and de-epoxy metabolites. *Food Chem. Toxicol.* 42 (4): 619–624.

10

Innovative Strategies in the Control of T-2 and HT-2 Toxins in Food and Feed

Thippeswamy Basaiah, Ankita B. Nayak, and Sowmya H. Veeranna

Department of Post-Graduate Studies and Research in Microbiology Jnanasahyadri, Kuvempu University, Shivamogga, Karnataka, India

CONTENTS

Abstract

Mycotoxins are widespread pollutants of food and feed that are created by certain fungi and have an impact on the well-being and productivity of farm animals. Particularly intriguing are the naturally occurring, extremely poisonous type A trichothecene (T-2) toxin and its deacetylated counterpart, HT-2 toxin, which are readily broken down in both acidic and alkaline environments. High quantities of T-2 and HT2 mycotoxins, which can cause hemorrhages and impair immunological function, are produced by *Fusarium langsethiae* in grains. Due to the global cultivation of commercially necessary crops, this is a significant public health concern. A promising, efficient, and affordable method for reducing mycotoxigenic fungus and

Anti-Mycotoxin Strategies for Food and Feed, First Edition. Edited by Deepa Nagaraju, Sreenivasa Marikunte Yanjarappa, Premila N. Achar, and Angel Medina Vaya.

mycotoxins is nanobiotechnology. Silver, zinc oxide, selenium, copper, nano clay, nano gel, nano binders, nanodiamonds, and green nano fungicides are examples of nanomaterials.

Keywords *Mycotoxin-binders, deacetylation, sequestering, hybrid nanomaterials, genetic modification*

Graphical Representation

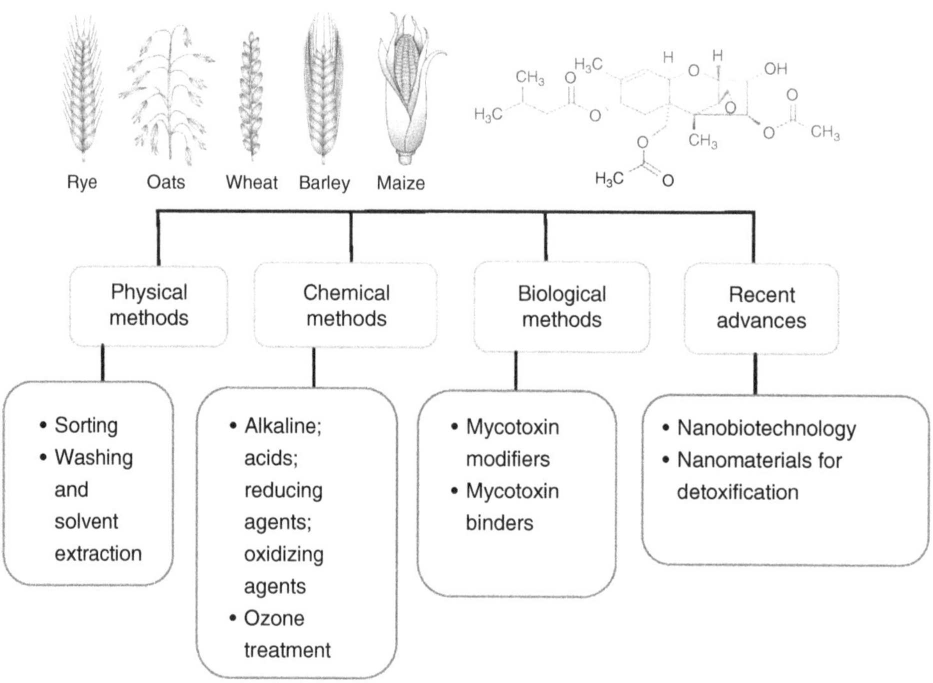

10.1 Introduction

Mycotoxins are toxic secondary metabolites with low molecular weight (Agriopoulou et al. 2020). A broad family of structurally similar secondary metabolites generated by numerous species of *Fusarium*, *Myrothecium*, *Trichoderma*, *Cephalosporium*, *Verticimonosporium*, and *Stachybotrys* are known as trichothecene (TCT) mycotoxins. One of the fungus genera with the most influence on food mycology, *Fusarium* species creates the majority of the significant TCT mycotoxins (Zhou et al. 2008). The most prevalent TCT is deoxynivalenol, T-2 toxin, HT-2 toxin, 4,15-diacetoxyscirpenol, and 15-monoacetoxyscirpenol (Diaz et al. 2005). *Fusarium sporotrichioides* and *F. langsethiae* are closely related species and have similar secondary metabolite spectra. The toxicity of TCTs is mainly due to their ability to inhibit protein synthesis and, at higher doses, they can also inhibit DNA and RNA synthesis acting, predominantly, on actively dividing tissues such as bone marrow, lymph nodes, thymus, and intestinal mucosa (Mateo et al. 2011). Warm and moist weather conditions favor plant infection with *Fusarium* species, while improper storage and handling of grain with high moisture content can lead to

T-2 toxin contamination. Among all grains tested so far, corn, wheat, barley, oat, and rye are most frequently contaminated with this mycotoxin (Afolabi et al. 2013).

10.2 Occurrence and Distribution

TCTs are cyclic sesquiterpenoid toxins characterized by a variable number of acetoxy and hydroxyl groups, an epoxide ring at positions C12–C13, and a double bond between C9 and C10. They are easily absorbed into the gastrointestinal membranes and are rapidly distributed to various organs and tissues of the body due to their low molecular weight and amphipathic nature. The most toxic groups of TCTs are type A (T-2 and HT-2) compared to type B analogues. The main fungal species producing HT-2 and T-2 toxins is *F. langsethiae* (Nagaraja et al. 2016; Agriopoulou et al. 2020). HT-2 and T-2 toxins show toxic effects such as growth retardation, myelotoxicity, hematotoxicity, and necrotic lesions on contact sites. Type A possesses some toxicity effects such as necrotic lesions, myelotoxicity, hematotoxicity, and growth retardation on the contact site, and mainly leads to hemorrhage, diarrhea, and vomiting, whereas type B effects are negligible. TCTs mainly occur in cereals like rice, rye, maize, barley, wheat, and oats, and some cereals-derived products (Deepa et al. 2016a,b; Zhang et al. 2020).

10.3 Toxicity and Its Effects

TCTs are characterized by an epoxide at the C12, 13 positions, produced by several fungal genera (Di Gregorio et al. 2014). HT-2 and T-2 toxins show toxic effects such as growth retardation, myelotoxicity, hematotoxicity, and necrotic lesions on contact sites (Agriopoulou et al. 2020). T-2/HT-2 toxin is a non-volatile, thermostable, and less light-reactive mycotoxin, but it can be easily degraded under strong acid and alkaline conditions (Deepa and Sreenivasa 2017). Over the years, several studies have elucidated the adverse consequences of dietary exposure to T-2 toxin, which leads to various nervous disorders and causes diarrhea. Recently, it was shown that the T-2 toxin is highly cardiotoxic (Figure 10.1).

Several other studies have shown that T-2 toxin can affect cell membrane permeability at low concentrations (4 pg/mL) and affects multiple metabolic pathways. T-2/HT-2 toxin-induced apoptosis signaling is independent of p53 and the Fas/Fas ligand-mediated pathway (Nagaraja et al. 2016). T-2 toxin exposure was observed to induce the ribotoxic stress response, which sequentially activated the c-Jun N-terminal kinase and T-2 toxin exposure to primary rat keratinocytes significantly increased c-fos and c-jun mRNA expression levels and elevated TNF- and IL-1 cytokine

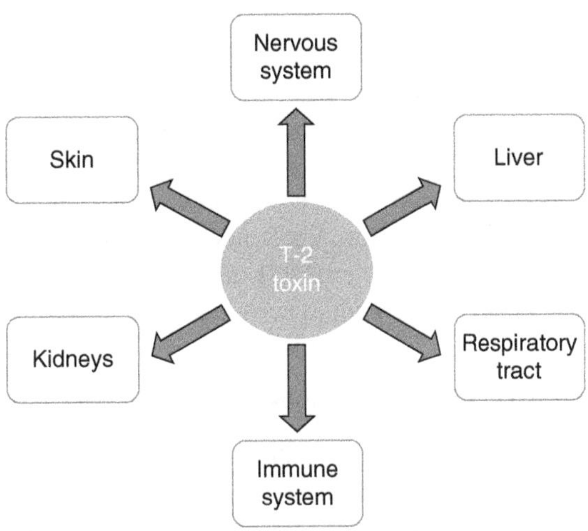

Figure 10.1 Toxicity of T-2 toxin.

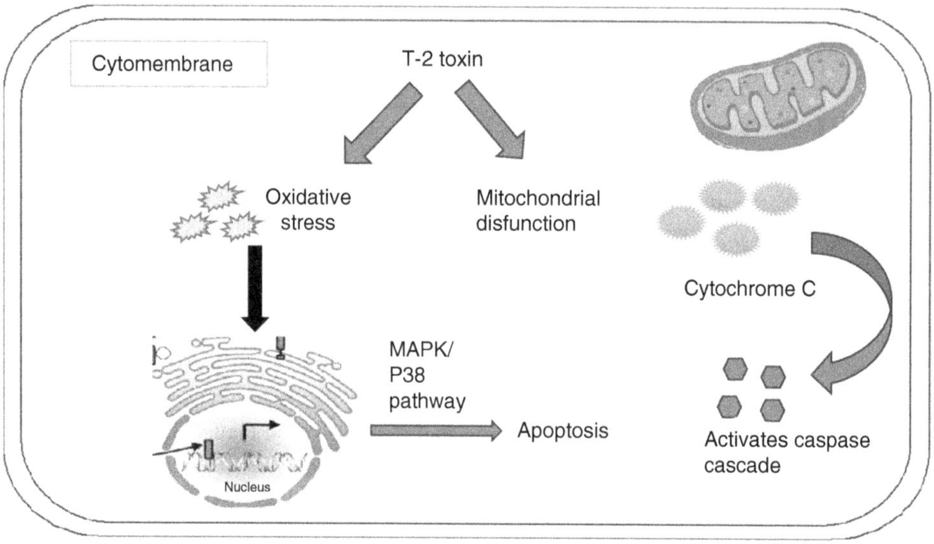

Figure 10.2 T-2 toxin mode of action.

secretion, suggesting activation of the inflammation-mediated apoptosis pathway. Bone malformation was also observed with irregular and shorter proliferative cell column arrangements in the bone (Dey et al. 2022) (Figure 10.2). Whereas type B TCT is the least toxic of the TCTs, and their occurrence is an indicator of the potential presence of other, more toxic TCTs (Agriopoulou et al. 2020).

10.4 Detoxification Strategies Against Trichothecene

Mycotoxin may be analyzed using a variety of analytical methods in various matrices. The most popular techniques for mycotoxin analysis are those utilizing HPLC and either MS/MS or fluorescence detection (FLD). For LC-MS/MS analysis and mycotoxin, the extraction methods: solid-phase extraction (SPE), solid-liquid extraction (SLE), and liquid-liquid extraction (LLE) are often employed (Pantano et al. 2021).

Integrated mycotoxin contamination preventive practices can minimize the presence of T-2/HT-2 toxin in food. Pre-harvest control, harvest control, and post-harvest strategies should mitigate mycotoxin production in agricultural commodities (Deepa and Sreenivasa 2019). However, it may not be possible to completely prevent the formation of T-2/HT-2 in agricultural products, and decontamination strategies involving physical, chemical, and biological techniques need to be used to decontaminate T-2/HT-2 toxin (Table 10.1).

10.4.1 Physical Methods

Segregation, cleaning, milling, boiling, roasting, irradiation, and microwave heating are commonly used physical methods for mycotoxin control. However, due to T-2's heat-stable nature, cooking processing such as boiling, baking, and extrusion cannot provide a 100%

Table 10.1 Strategies against T2 and HT-2 in food and feed.

Strategies		Methods	Percent of reduction (%)	References
Physical method	Sorting	Sieving, aspiration, gravity separation, photoelectric separation, image processing	63	Kabak et al. (2006) and Matumba et al. (2015)
	Washing and solvent extraction	Washing, solvent extraction (methanol, ethanol, hexane, acetonitrile, isopropanol, and aqueous acetone, etc.)	64–69	Kabak et al. (2006), Karlovsky et al. (2016), and Matumba et al. (2015)
Chemical method	Alkaline; acids; reducing agents; oxidizing agents	Ammonia, sodium hydroxide, potassium hydroxide, sodium carbonate, etc.	80–100	Janik et al. (2021) and Bretz et al. (2006)
	Ozone treatment	Ozone, hydrogen peroxide, chlorine, sodium, and calcium hypochlorite, etc.	70–90	Janik et al. (2021) and Young (1986)
Biological method	Mycotoxin modifiers	Lactic acid bacteria *Eggerthella* sp. DII-9	100	Haque et al. (2020) and Gao et al. (2018)
		Aspergillus, *Alternaria*, *Absidia*, *Armillariella*, *Candida*, *Dactylium*, *Mucor*, *Penicillium*,*Peniophora*, *Pleurotus*, *Trichosporon*, and *Rhizopus*	94.3	Haque et al. (2020) and Gao et al. (2018)
	Mycotoxin binders	Aluminosilicates, Bentonites, Montmorillonites, Zeolite, Activated carbons.	85.4	Di Gregorio et al. (2014)
		Saccharomyces cerevisiae	90	Nešić et al. (2021)
		Enzymes microfibers	80	Nešić et al. (2021) and Boudergue et al. (2009)
Recent advances	Nanobiotechnology	AgNPs, ZnO-NPs, SNP, CuNPs, SAMNs, nano clay, nano gel, nano binders, and nanodiamonds	75	Haque et al. (2020) and Shinde (2015)
	Nanomaterials for mycotoxin detoxification	Cholesterin, divinylbenzene-styrene polymers, polyvinylpyrrolidone, and humic acid polymers	Above 95	Thipe et al. (2020)
		Graphene/ZnO hybrids, g-C_3N_4, Fe_2O_3, and titanium dioxide	Above 90	Haque et al. (2020) and Shinde (2015)

degradation rate. Color sorting can reduce the mycotoxin level in end products of oat flake, and more than 90% of T-2 toxin can be removed during industrial processing (Deepa et al. 2021; Janik et al. 2021). Physical segregation of contaminated crops is an important option for producers, as detoxification of mycotoxins by chemical applications is not acceptable in some regions (Kabak et al. 2006) (Table 10.1).

10.4.1.1 Sorting

The segregation and sorting of damaged and discolored crops containing visible mold growth can lead to the removal of significant quantities of mycotoxins from these crops. Manual, mechanical, and electronic methods can all be used for the segregation of crops. Manual selection is the simplest way to physically remove contaminated grains, but it is a time-consuming procedure that limits its applicability (Kabak et al. 2006).

10.4.1.2 Heat Treatment

Mycotoxins are relatively heat-stable within the range of conventional food-processing temperatures (80–121 °C). So, little or no destruction occurs under normal cooking conditions. The sensitivity of mycotoxins to heat treatment is affected by many factors, such as the moisture content, pH, and ionic strength of food. Roasting or frying for periods of up to 30 minutes at temperatures between 150 and 200 °C can result in residual levels of between 20% and 60%. Degradation by heat treatment depends on the type of mycotoxin and its concentration, the extent of binding between mycotoxin and food constituents, the degree of heat penetration, the heating temperature, and the processing time (Kabak et al. 2006).

10.4.2 Chemical Methods

Chemical agents have been indicated as decontaminants dedicated to mycotoxins. Chemicals used nowadays for the decontamination of mycotoxins could be divided into the following categories: alkaline (ammonia gas, sodium hydroxide, calcium hydroxide); acids (acetic acid, phosphoric acid, formic acid, propionic acid); reducing agents (sodium bisulfite, sugars: D-glucose or D-fructose); oxidizing agents (ozone, hydrogen peroxide) (Janik et al. 2021). However, there are not many publications related to efficiency versus T-2 toxin. A wide range of chemicals have been shown to reduce, destroy, or inactivate mycotoxins (Kabak et al. 2006) (Table 10.1).

10.4.3 Biological Methods

Biological detoxification refers to mycotoxins' degradation or enzymatic transformation into less toxic compounds comprising acetylation, glycosylation, ring cleavage, hydrolysis, deamination, and decarboxylation (Table 10.1).

10.4.3.1 Mycotoxin Modifiers

Mycotoxin modifiers are microorganisms and enzymes that bio-transform mycotoxins into less toxic metabolites, leading to the reduction of mycotoxin (Achar et al. 2020; Haque et al. 2020).

Use of Microorganisms Biological approaches for mycotoxin decontamination have been used to manage them in food and feeds. Mechanisms in the removal of toxins by microorganisms are still being investigated, and successful results have been obtained in recent years. A wide range of microorganisms, including bacteria, fungi, and yeasts, have proven biodegradation capacity (Haque et al. 2020). Recently, *Azotobacter* with PGP activity has proved to degrade mycotoxin by more than 90% (Deepa et al. 2022).

Bacteria Mycotoxin-degrading bacteria have been isolated from different sources, including rumen and intestinal flora, soil, and water. Lactic acid bacteria (LAB) such as *Lactobacillus*, *Bifidobacterium*, *Propionibacterium*, and *Lactococcus* are important as they prevent the growth of molds and mycotoxins and improve feed utilization. *Eggerthella* sp. DII-9 has been isolated from chicken intestines and is capable of detoxifying TCTs with high de-epoxidation efficiency (Haque et al. 2020).

Fungi and Yeast TCTs are harmful to eukaryotes. Thus, organisms that produce them have defense systems. TCTs are produced by *Fusarium* through a succession of C-3 acetylated intermediates, whose acetylation is regulated by the acetyltransferase gene (Tri101). TCTs can be exposed to ascomycetes such as *Aspergillus*, *Saccharomyces*, *Blastobotrys*, and *Trichomonascus* because C-3 acetylation lessens their toxicity. To increase plant resistance to *Fusarium graminearum*, the *Fusarium* TCT acetyltransferase gene has been introduced into plants (McCormick 2013).

To boost cereals' resistance to *Fusarium* head blight, finding more trichothecene-detoxifying genes that can be expressed in cereals is necessary.

Three methods of T-2 toxin detoxification by yeast in the *Trichomonascus* clade have been identified: C-3 acetylation, hydrolysis of the C-8 isovaleryl group to neosolaniol, and C-3 glucosylation (McCormick 2013).

10.4.3.2 Mycotoxin Binders

Mycotoxin binders, also known as adsorbents or sequestering agents, are used to decontaminate animal feed by binding the mycotoxin and inhibiting its absorption in the gastrointestinal tract. They can be silica-based inorganic compounds or carbon-based organic polymers (Di Gregorio et al. 2014).

Aluminosilicates Silicate minerals are the largest class of mycotoxin-sequestering agents, and most studies have focused on aluminosilicates and tectosilicates, including zeolites (Di Gregorio et al. 2014).

Bentonites Bentonites are impure clay formed from volcanic ash weathering, consisting of montmorillonite (Di Gregorio et al. 2014). Bentonite feeding (5–10%) inhibits the toxic effects of T-2 by decreasing intestinal absorption and increasing fecal excretion of the toxin (Adhikari et al. 2017).

Montmorillonites Montmorillonite is a layered silicate that absorbs organic substances on its external surfaces or within its interlaminar spaces (Di Gregorio et al. 2014).

Zeolite Zeolites are crystalline hydrated aluminosilicates of alkali and alkaline-earth cations, with Clinoptilolite being a natural zeolite used for the adsorption of heavy metals from aqueous solutions (Di Gregorio et al. 2014).

Hydrated Sodium Calcium Aluminosilicate HSCAS is a naturally occurring and heat-processed calcium montmorillonite used as an anticaking additive in animal feed (Di Gregorio et al. 2014).

Activated Carbons Activated carbon (AC) is a non-soluble powder formed by the pyrolysis of organic compounds. Super-activated charcoal differs from AC in reducing particle size, increasing the surface area. The specific surface area of AC varies from 500 to 3500 m^2/g (Di Gregorio et al. 2014).

Yeasts *Saccharomyces cerevisiae* yeast cell walls are used as a dietary mycotoxin adsorbing agent, consisting of proteins and carbohydrates. Mannan chains are exposed on the external surface and linked to cell wall proteins (Nešić et al. 2021).

It has been demonstrated that broilers exposed to T-2 toxin benefit from the protection offered by esterified glucomannan. According to studies, adherence to cell wall components removes mycotoxins instead of covalent binding or metabolism. To determine the involvement of various cell wall components in mycotoxin binding, further kinetic investigations using live and physicochemically changed intact *S. cerevisiae* cells are required. T-2 toxin can also be bound by mannans (Shetty and Jespersen 2006).

Enzymes Recent efforts have been made to find enzymes that can degrade and metabolize mycotoxins. The main conversion paths are hydroxylation, hydrogenation, hydrolysis, oxidation, esterification, glucuronidation, glycosylation, de-epoxidation, methylation, sulfation, demethylation, and deamination, which depend on the type and nature of mycotoxin (Nešić et al. 2021).

- **Protease A:** Proteases are enzymes that hydrolyze the peptide bonds in polypeptide chains to degrade proteins. They function best in an acidic environment, and Protease A is produced by fermenting *Aspergillus niger* strains (Boudergue et al. 2009).
- **Pancreatin:** Trypsin, amylase, lipase, and protease make up the combination of pancreatic enzymes known as pancreatin, which is generated by the exocrine cells of the pancreas (Boudergue et al. 2009).
- **Carboxypeptidase A:** A pancreatic enzyme called carboxypeptidase A breaks down peptide bonds in C-terminal residues with aromatic or aliphatic side chains (Boudergue et al. 2009).
- **Epoxidase:** The enzymes known as epoxidase are capable of biotransforming epoxide groups into diene groups (Boudergue et al. 2009).
- **Lactonohydrolase:** The hydrolysis of lactone rings (intramolecular cyclic esters) by lactonohydrolases produces a hydroxyl and a carboxyl group (Boudergue et al. 2009).

Micronized Fibers Micronized fibers can be obtained from different plant materials such as cereals (wheat, barley, oat), pea hulls, apples, bamboo, etc. . . . They are constituted mainly of cellulose, hemicelluloses, and lignin and can be obtained in ultrafine (<100 μ) or less fine (>100 μ) fractions (Boudergue et al. 2009). Grape pomace has the potential to be used as a large-spectrum adsorbent material other than grape pomace and wheat fibers, the ability of food plants, and byproducts to absorb mycotoxins. The study's findings, which demonstrate that a variety of mycotoxins are present in various dietary fibers, are very inventive (Čolović et al. 2019).

10.4.3.3 Mechanism of Trichothecene Detoxification by Microorganism's

Ruminant Animals
Microorganisms from sheep rumen fluid were found to have a deacetylation function, transforming T-2 toxin into HT-2 toxin after incubation with rumen fluid under anerobic conditions. *Eubacterium* strain BBSH 797 was the most intensively studied bacterial isolate that was capable of transforming TCTs. Several single strains of rumen bacteria known to have esterase activity were tested for their capability of deacetylating T-2 toxin (Zhou et al. 2008).

Non-ruminant Animals TCT mycotoxins were incubated anerobically with suspensions of microorganisms from various nonruminant animals, resulting in different transformations. Deacetylation and deep oxidation were observed with microorganisms from rats and swine, resulting in deacetylated de-epoxy products. Intestinal microorganisms of chickens showed only deacetylation activity and transformation. It was found that the deep oxidation function of the intestinal microorganisms of chickens may vary greatly among the samples collected from different chicken varieties, individuals, and intestinal regions (Zhou et al. 2008).

Environments Environmental samples from soil, water, and plants have been used to select TCT-transforming microorganisms. A bacterial strain able to transform type A TCTs has been identified from the soil. *Curtobacterium* spp. strain 114-2, using T-2 toxin as its sole carbon source, transformed T-2 toxin into HT-2 toxin and T-2 triol in an aerobic condition. Microflora (microbial communities) of fresh water have also been found to be able to degrade T-2 toxin, but the microorganisms responsible for the biotransformation have not been identified (Zhou et al. 2008).

Plant Fungal Pathogens *Penicillium chrysogenum* deacetylated crotocin, and three TCT-producing species *F. nivale*, *F. roseum*, and *F. solani* were found to be able to transform TCTs into their acetylated or deacetylated products (Zhou et al. 2008).

10.5 Advances in Detoxification Strategies of Trichothecene

10.5.1 Nanobiotechnology

This technique is a promising, effective, and low-cost strategy to control mycotoxigenic fungi and mycotoxins in the agriculture and food industries. Nanomaterials such as silver nanoparticles (AgNPs), zinc oxide nanoparticles (ZnO-NPs), selenium nanoparticles (SNP), copper nanoparticles (CuNPs), magnetic nanoparticles like surface active maghemite nanoparticles (SAMNs), nano clay, nano gel, nano binders, and nanodiamonds can bind and remove mycotoxins or pathogens in food and feed. Another nano-based approach could be the use of green nano fungicide formulations developed by phytochemicals extracted from plant materials with antibacterial and antifungal activity. The advantage of this method is cheap to prepare from natural constituents of plants that present no toxicity to human and animal health (Haque et al. 2020).

10.5.2 Nanomaterials for Mycotoxin Detoxification

Hybrid nanomaterials have found applications as detoxifying agents for mycotoxins, acting as non-nutritive binders in feed to sequester them. It is important to consider the mycotoxins' structural diversity and chemical and physical properties when developing a detoxifying material. Mycotoxins can be polar, nonpolar, and amphipathic (HT-2 and T-2). Hybrid nanomaterials composed of silica-based inorganic compounds, carbon nanoforms, and other polymers can be used to sequester mycotoxins. Examples include cholestyramine, divinylbenzene-styrene polymers, polyvinylpyrrolidone, and humic acid polymers. Carbon nanoforms (graphene, graphene oxide, fullerenes, fibers, and nanotubes) are amphoteric and their protonable and deprotonable surfaces make them ideal candidates for incorporation in the adsorbents of mycotoxins (Thipe et al. 2020). Detoxification of mycotoxins is a challenge in the food industry, but chemical and physical methods still suffer from limitations. Photocatalytic degradation as a progressive oxidation technology has the potential to detoxify mycotoxins due to its low cost, environmentally friendly, easy operation at mild pressure, and temperature conditions, and no secondary pollution. Nanomaterials such as graphene/ZnO hybrids, g-C_3N_4, Fe_2O_3, and titanium dioxide (TiO_2) have been widely applied in the photocatalytic degradation of mycotoxins (Haque et al. 2020). Nanomaterials for packaging materials protect the integrity of food and feed commodities during storage and transportation against spoilage from fungal growth and mycotoxin production. Nanofibers have gained considerable interest in the packaging industry (Thipe et al. 2020).

10.5.3 Nanomaterials-Based Immunoassays

Immunoassays are based on the interaction of antibodies with antigens and the signal elements for labeling the interaction. They can be identified by bare eyes and simple analysis devices, and have been the most popular detection methods for rapid analysis in nonlaboratory conditions. Nanotechnology has provided great opportunities for the development of immunoassays. Nanomaterials, such as metal nanomaterials, carbon nanomaterials, metal-organic framework nanoparticles (MOFs), gold nanoparticles (AuNPs), covalent organic framework nanoparticles (COFs), upconversion NPs (UCNPs), magnetic particles, silica NPs, and quantum dots, have attracted increasing interest due to their unique properties such as enhanced surface reactivity, varying sizes, good electrical conductivity, and strong fluorescence. These nanomaterials have been widely applied in immunoassays due to their biocompatibility and large surface area, which benefit binding biomolecules and serve as electroactive signal labels. AuNPs, AgNPs, MOFs, COFs, and MNPs have good biocompatibility and large surface area, which benefit from binding the biomolecules and serve as electroactive signal labels (Zhang et al. 2020).

10.5.4 Antifungal Nanomaterials in Detoxification of Mycotoxin Production

Nanotechnology and antifungal nanomaterials have made it possible to use them as efficient antifungal agents. Nanomaterials have been widely used for antifungal and inhibition of mycotoxin production. Nanomaterial-based antifungal strategies are divided into two categories: one where an antifungal compound is encapsulated into the polymeric nanomaterials and released under appropriate conditions, and one where nanomaterials directly play a key role in the inhibition effect of fungi. Metal NPs (e.g. Fe_2O_3, SWCNTs, CuNPs, and AgNPs) have been widely used as efficient antifungal agents against fungal pathogens due to their outstanding antimicrobial properties. ZnO and copper oxide (CuO) have also been investigated as green and efficiently synergistic antifungal agents and can be used against different fungal pathogens, the cytotoxicity of which may be related to their surface charge. ZnO NPs possess outstanding antifungal activity without any photoactivation (Zhang et al. 2020).

10.5.5 Genetic Improvement of Crops

Mycotoxin contamination can be reduced by developing disease-resistant traits through more sophisticated biotechnological approaches during the pre-harvest stage. Modern transgenic techniques such as host-induced gene silencing (HIGS), RNA interference (RNAi), microRNA- or artificial microRNA-mediated gene silencing, designer transcription activator-like effector (dTALE)-mediated up- or down-regulation of gene expression, Zn-Finger nucleases, mega-nucleases, transcription activator-like effector nucleases (TALEN), clustered regularly interspaced short palindromic repeats (CRISPR)/Cas9, and oligonucleotide-directed mutagenesis (ODN)-based gene-editing techniques can be applied for the development of mycotoxin-resistant plant. In the HIGS method, pathogenic fungi are directed by the host plant to downregulate the expression of its genes, without requiring the host plant to express a remote protein. An RNAi-based approach for mycotoxin resistance in the crop is essential for fungus and toxin production. The transgenic crop was developed with self-complementary hairpin RNAs of antifungal genes resulting in small interfering RNAs (siRNAs) by the host plant's DICERlike enzymes. Dual silence Bc-Dcl1 and Bc-Dcl2 genes revealed a substantial decrease in fungal pathogenicity and growth in a wide range of plants. This method may be considered a promising target for control of mycotoxins (Haque et al. 2020).

10.6 Summary

TCTs are among the most prominent and dangerous toxins associated with food safety. They are important contaminants with a multitude of effects on both human and animal health, causing significant economic problems throughout the agri-food chain. Hazard analysis and critical control points are implemented across the food chain from farm to fork and at all stages of food handling, providing global food security. Prevention is an important strategy in the fight against mycotoxins and should be applied in the pre-harvest stages, in raw materials, and processed foods. Detoxification methods can also be applied without affecting the organoleptic characteristics of the foods. Continuous monitoring of mycotoxins in food products can prevent significant problems in the marketing, distribution, and consumption of foods.

Researchers are looking for innovative solutions such as gene editing of crops, rapid and cheap test technology, mycotoxin inhibit technology, nano antibody that reduces contamination in the food chain, and the development of fungi-resistant crops by genetic engineering technology. Nanotechnology has potential for agriculture, livestock, and the food industry.

10.7 Future Implications

The utilization of nanotechnology in the agricultural sector is still in its infancy, but a lot of work has been devoted to the development of sensors for the detection of mycotoxins. Hybrid nanomaterials, which are a relevantly new concept in plant science, are ideal for this detection through multiplexing technology. Hybrid nanomaterials have expanded into mycotoxin binders for the detoxification of mycotoxins in the gastrointestinal tract to limit the adverse toxicity of mycotoxins to key organs in the body. Management strategies also need to be implemented for food safety and security. Hybrid nanomaterials are of prime importance for a synergistic approach in tackling the problems of mycotoxins.

10.8 Study Questions

- Trichothecene and its types
- Effect of T-2 and HT-2 toxin on humans
- Detoxification of T-2 and HT-2 toxins
- Nanotechnology in the control of trichothecenes

Conflict of Interest

The authors confirm that they have no conflicts of interest.

Acknowledgments

The authors acknowledge one and all for their support in the successful completion of the chapter.

Author Contributions

Conceptualization and writing ABN; and SHV; Supervision, review, and editing TB.

References

Achar, P.N., Quyen, P., Adukwu, E.C. et al. (2020). Investigation of the antifungal and anti-aflatoxigenic potential of plant-based essential oils against *Aspergillus flavus* in peanuts. *J. Fungi* 6 (4): 383. https://doi.org/10.3390/jof6040383.

Agriopoulou, S., Stamatelopoulou, E., and Varzakas, T. (2020). Advances in occurrence, importance, and mycotoxin control strategies: prevention and detoxification in foods. *Foods* 9 (2): 137.

Adhikari, M., Negi, B., Kaushik, N. et al. (2017). T-2 mycotoxin: toxicological effects and decontamination strategies. *Oncotarget* 8 (20): 33933.

Afolabi, C.G., Ephraim, J., and Bandyopadhyay, R. (2013). Maize contamination by zearalenone and T-2 toxin and human exposure in Nigeria. *Mycotoxins* 63 (2): 143–149.

Boudergue, C., Burel, C., Dragacci, S. et al. (2009). Review of mycotoxin-detoxifying agents used as feed additives: mode of action, efficacy and feed/food safety. *EFSA Support. Publ.* 6 (9): 22E.

Bretz, M., Beyer, M., Cramer, B. et al. (2006). Thermal degradation of the fusarium mycotoxin deoxynivalenol. *J. Agric. Food Chem.* 54 (17): 6445–6451.

Čolović, R., Puvača, N., Cheli, F. et al. (2019). Decontamination of mycotoxin-contaminated feedstuffs and compound feed. *Toxins* 11 (11): 617.

Deepa, N., Achar, P.N., and Sreenivasa, M.Y. (2021). Current perspectives of biocontrol agents for management of *Fusarium verticillioides* and its Fumonisin in cereals—a review. *J. Fungi* 7: 776. https://doi.org/10.3390/jof7090776.

Deepa, N., Charith Raj, A.P., and Sreenivasa, M.Y. (2016). Multiplex PCR method for the early detection of fumonisin producing Fusarium verticillioides. *Food Biosci.* 13: 84–88.

Deepa, N., Chennappa, G., Deepthi, B.V. et al. (2022). Antifungal potential of *Azotobacter* species and its metabolites against *Fusarium verticillioides* and biodegradation of fumonisin. *J. Appl. Microbiol.* 133: 1–15.

Deepa, N., Nagaraja, H., and Sreenivasa, M.Y. (2016). Prevalence of fumonisin producing Fusarium verticillioides associated with cereals grown in Karnataka (India). *Food Science and Human Wellness*, 5 (3): 156–162.

Deepa, N. and Sreenivasa, M.Y. (2017). Fumonisins: a review on its global occurrence, epidemiology, toxicity and detection. *J. Vet. Med. Res.* 4 (6): 1093.

Deepa, N. and Sreenivasa, M.Y. (2019). Molecular methods and key genes targeted for the detection of fumonisin producing *Fusarium verticillioides* - an updated review. *Food Biosci.* 32: 100473. https://doi.org/10.1016/j.fbio.2019.100473.

Dey, D.K., Kang, J.I., Bajpai, V.K. et al. (2022). Mycotoxins in food and feed: toxicity, preventive challenges, and advanced detection techniques for associated diseases. *Crit. Rev. Food Sci. Nutr.* 21: 1–22. https://doi.org/10.1080/10408398.2022.2059650.

Di Gregorio, M.C., Neeff, D.V.D., Jager, A.V. et al. (2014). Mineral adsorbents for prevention of mycotoxins in animal feeds. *Toxin Rev.* 33 (3): 125–135.

Diaz, G.J., Cortes, A., and Roldan, L. (2005). Evaluation of the efficacy of four feed additives against the adverse effects of T-2 toxin in growing broiler chickens. *J. Appl. Poul. Res.* 14 (2): 226–231.

Gao, X., Mu, P., Wen, J. et al. (2018). Detoxification of trichothecene mycotoxins by a novel bacterium, *Eggerthella* sp. DII-9. *Food Chem. Toxicol.* 112: 310–319.

Haque, M.A., Wang, Y., Shen, Z. et al. (2020). Mycotoxin contamination and control strategy in human, domestic animal and poultry: a review. *Micr. Pathog.* 142: 104095.

Janik, E., Niemcewicz, M., Podogrocki, M. et al. (2021). T-2 toxin—the most toxic trichothecene mycotoxin: metabolism, toxicity, and decontamination strategies. *Molecules* 26 (22): 6868.

Kabak, B., Dobson, A.D., and Var, I.I.L. (2006). Strategies to prevent mycotoxin contamination of food and animal feed: a review. *Crit. Rev. Food Sci. Nutr.* 46 (8): 593–619.

Karlovsky, P., Suman, M., Berthiller, F. et al. (2016). Impact of food processing and detoxification treatments on mycotoxin contamination. *Mycotoxin Res.* 32: 179–205.

Mateo, E.M., Valle-Algarra, F.M., Mateo, R. et al. (2011). Effect of fenpropimorph, prochloraz and tebuconazole on growth and production of T-2 and HT-2 toxins by *Fusarium langsethiae* in oat-based medium. *Intern. J. Food Microbiol.* 151 (3): 289–298.

Matumba, L., Van Poucke, C., Njumbe Ediage, E. et al. (2015). Effectiveness of hand sorting, flotation/washing, dehulling, and combinations thereof on the decontamination of mycotoxin-contaminated white maize. *Food Addit. Contam. Part A* 32 (6): 960–969.

McCormick, S.P. (2013). Microbial detoxification of mycotoxins. *J. Chem. Ecol.* 39: 907–918.

Nagaraja, H., Chennappa, G., Rao, P.C.R.K. et al. (2016). Diversity of toxic and phytopathogenic *Fusarium* species occurring on cereals grown in Karnataka state, India. *3 Biotech* 6: 57.

Nešić, K., Habschied, K., and Mastanjević, K. (2021). Possibilities for the biological control of mycotoxins in food and feed. *Toxins* 13 (3): 198.

Pantano, L., La Scala, L., Olibrio, F. et al. (2021). QuEChERS LC–MS/MS screening method for mycotoxin detection in cereal products and spices. *Int. J. Environ. Res. Public Health* 18 (7): 3774.

Shinde, S.S. (2015). Antimicrobial activity of ZnO nanoparticles against pathogenic bacteria and fungi. *Sci. Med. Central* 3: 1033.

Shetty, P.H. and Jespersen, L. (2006). Saccharomyces cerevisiae and lactic acid bacteria as potential mycotoxin decontaminating agents. *Trends Food Sci. Technol.* 17 (2): 48–55.

Thipe, V.C., Thatyana, M., Ajayi, F.R. et al. (2020). Hybrid nanomaterials for detection, detoxification, and management of mycotoxins. In: Abd-Elsalam, K.A. (ed.) *Multifunctional Hybrid Nanomaterials for Sustainable Agri-Food and Ecosystems*, 271–285. Elsevier.

Young, J.C. (1986). Reduction in levels of deoxynivalenol in contaminated corn by chemical and physical treatment. *J. Agric. Food Chem.* 34 (3): 465–467.

Zhang, X., Li, G., Wu, D. et al. (2020). Recent advances on emerging nanomaterials for controlling the mycotoxin contamination: from detection to elimination. *Food Front.* 1 (4): 360–381.

Zhou, T., He, J., and Gong, J. (2008). Microbial transformation of trichothecene mycotoxins. *World Mycotoxin J.* 1 (1): 23–23.

11

Ergot Alkaloids and Anti-Mycotoxin Strategies in Food and Feed

Agriopoulou Sofia

Department of Food Science and Technology, University of the Peloponnese, Kalamata, Greece

CONTENTS

Abstract

Ergot alkaloids are comprised of a complex family of the derivatives of indole produced by the Clavicipitaceae (such as *Neotyphodium* and *Claviceps*) and Trichocomaceae (such as *Penicillium* and *Aspergillus*) families. *Claviceps purpurea* is the dominant producer. They cause ergotism; ergot alkaloids are both harmful and beneficial to humans; can cause delirious seizures, fits, St. Anthony's Fire, etc.; while the beneficial pharmacological effects of ergot alkaloids have led to the production of natural and semi-synthetic drugs aimed at inhibiting prolactin, treating parkinsonism, cerebrovascular insufficiency, migraine, and others. Rye, barley, wheat, triticale

Anti-Mycotoxin Strategies for Food and Feed, First Edition. Edited by Deepa Nagaraju, Sreenivasa Marikunte Yanjarappa, Premila N. Achar, and Angel Medina Vaya.

and oats, are the main crops affected by ergot alkaloids, with rye having the highest rates of fungal infection. Specific good pre- and post-harvest practices, as well as detoxification/removal strategies during agrofood and feed production, are examined in this chapter in order to protect general public health.

Keywords *Ergot alkaloids, prevention measures, decontamination, detoxification, good agricultural practices, emerging strategies, Graphical Representation*

Graphical Representation

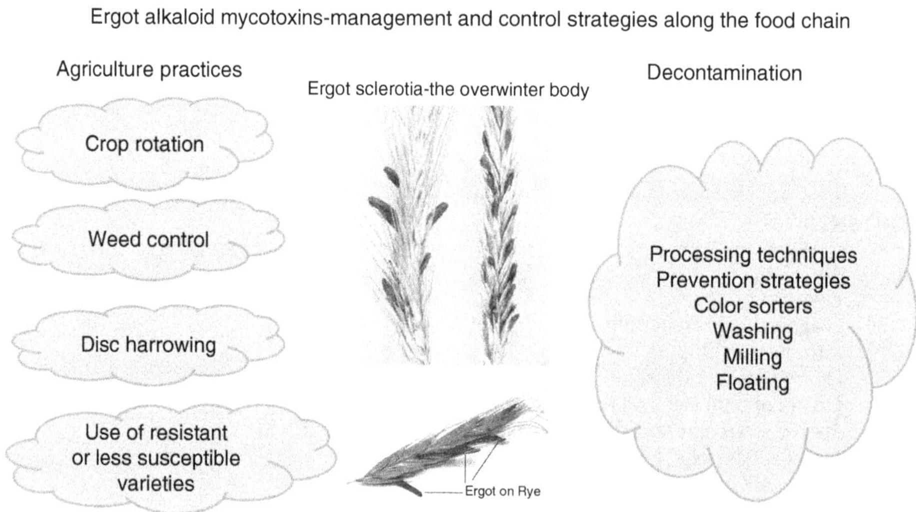

11.1 Introduction

Mycotoxins are hazardous contaminants found in both food and animal feed, causing many significantly negative effects on humans and animals. The most important genera from which these secondary metabolites originate are *Aspergillus*, *Fusarium*, *Penicillium*, *Alternaria*, and *Claviceps* spp. Among the known mycotoxins are aflatoxins (AFs), ochratoxins (OTs), fumonisins (FUMs), trichothecenes (TCTs), enniatins (ENNs), ergot alkaloids (EAs), *Alternaria* toxins, and patulin (PAT). AFs have received the most attention as they are responsible for many cases of significant human and livestock health problems (Sreenivasa et al. 2011a, b; Agriopoulou 2016; Deepa et al. 2016a, 2021; Agriopoulou et al. 2016, 2020a, b; Varzakas 2016; Agriopoulou 2021; Kumar et al. 2022; Smaoui et al. 2022). The totality of the toxic effects of mycotoxins on human and animal health are attributed to the term "mycotoxicosis" (Kaushik 2015).

EAs are toxic secondary metabolites, belonging to the family of indole alkaloids, mainly produced by Claviceps fungal species which contain approximately 80 compounds, whose effects have been known since the fifth century AD (Agriopoulou et al. 2020a). EAs produce ergotism disease, one of the oldest known human diseases caused by mycotoxins. Saint Anthony's fire or holy fire are synonyms used for this disease (Agriopoulou et al. 2020a). For this disease, there are testimonies from the Middle Ages, where symptoms of intense inflammation are described after eating rye-prepared foods contaminated with EAs.

There are two classical forms of ergot poisoning, namely the convulsive (neurological and abortogenic) and gangrenous (vasoconstrictive) forms (Cowan et al. 2023). People who consumed EA-contaminated food exhibited disorders such as hallucinations, convulsions, agalactia, burning sensation, vasoconstriction, and gangrene loss of limbs (Tittlemier et al. 2015; Grusie et al. 2018; Waret-Szkuta et al. 2019). Pigs, cattle, sheep, rabbits, and poultry are the most affected livestock (Craig et al. 2015). Symptoms such as reduced prolactin secretion, reduced progesterone secretion, altered ovarian function, reduced birth weight, reduced birth rate, and abortion may occur in cows consuming EA-contaminated feed (Cowan et al. 2023).

Cool and damp climatic conditions are favorable for the pathogen *Claviceps purpurea* (Leslie et al. 2021). Clavines (e.g. chanoclavine, agroclavine), lysergic acid, lysergic acid amides, and ergopeptines (e.g. ergovaline (Erv), ergotamine (Et), ergocornine (Eco), ergocristine (Ecr), ergosine (Es), ergocryptine) constitute the four groups of EAs depending on their chemical structure (Shahid et al. 2020; Caradus et al. 2022). A tetracyclic ergoline ring is a characteristic ring in the chemical structure of the most common EAs (Kifer et al. 2021), which is similar to the structure of biogenic amines (Craig et al. 2015). Ergometrine (Em), Et, Ecr, ergokryptine (Ekr), Es, and Eco, and their inline-epimeric forms ergotaminine (Etn), egometrinine (Emn), egocristinine (Ecrn), ergokryptinine (Ekrn), ergocroninine (Econ), and ergosinine (Esn) are the most commonly produced EAs for *Claviceps* species

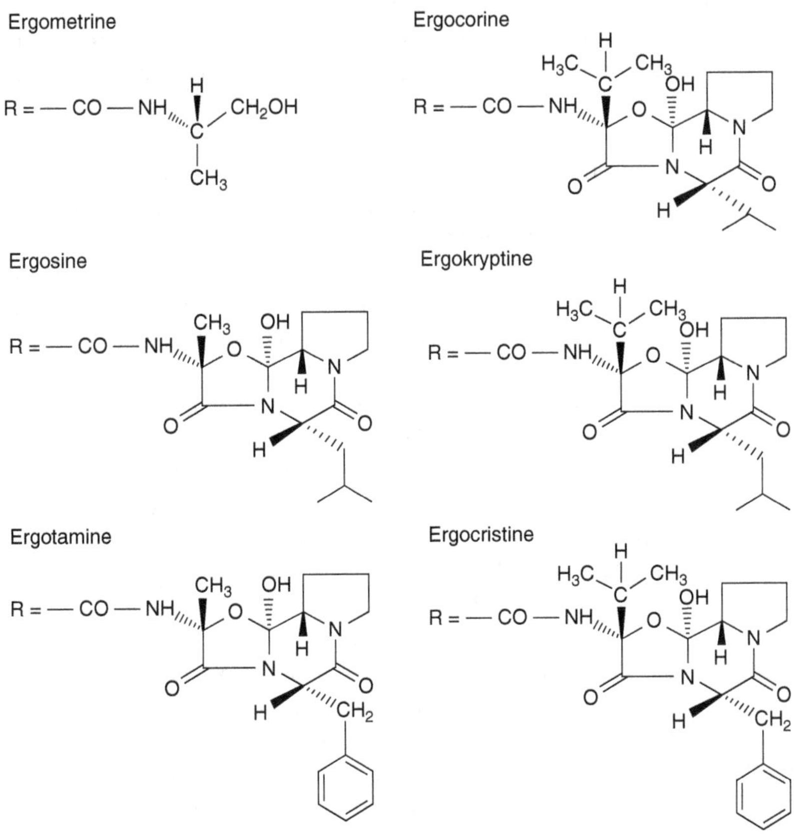

Figure 11.1 Chemical structure of the most common ergot alkaloids.

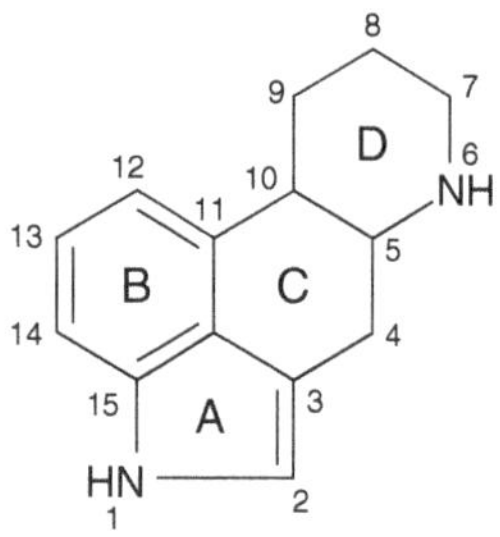

Figure 11.2 The structure of the tetracyclic ergoline ring system.

(Khaneghah et al. 2020). The chemical structure of the most common EAs and the structure of the tetracyclic ergoline ring system are presented (Figures 11.1 and 11.2).

In the United States, no regulatory limit has been established for EAs in grains (Craig et al. 2015). In a recent revision made by the European Commission in 2021 for milled products such as wheat, barley, and oats with an ash content of less than 0.9%, the EA level for refined white flour was limited to 100 ng/g. In addition, for milled products with an ash content of more than 0.9%, EA levels for wholemeal flour were limited to 150 ng/g (Commission Regulation (EU) 2021).

11.2 Occurrence and Distribution

The families Convolvulaceae, Poaceae, and Polygalaceae are the main target families for EAs (Wallwey and Li 2011). *C. purpurea*, *Claviceps fusiformis*, *Claviceps africana*, *Epichloë* spp., and *Neotyphodium* spp. produce significant quantities of EAs (Sreenivasa et al. 2008; Shimshoni et al. 2017; Eady 2021). As cereal kernels are infected by the pathogen *C. purpurea*, sclerotia with purplish or black color, also called ergots, or ergot bodies, appear, producing significant amounts of EAs (Babič et al. 2020). The alkaloid content displayed by sclerotia varies between 0.01% and 0.05% (Craig et al. 2015). The Poaceae family is very favorable for the fungus *C. purpurea* as more than 400 of its members have been found infected. Among the cultivated plants, there are also many weeds that are infected by *C. purpurea*. Cereals such as rye, wheat, triticale, barley, millet, and oats are infected with greater frequency, with rye and triticale being more susceptible to ergot than wheat and maize, due to the time difference in flowering and pollination (Debegnach et al. 2019; Králová et al. 2021; Liu et al. 2021; Alaoufi et al. 2023). Significant damages and losses can be observed in EA-infected cereal crops. Among these, lower seed quality and yield are the most common losses, making harvesting and threshing more difficult and complicating the international trade of contaminated seeds (El-Sayed et al. 2022) (Table 11.1).

The families Clavicipitaceae (such as *Neotyphodium* and *Claviceps*) and Trichocomaceae (such as *Penicillium* and *Aspergillus*) are the main EA-producing families (Florea et al. 2017). *C. purpurea* in the United States has been colonized by more than 160 different grass species (Leslie et al. 2021) and in the last 10 years, many cases of EA infection have been observed both in Canada (Menzies et al. 2017; Xue et al. 2017) and the United States (Wyka et al. 2020). Surveys conducted in China (Guo et al. 2016), Brazil (Ilha et al. 2003), and Australia (Blaney et al. 2009) indicated the EAs in cereal samples. Moreover, studies were conducted for EAs in many European countries by the European Food Safety Authority (EFSA). Between 2011 and 2016 EFSA collected data on EAs in food and feedstuffs from 15 different European countries, in order to express its scientific opinion. According to the results of its data "rye milling products," "mixed wheat and rye bread and rolls," "rye bread and rolls," and "rye flakes" were the most contaminated foods (Deepa et al. 2016b; European Food Safety Authority et al. 2017). The sampling countries were the United Kingdom, Sweden, Slovenia, the Netherlands, Malta, Lithuania, Italy, Ireland, Hungary, France, Finland, Germany, Croatia, Czech Republic, and Belgium.

Table 11.1 Recent studies of the presence of EAs in different food products in different countries.

Product	Country	No. of samples	Positive samples (%)	Range (μg/kg)	Method	References
Rye-based products Wheat-based products	Italy	16 55	85	2.6–188.6 2.5–1142.6	LC MS/MS	Debegnach et al. (2019)
Cereals	Canada	228	n.a.[a]	65–1140	LC-MS/MS	Tittlemier et al. (2015)
Cereal products	China	123	n.d.[b]	n.d.[b]	LC-MS/MS	Guo et al. (2016)
Cereal grains	Slovenia	517	17	14–4217	LC-MS/MS	Babič et al. (2020)
Rye grain	Poland	18	83	0.8–25		Bryła et al. (2015)
Rye flour		34	94	0.9–1215.5	LC-IT-MS/MS	
Rye bran		12	100	1.5–46		
Rye flakes		1	100	114–136.5		
Cereals-based food	The Netherlands	113	54	n.a.-115.4	LC-MS/MS	Mulder et al. (2015)

[a] n.a.: not available in the publication.
[b] n.d.: not detected.

Italy (Debegnach et al. 2019), France (Orlando et al. 2017), Slovenia (Babič et al. 2020), the United Kingdom (Crews et al. 2009), Albania (Topi et al. 2017), Poland (Bryła et al. 2015; Bryła et al. 2018), the Netherlands (Mulder et al. 2015), Croatia (Pleadin et al. 2022), and Germany (Appelt and Ellner 2009) are some European countries which have conducted studies for EAs and sclerotia occurrence in the last 15 years.

For the separation of EA isomers, the widely used technique is liquid chromatography. Ultraviolet (UV) and FLD detectors have been coupled with LC for analyzing EAs. LC-MS has also been used to quantify EAs in the last decade although effects of different magnitudes are shown for each EA epimer, especially ergometrine/ergometrinine, even after different purification procedures. This has the consequence of underestimating or overestimating EA levels (Chung 2021).

11.3 Effects of both Pre- and Post-Harvest Stages

The fields with EAs and mycotoxin-contaminated perennial cereals continue to be contaminated with a significant amount of sclerotia as these organs remain in the soil and produce a big number of ascospores (Alderman et al. 2015; Dung et al. 2016; Deepa and Sreenivasa 2017a, b). Critical periods for the fungus parasitizing plants (crops and weeds) are the rainy season and the flowering season (Guo et al. 2016). Even removal of ergots by hand does not guarantee the detection of EAs in cereal kernels (Shi et al. 2019).

Table 11.2 Represents various effects of ergot alkaloids on animals.

Ergot alkaloids in the food chain	Effects	Ergot alkaloids	References
Effects on animals	Elevated body temperature and respiration rates feed deterrent effect, poor animal live weight production gains, milk production, and growth rates	Ergovaline	Caradus et al. (2022)
Effects on sheep	Reduced ability to regulate body temperature, reduced fetal growth, and muscle development	Ergovaline	Duckett et al. (2014)
Effects on cattle	High rectal temperatures, high respiration rate, panting, drooling of clear mucus from the mouth and nose, extrusion of the tongue, and searching for shade and cool	Ergovaline	Caradus et al. (2022)
Effects on dairy cows	Reduced liveweight gain and milk yield	Ergovaline	Nicol and Klotz (2016)

Simultaneous harvesting of sclerotia with cereal grains or weeds leads to the production of EAs-contaminated food and feed (Agriopoulou 2021). Furthermore, during post-harvest milling of cereals, the separation of sclerotia from healthy grains is difficult and their inevitable fragmentation results in contaminated products (Pitt and Miller 2017). The removal and separation of sclerotia is more difficult in cases where these fungal sclerotia are produced in dry heat conditions, and are similar in size to cereal grains (Janik et al. 2020). Cleaning and removal of up to 82% of sclerotia has been achieved but this does not mean that total clearance can be achieved, as in the literature, there are cases with quite high levels of contamination (Agriopoulou 2021). Heat and UV light have been used for physical reduction of EAs (Schummer et al. 2020) (Table 11.2).

11.4 Recent Strategies Against Ergot Alkaloid Mycotoxins

The contamination that occurs from fungi each year is difficult to predict, as it depends on many conditions that vary from year to year. Cultivation technique, host plants, harvesting, fungal growth conditions, climate conditions or specific meteorological events and crop management vary and contribute differently in mycotoxin contamination (Deepa and Sreenivasa 2019a, b). Moreover, the same fungal strain can produce different mycotoxins in similar environments (Hao et al. 2023). Crops are contaminated by mycotoxins both pre-harvest during the growing season and post-harvest during the transport and storage of the produced food and feed, without this necessarily meaning the production of mycotoxins (Mahato et al. 2021) (Table 11.3).

11.5 Physical Control

Good storage practices (GSP), good agricultural practices (GAP), good hygiene practices (GHP), good manufacturing practices (GMP), and hazard analysis and critical control points (HACCP) practices are all significant mycotoxin management policies, although the

Table 11.3 Physical, chemical, and biological methods of ergot alkaloids management.

S. No.	Anti-mycotoxin strategy		Methodology	Percent of reduction (%)	References
1	Physical	Sorting and separation	Sclerotia loaded with alkaloids can be efficiently removed from the rye by opto-electronic sorting	70–80	Miedaner and Geiger 2015
		Heating	Exposure to both steam (100 °C) and 40 bar mechanical pressure caused degradation of alkaloids	11	Merkel et al. (2012)
		Cleaning	Cleaning and processing of cereals can remove the sclerotia	82	Krska and Crews (2023)
2	Chemical	A combination of prothioconazole and fluoxastrobin and galmano	Reductions in the percentage of ergot germination	95	Puhl et al. (2007)
		Ammonia treatment	The total concentration of ergot alkaloids (R- and S-epimers) decreased	8–29	Cherewyk et al. (2022)
		Chlorine	Treatment with chlorine and heat (150 and 200 °C)	90	Young et al. (1983)
3	Biological	Resistant varieties	Hybrid rye versus open-pollinated cultivars	The susceptibility was more than three times higher	Menzies and Turkington (2015)

presence of mycotoxins even with the implementation of these procedures should be considered unavoidable (Hamad et al. 2022). Geographical region, time of harvest, type of crop as well as variety have been shown to be important factors determining the content of EAs and the proportion of individual EAs within ergot bodies (Shi and Yu 2023). Ergot sclerotia can be physically separated by size, density, and color from healthy grain kernels (Cherewyk et al. 2022). During sorting, impurities are removed from the cereals, and it is applied before processing or after harvest (Shanakhat et al. 2018). Sclerotia loaded with alkaloids can be efficiently removed from the rye by optoelectronic sorting (Miedaner and Geiger 2015).

Nada et al. (2022) have recently shown several preharvest practices related to the production of mycotoxins. Among them, practices related to soil preparation such as plowing and crop rotation seem to be directly related. Moreover, application of botanical extracts and fungal biocontrol agents are also important preharvest practices (Nada et al. 2022). As the overwintering organs of Claviceps are sclerotia, their survival is considered particularly important. In addition, the low temperatures favor their germination in the coming spring (Uppala et al. 2016). Burying sclerotia in depth can help reduce their amounts while growing varieties with greater resistance or less susceptibility to the disease also impart smaller amounts of sclerotia to the final product (Battilani et al. 2009). The contribution of weeds to the maintenance of the inoculum of *C. purpurea* was studied by Wyka and Broders (2023). The results of the study indicated that brome grasses represented the primary source of *C. purpurea* inoculum associated with barley fields in Colorado's San Luis Valley (Wyka and Broders 2023).

Kernels damaged by mold show different physical properties to undamaged kernels. These properties are used to separate damaged from undamaged kernels by density segregation or by fractionation on gravity tables. These techniques are more effective in separating infected kernels from a set of fungi than from a specific toxin. NaCl solution efficiently separated Ergot-containing EAs from rye grains by flotation (Karlovsky et al. 2016).

11.6 Chemical Control

In the chemical breakdown of mycotoxins, what is achieved is their degradation into compounds with less toxicity than the corresponding parent (Misra et al. 2019). A strong oxidizing agent that has been reported to degrade several mycotoxins is ozone (O_3) (Sachadyn-Król and Agriopoulou 2020; Pandiselvam et al. 2022). Chemical treatments such as ammoniation, neutral electrolyzed oxidizing water, citric acid, sodium hydrosulfite, antioxidants, alkaline solutions, and salts had been tested for mycotoxin detoxification (Afsah-Hejri et al. 2020). Chlorine, O_3, sulfur dioxide, bleach, hydrogen peroxide, and ammonia have been used for the detoxification of EAs (Koester et al. 2020).

Cultivation practices that keep a crop healthy could control the production of EA mycotoxins. The application of fertilizers, as well as herbicides, aim at a resistant crop. The use of calcium cyanamide as a fertilizer in the spring caused a 40–50% reduction in the germination of sclerotia that were present in the soil (Battilani et al. 2009).

Alaoufi and co-workers in a very recent study evaluated the effect of field-applied fungicides on ergot weight, EA concentrations, other toxin concentrations, sclerotia composition, and sclerotia components in wheat (Alaoufi et al. 2023). Four fungicides (prothioconazole + metconazole, pydiflumetofen + propiconazole, azoxystrobin + propiconazole, and fluxapyroxad + pyraclostrobin) were evaluated. Fungicides had a significant ($p < 0.05$) impact on total ergot body weight (EBW), with all fungicides having lower EBW than the nontreated control. The fungicide premixture of pydiflumetofen + propiconazole had the lowest EBW among all treatments. Fluxapyroxad + pyraclostrobin had the lowest levels of EAs among fungicides, although none of the fungicide premixtures provided complete inhibition of ergot development nor reduction of EAs, and this could be related to fungicide application timing or the genotype of wheat used.

11.7 Biological Control

Biological detoxification is an alternative approach to mycotoxin management as it can lead to the production of less hazardous products (Sarrocco and Vannacci 2018). Inhibition of fungal growth and prevention of mycotoxin formation in food is achieved by biological

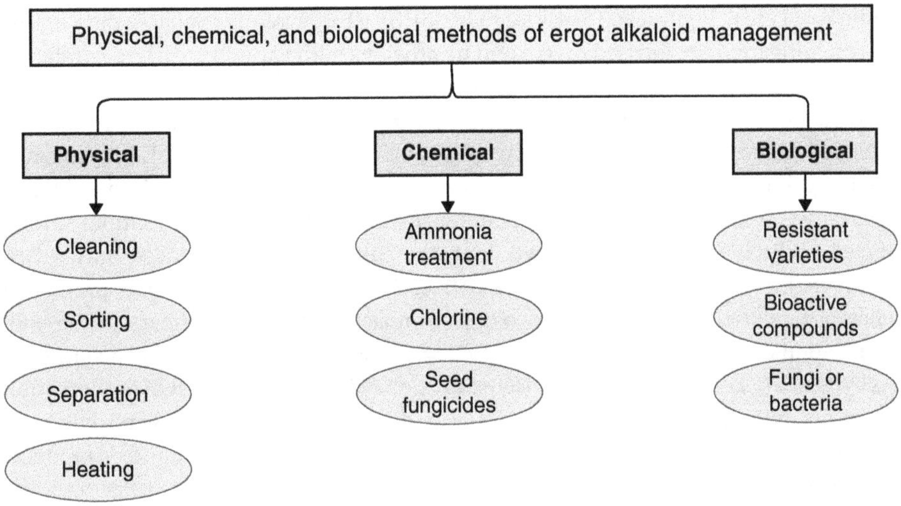

Figure 11.3 Physical, chemical, and biological methods of ergot alkaloid management.

means through the production of bioactive compounds, such as acetic and lactic acid, hydrogen peroxide, hydroxyl fatty acids, and phenolic compounds (Smaoui et al. 2022). Lactic acid bacteria (LAB) are microorganisms that produce all of the above compounds that have been widely studied for the degradation of mycotoxins due to their high safety in food applications (Agriopoulou et al. 2020c; Li et al. 2021). Plant growth-promoting rhizobacteria or plant growth-promoting microbes are playing a major role as a biological strategy against mycotoxins with their PGP activity (Chennappa et al. 2014, 2016, 2019). Yeast, fungi, essential oils, and enzymes are also used for the biological management of mycotoxins (Battilani et al. 2009; Prasad et al. 2010; Hahn et al. 2015; Yooussef et al. 2016; Achar et al. 2020; Nešić et al. 2021).

Recent studies on the biological control of EAs have shown that the use of certain fungi or bacteria resulted in their degradation. *Rhodococcus erythropolis* bacteria were used to degrade EAs, with the products of Et degradation to be cyclic dipeptide R-Pro-S-Phe and assumed unstable hemiaminal intermediate, ergine pyruvate (Lyagin and Efremenko 2019). The fungus *Fusarium roseum* had an effective effect when applied against sclerotia in wheat (Battilani et al. 2009). Also, the bacteria *Pseudomonas aureofaciens* and the fungus *Trichoderma lignorum* were tested as biological agents against EAs. The results of these studies did not show a significant effect on the germination of sclerotia (Dabkevicius and Semaskiene 2002) (Figure 11.3).

11.8 Detoxification Methods of Ergot Alkaloids

Grain processing technique is an approach by which EA mycotoxins could possibly eliminate (Merkel et al. 2012; Bryła et al. 2019; Tittlemier et al. 2019). The binders also show a great capacity to adsorb mycotoxins, preventing their absorption in the digestive system and helping to reduce the potential harm resulting from the consumption of contaminated cereal Ergot feed (Stanford et al. 2018). The currently available data on EA mycotoxin mitigation are focused on rye and its products with varying rates of degradation as this depends on the different nature of the contamination (Tittlemier et al. 2019). In a study, Tittlemier et al. studied the fate of EAs during laboratory-scale durum processing and production and cooking of pasta. The results of the research showed that EA mycotoxins were reduced, but not in a stable way since the amounts of R-enantiomers and S-enantiomers changed between each other during the treatment (Tittlemier et al. 2019). In similar studies conducted by Bryła et al. (2019) for rye flour, the baking process produced only a 22% reduction in EA mycotoxins (Bryła et al. 2019). This has to be considered promising evidence of potential reduction of toxicological impact for pasta consumers in the end. Ammonization of the R- and S-epimers of EAs was able to reduce the total concentration of EAs by 8–29% (Cherewyk et al. 2022). Detoxification of EAs as a side effect of fermentation has been documented. The loss of most of EAs during malting and brewing has been recorded proving that some enzymatic activities may transform EAs into non-toxic products (Karlovsky et al. 2016).

Recent advanced methods like genetic engineering have also been used for EA management. Hudson et al. studied the genetic manipulation of the EA pathway in *Epichloë festucae* var. *lolii* and its effect on black beetle feeding deterrence. They genetically modified *E. festucae* var. *lolii* strain AR5 to eliminate key enzymatic steps in the ergovaline pathway to determine if intermediate EA compounds can still provide insecticidal benefits in the absence of the toxic end product Ergovaline. Ergovaline was not detected in any of the deletion associations, indicating that bioactivity toward black beetle can be obtained in the absence of this mammalian toxin (Hudson et al. 2021).

11.9 Summary

The occurrence and contamination of mycotoxins concern the entire food chain since these are confirmed important contaminants that cause damage to both human and animal health. The contamination of food and feed by EA mycotoxins varies significantly from year to year as many factors are involved in the production and dispersion of sclerotia which are the responsible organs for the production of these mycotoxins. The prevalence of low temperatures as well as increased humidity before and during flowering have a significant effect on the production of EA mycotoxins. Physical, chemical, and biological means have been used for EA mycotoxin management, as well as different detoxification/degradation/and binding methods in order to avoid contamination. In order to achieve a satisfactory reduction in contamination by these mycotoxins, an integrated management system that would include all available means could contribute significantly.

11.10 Future Perspective

Contamination by mycotoxin EAs in food and feed is closely related to the presence of the fungus *C. purpurea*. Although control of this fungus is a key priority for the main crop at both pre- and post-harvest levels, future management strategies for this infection in the main crops should take into account the large inoculum reservoir in the grass population near the field production, as it is proven that they contribute significantly to the spread of the disease. Therefore, the ecology of ergot disease should be studied for both cultivated and non-cultivated grass species. Given that none of the existing practices and means provides a complete inhibition of the growth of sclerotia nor a complete reduction of EA mycotoxins, it is still requested to find the optimal conditions for the development of future management tools in the field.

11.11 Study Questions

1) To which category of contaminants do EA mycotoxins belong and why do they pose a risk to human and animal health?
2) What are the main foods in which EA mycotoxins are mainly found?
3) How does the presence of sclerotia relate to the detection and recognition of EA mycotoxins?
4) How to control EA mycotoxins in food and feed before harvest?
5) How to control EA mycotoxins in food and feed after harvest?

Acknowledgments

Acknowledge one and all supported to successfully publish the chapter.

Conflict of Interest

Author has no conflict of interest as I am the sole author.

Author Contributions

Overall writing S.A.

References

Achar, P.N., Quyen, P., Adukwu, E.C. et al. (2020). Investigation of the antifungal and anti-aflatoxigenic potential of plant-based essential oils against *Aspergillus flavus* in peanuts. *J. Fungi* 6 (4): 383. https://doi.org/10.3390/jof6040383.

Afsah-Hejri, L., Hajeb, P., and Ehsani, R.J. (2020). Application of ozone for degradation of mycotoxins in food: a review. *Compr. Rev. Food Sci. Food Saf.* 19 (4): 1777–1808.

Agriopoulou, S. (2016). Enniatins: an emerging food safety issue. *EC Nutr.* 3: 1142–1146.

Agriopoulou, S. (2021). Ergot alkaloids mycotoxins in cereals and cereal-derived food products: characteristics, toxicity, prevalence, and control strategies. *Agronomy* 11 (5): 931.

Agriopoulou, S., Koliadima, A., Karaiskakis, G., and Kapolos, J. (2016). Kinetic study of aflatoxins' degradation in the presence of ozone. *Food Control* 61: 221–226.

Agriopoulou, S., Stamatelopoulou, E., and Varzakas, T. (2020a). Advances in occurrence, importance, and mycotoxin control strategies: prevention and detoxification in foods. *Foods* 9: 137.

Agriopoulou, S., Stamatelopoulou, E., and Varzakas, T. (2020b). Advances in analysis and detection of major mycotoxins in foods. *Foods* 9: 518.

Agriopoulou, S., Stamatelopoulou, E., Sachadyn-Król, M., and Varzakas, T. (2020c). Lactic acid bacteria as antibacterial agents to extend the shelf life of fresh and minimally processed fruits and vegetables: quality and safety aspects. *Microorganisms* 8: 952.

Alaoufi, S., Friskop, A., and Simsek, S. (2023). Effect of field-applied fungicides on *Claviceps purpurea* sclerotia and associated toxins in wheat. *J. Food Protect.* 86 (3): 100046.

Alderman, S.C., Walenta, D.L., Hamm, P.B. et al. (2015). Afternoon ascospore release in *Claviceps purpurea* optimizes perennial ryegrass infection. *Plant Dis.* 99 (10): 1410–1415.

Appelt, M. and Ellner, F.M. (2009). Investigations into the occurrence of alkaloids in ergot and single sclerotia from the 2007 and 2008 harvests. *Mycotoxin Res.* 25 (2): 95–101.

Babič, J., Tavčar-Kalcher, G., Celar, F.A. et al. (2020). Ergot and ergot alkaloids in cereal grains intended for animal feeding collected in Slovenia: occurrence, pattern and correlations. *Toxins* 12 (11): 730.

Battilani, P., Costa, L.G., Dossena, A. et al. (2009). Scientific information on mycotoxins and natural plant toxicants. *EFSA Support. Publ.* 6 (9): 24E.

Blaney, B.J., Molloy, J.B., and Brock, I.J. (2009). Alkaloids in Australian rye ergot (*Claviceps purpurea*) sclerotia: implications for food and stockfeed regulations. *Anim. Product. Sci.* 49 (11): 975–982.

Bryła, M., Szymczyk, K., Jędrzejczak, R., and Roszko, M. (2015). Application of liquid chromatography/ion trap mass spectrometry technique to determine ergot alkaloids in grain products. *Food Technol. Biotechnol.* 53 (1): 18–28.

Bryła, M., Ksieniewicz-Woźniak, E., Podolska, G. et al. (2018). Occurrence of ergot and its alkaloids in winter rye harvested in Poland. *World Mycotoxin J.* 11 (4): 635–646.

Bryła, M., Ksieniewicz-Woźniak, E., Waśkiewicz, A. et al. (2019). Stability of ergot alkaloids during the process of baking rye bread. *LWT* 110: 269–274.

Caradus, J.R., Card, S.D., Finch, S.C. et al. (2022). Ergot alkaloids in New Zealand pastures and their impact. *New Zeal. J. Agric. Res.* 65 (1): 1–41.

Chennappa, G., Adkar-Purushothama, C.R., Umdale Suraj, K. et al. (2014). Impact of pesticides on PGPR activity of *Azotobacter* sp. isolated from pesticide flooded paddy soils. *Greener J. Agric. Sci.* 4 (4): 117–129.

Chennappa, G., Naik, M.K., Adkar-Purushothama, C.R. et al. (2016). PGP, abiotic stress tolerant and antifungal activity of *Azotobacter* sp. isolated from paddy soils. *Indian J. Exp. Biol.* 54 (5): 322–331.

Chennappa, G., Udaykumar, N., Vidya, M. et al. (2019). *Azotobacter*—a natural resource for bioremediation of toxic pesticides in soil ecosystems. In: *New and Future Developments in Microbial Biotechnology and Bioengineering* (ed. J.S. Singh and D.P. Singh), 267–279. Elsevier.

Cherewyk, J.E., Grusie-Ogilvie, T.J., Parker, S.E. et al. (2022). Ammonization of the R-and S-epimers of ergot alkaloids to assess detoxification potential. *J. Agric. Food. Chem.* 70 (29): 8931–8941.

Chung, S.W. (2021). A critical review of analytical methods for ergot alkaloids in cereals and feed and in particular suitability of method performance for regulatory monitoring and epimer-specific quantification. *Food Addit. Contam. Part A* 38 (6): 997–1012.

Commission Regulation (EU) (2021). 2021/1399 of 24 August 2021 amending Regulation (EC) No 1881/2006 as regards maximum levels of ergot sclerotia and ergot alkaloids in certain foodstuffs (Text with EEA relevance). *Off. J. Eur. Union* L 301: 1, ELI: http://data.europa.eu/eli/reg/2021/1399/oj. https://op.europa.eu/en/publicationdetail/-/publication/a4c8ffba-053e-11ec-b5d3-01aa75ed71a1.

Cowan, V.E., Chohan, M., Blakley, B.R. et al. (2023). Chronic ergot exposure in adult bulls suppresses prolactin but minimally impacts results of typical breeding soundness exams. *Theriogenology* 197: 71–83.

Craig, A.M., Klotz, J.L., and Duringer, J.M. (2015). Cases of ergotism in livestock and associated ergot alkaloid concentrations in feed. *Front. Chem.* 3: 8.

Crews, C., Anderson, W.A.C., Rees, G., and Krska, R. (2009). Ergot alkaloids in some rye-based UK cereal products. *Food Addit. Contam. Part B* 2 (1): 79–85.

Dabkevicius, Z. and Semaskiene, R. (2002). Control of ergot (*Claviceps purpurea* (FR.) Tul.) ascocarpus formation under the impact of chemical and biological seed dressing. In: *Plant Protection Science* (ed. V. Taborsky, J. Polak, A. Lebede, and V. Kudela). Kėdainiai: Lithuanian Institute of Agriculture.

Debegnach, F., Patriarca, S., Brera, C. et al. (2019). Ergot alkaloids in wheat and rye derived products in Italy. *Foods* 8 (5): 150.

Deepa, N. and Sreenivasa, M.Y. (2017a). *Fusarium verticillioides*, a globally important pathogen of agriculture and livestock: a review. *J. Vet. Med. Res.* 4 (4): 1084.

Deepa, N. and Sreenivasa, M.Y. (2017b). Fumonisins: a review on its global occurrence, epidemiology, toxicity and detection. *J. Vet. Med. Res.* 4 (6): 1093.

Deepa, N. and Sreenivasa, M.Y. (2019a). Biocontrol strategies for effective management of phytopathogenic fungi associated with cereals. In: *New and Future Developments in Microbial Biotechnology and Bioengineering* (ed. J.S. Singh and D.P. Singh), 177–189. Elsevier. ISBN: 9780444641915 10.1016/B978-0-444-64191-5.00013-4.

Deepa, N. and Sreenivasa, M.Y. (2019b). Molecular methods and key genes targeted for the detection of fumonisin producing *Fusarium verticillioides* - an updated review. *Food Biosci.* 32: 100473. https://doi.org/10.1016/j.fbio.2019.100473.

Deepa, N., Nagaraja, H., and Sreenivasa, M.Y. (2016a). Prevalence of fumonisin producing *Fusarium verticillioides* associated with cereals grown in Karnataka (India). *Food Sci. Human Well.* 5: 156–162. https://doi.org/10.1016/j.fshw.2016.07.001.

Deepa, N., Charith Raj, A.P., and Sreenivasa, M.Y. (2016b). Multiplex PCR method for the early detection of fumonisin producing *Fusarium verticillioides*. *Food Biosci.* 13: 84–88.

Deepa, N., Achar, P.N., and Sreenivasa, M.Y. (2021). Current perspectives of biocontrol agents for management of *Fusarium verticillioides* and its Fumonisin in cereals—a review. *J. Fungi* 7: 776. https://doi.org/10.3390/jof7090776.

Duckett, K.S., Andrae, J.G., and Pratt, S.L. (2014). Exposure to ergot alkaloids during gestation reduces fetal growth in sheep. *Front. Chem.* 2: 68.

Dung, J.K., Alderman, S.C., Walenta, D.L., and Hamm, P.B. (2016). Spatial patterns of ergot and quantification of sclerotia in perennial ryegrass seed fields in eastern Oregon. *Plant Dis.* 100 (6): 1110–1117.

Eady, C. (2021). The impact of alkaloid-producing *Epichloë* endophyte on forage ryegrass breeding: a New Zealand perspective. *Toxins* 13 (2): 158.

El-Sayed, R.A., Jebur, A.B., Kang, W. et al. (2022). An overview on the major mycotoxins in food products: characteristics, toxicity, and analysis. *J. Future Foods* 2 (2): 91–102.

European Food Safety Authority, Arcella, D., Gómez Ruiz, J.Á. et al. (2017). Human and animal dietary exposure to ergot alkaloids. *EFSA J.* 15 (7): e04902.

Florea, S., Panaccione, D.G., and Schardl, C.L. (2017). Ergot alkaloids of the family Clavicipitaceae. *Phytopathology* 107 (5): 504–518.

Grusie, T., Cowan, V., Singh, J. et al. (2018). Proportions of predominant Ergot alkaloids (*Claviceps purpurea*) detected in Western Canadian grains from 2014 to 2016. *World Mycotoxin J.* 11 (2): 259–264.

Guo, Q., Shao, B., Du, Z., and Zhang, J. (2016). Simultaneous determination of 25 ergot alkaloids in cereal samples by ultraperformance liquid chromatography–tandem mass spectrometry. *J. Agric. Food. Chem.* 64 (37): 7033–7039.

Hahn, I., Thamhesl, M., Apfelthaler, E. et al. (2015). Characterisation and determination of metabolites formed by microbial and enzymatic degradation of ergot alkaloids. *World Mycotoxin J.* 8 (4): 393–404.

Hamad, G.M., Mehany, T., Simal-Gandara, J. et al. (2022). A review of recent innovative strategies for controlling mycotoxins in foods. *Food Control* 144: 109350.

Hao, W., Guan, S., Li, A. et al. (2023). Mycotoxin occurrence in feeds and raw materials in China: a five-year investigation. *Toxins* 15 (1): 63.

Hudson, D., Mace, W., Popay, A. et al. (2021). Genetic manipulation of the ergot alkaloid pathway in *Epichloë festucae* var. lolii and its effect on black beetle feeding deterrence. *Toxins* 13: 76.

Ilha, M.R., Loretti, A.P., and Barros, C.S. (2003). Hyperthermic syndrome in dairy cattle associated with consumption of ergots of *Claviceps purpurea* in southern Brazil. *Vet. Human Toxicol.* 45 (3): 140–145.

Janik, E., Niemcewicz, M., Ceremuga, M. et al. (2020). Molecular aspects of mycotoxins—a serious problem for human health. *Int. J. Mol. Sci.* 21 (21): 8187.

Karlovsky, P., Suman, M., Berthiller, F. et al. (2016). Impact of food processing and detoxification treatments on mycotoxin contamination. *Mycotoxin Res.* 32: 179–205.

Kaushik, G. (2015). Effect of processing on mycotoxin content in grains. *Crit. Rev. Food Sci. Nutr.* 55 (12): 1672–1683.

Khaneghah, A.M., Farhadi, A., Nematollahi, A. et al. (2020). A systematic review and meta-analysis to investigate the concentration and prevalence of trichothecenes in the cereal-based food. *Trends Food Sci. Technol.* 102: 193–202.

Kifer, D., Sulyok, M., Jakšić, D. et al. (2021). Fungi and their metabolites in grain from individual households in Croatia. *Food Addit. Contam. Part B* 14 (2): 98–109.

Koester, L.R., Poole, D.H., Serão, N.V., and Schmitz-Esser, S. (2020). Beef cattle that respond differently to fescue toxicosis have distinct gastrointestinal tract microbiota. *PLoS One* 15 (7): e0229192.

Králová, M., Frébortová, J., Pěnčík, A., and Frébort, I. (2021). Overexpression of Trp-related genes in *Claviceps purpurea* leading to increased ergot alkaloid production. *New Biotechnol.* 61: 69–79.

Krska, R. and Crews, C. (2023). HPLC/MS/MS Method for the determination of Ergot Alkaloids in cereals. http://www.food.gov.uk/sites/default/files/C03057.pdf (accessed 17 April 2023).

Kumar, P., Mahato, D.K., Gupta, A. et al. (2022). Nivalenol mycotoxin concerns in foods: an overview on occurrence, impact on human and animal health and its detection and management strategies. *Toxins* 14 (8): 527.

Leslie, J.F., Moretti, A., Mesterházy, Á. et al. (2021). Key global actions for mycotoxin management in wheat and other small grains. *Toxins* 13 (10): 725.

Li, C., Kong, Q., Mou, H. et al. (2021). Biotransformation of alkylamides and alkaloids by lactic acid bacteria strains isolated from Zanthoxylum bungeanum meal. *Bioresour. Technol.* 330: 124944.

Liu, M., Shoukouhi, P., Bisson, K.R. et al. (2021). Sympatric divergence of the ergot fungus, *Claviceps purpurea*, populations infecting agricultural and nonagricultural grasses in North America. *Ecol. Evol.* 11 (1): 273–293.

Lyagin, I. and Efremenko, E. (2019). Enzymes for detoxification of various mycotoxins: origins and mechanisms of catalytic action. *Molecules* 24 (13): 2362.

Mahato, D.K., Devi, S., Pandhi, S. et al. (2021). Occurrence, impact on agriculture, human health, and management strategies of zearalenone in food and feed: a review. *Toxins* 13 (2): 92.

Menzies, J.G. and Turkington, T.K. (2015). An overview of the ergot (*Claviceps purpurea*) issue in western Canada: challenges and solutions. *Can. J. Phytopathol.* 37: 40–51.

Menzies, J.G., Klein-Gebbinck, H.W., Gordon, A., and O'Sullivan, D.M. (2017). Evaluation of *Claviceps purpurea* isolates on wheat reveals complex virulence and host susceptibility relationships. *Can. J. Plant. Pathol.* 39 (3): 307–317.

Merkel, S., Dib, B., Maul, R. et al. (2012). Degradation and epimerization of ergot alkaloids after baking and in vitro digestion. *Anal. Bioanal. Chem.* 404: 2489–2497.

Miedaner, T. and Geiger, H.H. (2015). Biology, genetics, and management of ergot (*Claviceps* spp.) in rye, sorghum, and pearl millet. *Toxins* 7 (3): 659–678.

Misra, N.N., Yadav, B., Roopesh, M.S., and Jo, C. (2019). Cold plasma for effective fungal and mycotoxin control in foods: mechanisms, inactivation effects, and applications. *Compr. Rev. Food Sci. Food Saf.* 18 (1): 106–120.

Mulder, P.P., Pereboom-de Fauw, D.P., Hoogenboom, R.L. et al. (2015). Tropane and ergot alkaloids in grain-based products for infants and young children in the Netherlands in 2011–2014. *Food Addit. Contam. Part B* 8 (4): 284–290.

Nada, S., Nikola, T., Bozidar, U. et al. (2022). Prevention and practical strategies to control mycotoxins in the wheat and maize chain. *Food Control* 136: 108855.

Nešić, K., Habschied, K., and Mastanjević, K. (2021). Possibilities for the biological control of mycotoxins in food and feed. *Toxins* 13 (3): 198.

Nicol, A.M. and Klotz, J.L. (2016). Ergovaline, an endophytic alkaloid. 2. Intake and impact on animal production, with reference to New Zealand. *Anim. Prod. Sci.* 56: 1775–1786.

Orlando, B., Maumené, C., and Piraux, F. (2017). Ergot and ergot alkaloids in French cereals: occurrence, pattern and agronomic practices for managing the risk. *World Mycotoxin J.* 10 (4): 327–338.

Pandiselvam, R., Singh, A., Agriopoulou, S. et al. (2022). A comprehensive review of impacts of ozone treatment on textural properties in different food products. *Trends Food Sci. Technol.* 127: 74–86.

Pitt, J.I. and Miller, J.D. (2017). A concise history of mycotoxin research. *J. Agric. Food. Chem.* 65 (33): 7021–7033.

Pleadin, J., Kudumija, N., Škrivanko, M. et al. (2022). Ergot sclerotia and ergot alkaloids occurrence in wheat and rye grains produced in Croatia. *Veterinarska Stanica* 53 (5): 503–511.

Prasad, M.N.N., Shankara Bhat, S., and Sreenivasa, M.Y. (2010). Antifungal activity of essential oils against *Phomopsis azadirachtae*- the causative agent of die-back disease of neem. *J. Agric. Technol.* 6 (1): 127–133.

Puhl, T., Suty, H.A., and Adam, N. (2007). Control of ergot by seed treatment. *Gesunde Pflanzen* 59 (4): 147–150.

Sachadyn-Król, M. and Agriopoulou, S. (2020). Ozonation as a method of abiotic elicitation improving the health-promoting properties of plant products—a review. *Molecules* 25 (10): 2416.

Sarrocco, S. and Vannacci, G. (2018). Preharvest application of beneficial fungi as a strategy to prevent postharvest mycotoxin contamination: a review. *Crop Protect.* 110: 160–170.

Schummer, C., Zandonella, I., van Nieuwenhuyse, A., and Moris, G. (2020). Epimerization of ergot alkaloids in feed. *Heliyon* 6 (6): e04336.

Shahid, M.G., Nadeem, M., Gulzar, A. et al. (2020). Novel ergot alkaloids production from *Penicillium citrinum* employing response surface methodology technique. *Toxins* 12 (7): 427.

Shanakhat, H., Sorrentino, A., Raiola, A. et al. (2018). Current methods for mycotoxins analysis and innovative strategies for their reduction in cereals: an overview. *J. Sci. Food Agric.* 98 (11): 4003–4013.

Shi, H. and Yu, P. (2023). Using molecular sectroscopic techniques (NIR and ATR-FT/MIR) coupling with various chemometrics to test possibility to reveal chemical and molecular response of cool-season adapted wheat grain to ergot alkaloids. *Toxins* 15 (2): 151.

Shi, H., Schwab, W., Liu, N., and Yu, P. (2019). Major ergot alkaloids in naturally contaminated cool-season barley grain grown under a cold climate condition in western Canada, explored with near-infrared (NIR) and fourier transform mid-infrared (ATR-FT/MIR) spectroscopy. *Food Control* 102: 221–230.

Shimshoni, J.A., Cuneah, O., Sulyok, M. et al. (2017). Newly discovered ergot alkaloids in sorghum ergot *Claviceps africana* occurring for the first time in Israel. *Food Chem.* 219: 459–467.

Smaoui, S., Agriopoulou, S., D'Amore, T. et al. (2022). The control of *Fusarium* growth and decontamination of produced mycotoxins by lactic acid bacteria. *Crit. Rev. Food Sci. Nutr.* 62: 1–28.

Sreenivasa, M.Y., Dass, R.S., Charith Raj, A.P., and Janardhana, G.R. (2008). PCR-based detection of genus *Fusarium* and Fumonisin-producing isolates from freshly harvested sorghum grains grown in Karnataka, India. *J. Food Saf.* 28: 236–237.

Sreenivasa, M.Y., Dass, R.S., Adkar-Purushothama, C.R. et al. (2011a). Assessment of the growth inhibiting effect of some plant essential oils on different *Fusarium* species isolated from sorghum and maize grains. *J. Plant Dis. Protect.* 118 (6): 208–213.

Sreenivasa, M.Y., Dass, R.S., Charith Raj, A.P., and Janardhana, G.R. (2011b). Mycological evaluation of maize grains produced in Karnataka (India) for the post harvest fungal contamination. *World Appl. Sci. J.* 13 (4): 688–692.

Stanford, K., Swift, M., Wang, Y. et al. (2018). Effects of feeding a mycotoxin binder on nutrient digestibility, alkaloid recovery in feces, and performance of lambs fed diets contaminated with cereal ergot. *Toxins* 10: 312.

Tittlemier, S.A., Drul, D., Roscoe, M., and McKendry, T. (2015). Occurrence of ergot and ergot alkaloids in western Canadian wheat and other cereals. *J. Agric. Food. Chem.* 63 (29): 6644–6650.

Tittlemier, S.A., Drul, D., Roscoe, M. et al. (2019). Fate of ergot alkaloids during laboratory scale durum processing and pasta production. *Toxins* 11 (4): 195.

Topi, D., Jakovac-Strajn, B., Pavšič-Vrtač, K., and Tavčar-Kalcher, G. (2017). Occurrence of ergot alkaloids in wheat from Albania. *Food Addit. Contam. Part A* 34 (8): 1333–1343.

Uppala, S.S., Wu, B.M., and Alderman, S.C. (2016). Effects of temperature and duration of preconditioning cold treatment on sclerotial germination of *Claviceps purpurea*. *Plant Dis.* 100 (10): 2080–2086.

Varzakas, T. (2016). Quality and safety aspects of cereals (wheat) and their products. *Crit. Rev. Food Sci. Nutr.* 56: 2495–2510.

Wallwey, C. and Li, S.M. (2011). Ergot alkaloids: structure diversity, biosynthetic gene clusters and functional proof of biosynthetic genes. *Nat. Prod. Rep.* 28 (3): 496–510.

Waret-Szkuta, A., Larraillet, L., Oswald, I.P. et al. (2019). Unusual acute neonatal mortality and sow agalactia linked with ergot alkaloid contamination of feed. *Porcine Health Manag.* 5 (1): 1–5.

Wyka, S. and Broders, K. (2023). Brome grasses represent the primary source of *Claviceps purpurea* inoculum associated with barley fields in the San Luis Valley of Colorado. *Can. J. Plant Pathol.* 45 (1): 15–29.

Wyka, S.A., Mondo, S.J., Liu, M. et al. (2020). A large accessory genome, high recombination rates, and selection of secondary metabolite genes help maintain global distribution and broad host range of the fungal plant pathogen *Claviceps purpurea*. *BioRxiv* https://doi.org/10.1101/2020.05.20.106880.

Xue, A.G., Chen, Y., and Ai-Rewashdy, Y. (2017). Diseases of spring wheat in central and eastern Ontario in 2017. *Can. Plant Dis. Survey* 98: 148–149.

Yooussef, M.M., Pham, Q., Achar, P.N., and Sreenivasa, M.Y. (2016). Antifungal activity of essential oils on *Aspergillus parasiticus* isolated from peanuts. *J. Plant Protect. Res.* 56 (2): 139–142. https://doi.org/10.1515/jppr-2016-0021.

Young, J.C., Chen, Z.J., and Marquardt, R.R. (1983). Reduction in alkaloid content of ergot sclerotia by chemical and physical treatment. *J. Agric. Food. Chem.* 31 (2): 413–415.

Further Reading

Caradus, J.R., Card, S.D., Finch, S.C. et al. (2022). Ergot alkaloids in New Zealand pastures and their impact. *New Zeal. J. Agric. Res.* 65 (1): 1–41.

Chen, J.J., Han, M.Y., Gong, T. et al. (2017). Recent progress in ergot alkaloid research. *RSC Adv.* 7 (44): 27384–27396.

Cowan, V.E., Chohan, M., Blakley, B.R. et al. (2023). Chronic ergot exposure in adult bulls suppresses prolactin but minimally impacts results of typical breeding soundness exams. *Theriogenology* 197: 71–83.

Höfs, S., Jaut, V., and Schneider, R.J. (2023). Ergometrine sensing in rye flour by a magnetic bead-based immunoassay followed by flow injection analysis with amperometric detection. *Talanta* 254: 124172.

Panaccione, D.G. (2023). Derivation of the multiply-branched ergot alkaloid pathway of fungi. *Microbial Biotechnol.* 16: 742–756.

Websites

BfR FAQ. (2013). Frequently asked questions on ergot alkaloids in cereal products. https://www.bfr.bund.de/cm/349/frequently-asked-questions-on-ergot-alkaloids-in-cereal-products.pdf.

Commission Regulation (EU) (2021). 2021/1399 of 24 August 2021 amending Regulation (EC) No 1881/2006 as regards maximum levels of ergot sclerotia and ergot alkaloids in certain foodstuffs (Text with EEA relevance). *Off. J. Eur. Union* L 301: 1, ELI: http://data.europa.eu/eli/reg/2021/1399/oj. https://op.europa.eu/en/publicationdetail/-/publication/a4c8ffba-053e-11ec-b5d3-01aa75ed71a1.

European Food Safety Authority, Arcella, D., Gómez Ruiz, J.Á. et al. (2017). Human and animal dietary exposure to ergot alkaloids. *EFSA J.* 15 (7): e04902. https://efsa.onlinelibrary.wiley.com/doi/full/10.2903/j.efsa.2017.4902.

Gordon, A., Delamare, G., Tente, E. and Boyd, L. (2019). Determining the routes of transmission of ergot alkaloids in cereal grains (No. 603). AHDB Project Report. https://ahdb.org.uk/determining-the-routes-of-transmission-of-ergot-alkaloids-in-cereal-grains.

Titley, M. and Prescott, L.-A. 2018). Validation of ergot alkaloids in feeds by LC-MS/MS AAFCO annual meeting. Carling: Ottawa Laboratory. https://www.aafco.org/wp-content/uploads/2023/01/201808_AAFCO_Validation_of_Ergot_Alkaloids_in_Feeds_by_LC-MS_MS.pdf.

Index

[Note: Numbers mentioned is Page numbers; Italicized page numbers figures; Bold page numbers table]

Anti-Mycotoxin Strategies for Food and Feed, First Edition. Edited by Deepa Nagaraju, Sreenivasa Marikunte Yanjarappa, Premila N. Achar, and Angel Medina Vaya.

b

c

www.ingramcontent.com/pod-product-compliance
Lightning Source LLC
LaVergne TN
LVHW062208200926
848484LV00006B/1348